DYING TO COUNT

MEDICAL ANTHROPOLOGY: HEALTH, INEQUALITY, AND SOCIAL JUSTICE

Series editor: Lenore Manderson

Books in the Medical Anthropology series are concerned with social patterns of and social responses to ill health, disease, and suffering, and how social exclusion and social justice shape health and healing outcomes. The series is designed to reflect the diversity of contemporary medical anthropological research and writing, and will offer scholars a forum to publish work that showcases the theoretical sophistication, methodological soundness, and ethnographic richness of the field.

Books in the series may include studies on the organization and movement of peoples, technologies, and treatments, how inequalities pattern access to these, and how individuals, communities, and states respond to various assaults on well-being, including from illness, disaster, and violence.

Carina Heckert, *Fault Lines of Care: Gender, HIV, and Global Health in Bolivia*
Joel Christian Reed, *Landscapes of Activism: Civil Society and HIV and AIDS Care in Northern Mozambique*
Alison Heller, *Fistula Politics: Birthing Injuries and the Quest for Continence in Niger*
Jessica Hardin, *Faith and the Pursuit of Health: Cardiometabolic Disorders in Samoa*
Beatriz M. Reyes-Foster, *Psychiatric Encounters: Madness and Modernity in Yucatan, Mexico*
Sonja van Wichelen, *Legitimating Life: Adoption in the Age of Globalization and Biotechnology*
Andrea Whittaker, *International Surrogacy as Disruptive Industry in Southeast Asia*
Lesley Jo Weaver, *Sugar and Tension: Diabetes and Gender in Modern India*
Ellen Block and Will McGrath, *Infected Kin: Orphan Care and AIDS in Lesotho*
Nolan Kline, *Pathogenic Policing: Immigration Enforcement and Health in the U.S. South*
Ciara Kierans, *Chronic Failures: Kidneys, Regimes of Care, and the Mexican State*
Stéphanie Larchanché, *Cultural Anxieties: Managing Migrant Suffering in France*
Dvera I. Saxton, *The Devil's Fruit: Farmworkers, Health, and Environmental Justice*
Siri Suh, *Dying to Count: Post-Abortion Care and Global Reproductive Health Politics in Senegal*

CONTENTS

Illustrations   ix

Foreword by Lenore Manderson   xi

Abbreviations   xv

Note on Anonymity and Language   xvii

Introduction: PAC as Reproductive Governance   1

1   A "Transformative" Intervention   25

2   A Troublesome Technology: The Multiple Lives of MVA in Senegal   52

3   "We Wear White Coats, Not Uniforms": Abortion Surveillance in Hospitals   82

4   When Abortion Does Not Count: Interpreting PAC Data   109

Conclusion: Evidence, Harm Reduction, and Reproductive Justice   141

Appendix A: Methodology   153

Appendix B: Cases of Admitted and Suspected Induced Abortions   159

Acknowledgments   163

Notes   167

References   175

Index   199

ILLUSTRATIONS

FIGURES

	Map of Senegal and its administrative regions	xx
Figure I.1	Manual vacuum aspiration	5
Figure 1.1	Abortion as a percentage of admissions to the maternity ward in three hospitals, 2006–2010	45
Figure 1.2	Delivery room at l'Hôpital Médina	47
Figure 2.1	MVA room at l'Hôpital de Ville	53
Figure 2.2	Percentage of PAC cases treated with MVA, digital evacuation (DE) and dilation and curettage (D&C) at three hospitals, 2004–2010	73
Figure 2.3	MVA kit at l'Hôpital Médina	74
Figure 3.1	Ultrasound report, retrieved from the archives of a prosecuted abortion case, confirming the defendant had "attempted abortion."	92
Figure 4.1	Abortions treated in three hospitals over twenty-four months between 2009 and 2010	132

TABLES

Table 2.1	Treatment of PAC cases by type of provider at l'Hôpital de Ville, 2009–2010	76
Table 3.1	Types of abortions treated at three hospitals, 2009–2010	101
Table 4.1	Total abortions and percentage treated with MVA in three hospitals, 2004–2010	129
Table A.1	Number, profession, and institutional affiliation of health professionals interviewed in three regions	155
Table B.1	Cases of admitted and suspected induced abortions in six months of PAC register data in three hospitals, 2009–2010	160

FOREWORD

LENORE MANDERSON

Medical Anthropology: Health, Inequality, and Social Justice aims to capture the diversity of contemporary medical anthropological research and writing. The beauty of ethnography is its capacity, through storytelling, to make sense of suffering as a social experience and to set it in context. Central to our focus in this series, therefore, is the way in which social structures, political-economic systems, and ideologies shape the likelihood and impact of infections, injuries, bodily ruptures and disease, chronic conditions and disability, treatment and care, and social repair and death.

Health and illness are social facts; the circumstances of the maintenance and loss of health are always and everywhere shaped by structural, local, and global relations. Social formations and relations, culture, economy, and political organization as much as ecology shape the variance of illness, disability, and disadvantage. The authors of the monographs in this series are concerned centrally with health and illness, healing practices, and access to care, but in each case they highlight the importance of such differences in context as expressed and experienced at individual, household, and wider levels: health risks and outcomes of social structure and household economy, health systems factors, and national and global politics and economics all shape people's lives. In their accounts of health, inequality, and social justice, the authors move across social circumstances, health conditions, and geography, and their intersections and interactions, to demonstrate how individuals, communities, and states manage assaults on people's health and well-being.

As medical anthropologists have long illustrated, the relationships of social context and health status are complex. In addressing these questions, the authors in this series showcase the theoretical sophistication, methodological rigor, and empirical richness of the field, while expanding a map of illness, social life, and institutional life to illustrate the effects of material conditions and social meanings in troubling and surprising ways. The books reflect medical anthropology as a constantly changing field of scholarship, drawing on research diversely in residential and virtual communities, in clinics and laboratories, in emergency care and public health settings, with service providers, individual healers, and households, and with social bodies, human bodies, and biologies. While medical anthropology once concentrated on systems of healing, particularly diseases and embodied experiences, today the field has expanded to include environmental disaster and war, science, technology and faith, and gender-based violence and forced migration. Curiosity about the body and its vicissitudes remains a pivot of our work, but our concerns are with the location of bodies in social life, and with how social structures, temporal imperatives, and shifting exigencies shape life courses. This dynamic field reflects an ethics of the discipline to address these pressing issues of our time.

Globalization has contributed to and adds to the complexity of influences on health outcomes; it (re)produces social and economic relations that institutionalize poverty, unequal conditions of everyday life and work, and environments in which diseases increase or subside. Globalization patterns the movement and relations of peoples, technologies and knowledge, and programs and treatments; it shapes differences in health experiences and outcomes across space; it informs and amplifies inequalities at individual and country levels. Global forces and local inequalities compound and constantly load on individuals to impact on their physical and mental health, and on their households and communities. At the same time, as the subtitle of this series indicates, we are concerned with questions of social exclusion and inclusion, social justice and repair, again both globally and in local settings. The books will challenge readers to reflect not only on sickness and suffering, deficit and despair, but also on resistance and restitution—on how people respond to injustices and evade the fault lines that may seem to predetermine life outcomes. The aim is to widen the frame within which we conceptualize embodiment and suffering.

Worldwide, abortion remains politicized, subject to harsh disapproval, criminalization, moralization, and rebuke, just as it was three decades ago when it was the subject of fierce international debate. Abortion continues to be a signal matter of reproductive health, women's rights, and human rights. The national and local contexts in which it is sought and provided have an enormous impact on women's lives. For those who survive, it can have continuing harsh and violent repercussions for their health, reproductive potential, and well-being.

Yet data on abortion and abortion care needs are scanty and unreliable, reflecting legal constraints. Depending on the methods of estimating, around 75 million abortions are induced yearly owing to unintended pregnancy, with little difference among countries despite variations in legal access to abortion and level of restrictions. A significant proportion of these abortions are categorized as unsafe—self-induced or performed by unskilled practitioners, often in unhygienic environments without access to medical interventions in an emergency, or conducted in settings where post-abortion care (medical and surgical intervention following abortion) is absent or delivered in stealth, in an atmosphere of fear, violence, and judgment. As a result, around 13 percent of maternal deaths worldwide are estimated to occur annually as a result of abortion. The scandal is not only these deaths and the lack of women's autonomy and access to contraception that are their backdrop; the scandal is the continued silence on abortion, the global politics and economics that drive this, and the condemnation of those who advocate for change.

The other scandal is this: the numbers of women who lack access to contraception; the numbers of unintended pregnancies, attempted abortions, and deaths from abortion; and the outcomes of post-abortion care are all largely guestimates. In a climate of reprobation, stigmatization, and censure, the statistics from modeling are the best we have.

In *Dying to Count: Post-Abortion Care and Global Reproductive Health Politics in Senegal*, Siri Suh weaves together the history and politics of post-abortion care, technology, and field research conducted in Senegal over a decade. Suh illustrates how women's experiences of abortion, post-abortion care, and obstetric violence are shaped by global systems of governance, whereby states, religious authorities, donor agencies, nongovernmental organizations, and privatized health services manipulate and control women's health, obstetric care, and technologies.

In Senegal, induced abortion is illegal under any circumstance. Those who provide this procedure, despite this, are at risk of being reported and apprehended. They face fines, imprisonment, and, for health practitioners, revocation of certification and loss of (professional) livelihood. Between a third and a quarter of women in Senegalese prisons are there because they have acted outside the abortion law. Providers continue to meet the needs of desperate women covertly, contributing to what we know or guess about abortion, post-abortion care, and maternal morbidity and mortality.

Suh argues that post-abortion care is a means of harm reduction for the poorest, most vulnerable women, whose abortions are conducted in environments of restriction and violence. However, as she teases out in this extraordinary book, the statistics that tie post-abortion care to fewer deaths are hidden in the silence on the circumstances in which women present to hospitals, in incomplete hospital records, and in the reluctance of providers to identify abortion as a cause of death. And inaccurate records fail to provide acceptable evidence to support interventions such as post-abortion care. Women continue to die, in other words, for lack of data on ways to prevent their deaths.

Dying to Count is wonderfully written and beautifully paced, like a gripping detective story. It is both superb scholarship of data, record keeping, metrics, and politics, and a book that will impassion those who are wary of statistics as well as those who need no convincing.

ABBREVIATIONS

AJS	l'Association des Juristes Sénégalaises / Senegalese Association of Women Lawyers
AMDD	Averting Maternal Death and Disability
AMIU	l'aspiration manuelle intra-utérine / manual vacuum aspiration
ASBEF	L'Association Sénégalaise pour le Bien-Être Familial / Senegalese Association for Familial Well-Being
AVSC	Association for Voluntary Surgical Contraception
CEDAW	Convention on the Elimination of all Forms of Discrimination Against Women
CEFOREP	Centre Régionale de Formation, de Recherche, et de Plaidoyer en Santé de la Reproduction / Regional Center for Training, Research, and Advocacy in Reproductive Health
CHU	Centre Hospitalier Universitaire / University Hospital Center
CRR	Center for Reproductive Rights
DHS	Demographic and Health Surveys
DSR	Division de la Santé de la Reproduction / Division of Reproductive Health
EmOC	emergency obstetric care
EVA	electric vacuum aspiration
FP 2020	Family Planning 2020 Initiative
FIGO	International Federation of Gynecology and Obstetrics
ICPD	International Conference on Population and Development
IHME	Institute for Health Metrics and Evaluation
IMF	International Monetary Fund
IPPF	International Planned Parenthood Federation
IRH	Institute for Reproductive Health
LARC	long-acting reversible contraceptive
LEM	List of Essential Medications
MDG	Millennium Development Goal
MSAS	Ministère de la Santé et de l'Action Sociale / Ministry of Health and Social Action
MSF	Médecins Sans Frontières / Doctors Without Borders
MSH	Management Sciences for Health
MSI	Marie Stopes International
MVA	manual vacuum aspiration
NGO	nongovernmental organization
PAC	post-abortion care

PNA	Pharmacie Nationale d'Approvisionnement / National Pharmacy Supply
PPH	postpartum hemorrhage
PREMOMA	Prevention of Maternal Mortality and Morbidity Project
RCT	randomized controlled trial
SDG	Sustainable Development Goal
SDM	Standard Days Method
SMI	Safe Motherhood Initiative
STS	science and technology studies
TFR	total fertility rate
UCAD	L'Université Cheikh Anta Diop / Cheikh Anta Diop University
UN	United Nations
UNFPA	United Nations Population Fund
USAID	United States Agency for International Development
WHO	World Health Organization

NOTE ON ANONYMITY AND LANGUAGE

Most of the individuals and health facilities mentioned in this book have been given pseudonyms. Exceptions include individuals, health facilities, and organizations identified by name in public documents such as newspapers, reports, books, or articles. Throughout the book, I use my interlocutors' words in French (and in a few instances, Wolof). For example, research participants used the French term *l'interrogation* to describe the practice of questioning post-abortion care patients. While the equivalent in English would be "the medical interview," during which the health worker gathers information from the patient for the purposes of diagnosis and therapy, in the Senegalese context the possibility of illegal induced abortion injected an investigative quality into this practice. I discuss l'interrogation in greater detail in chapter 3. In American English, the term "abortion" almost always refers to induced abortion or voluntary pregnancy termination. In French, the term *avortement* may refer to either spontaneous abortion (miscarriage) or induced abortion. When discussing post-abortion care, my interlocutors did not always distinguish between spontaneous abortion (*avortement spontané* or *fausse couche*) and induced abortion (*avortement provoqué*).

DYING TO COUNT

Map of Senegal and its administrative regions. Source adapted on June 22, 2020 from Wikimedia. File:Senegal, administrative divisions in colour. https://commons.wikimedia.org/wiki/File:Senegal_administrative_divisions_in_colour_2.svg. This file is licensed under the Creative Commons Attribution-Share Alike 4.0 International license.

INTRODUCTION
PAC as Reproductive Governance

Maimouna Diallo lay weak and feverish on a bed in the busy maternity ward of l'Hôpital de Ville, a large district hospital in Senegal, surrounded by a cluster of doctors, midwives, nurses, and auxiliary staff in white coats. She had arrived, alone, very late into the night shift and was now being examined by the senior gynecologist, Dr. Fall, during his early-morning rounds. As he performed the manual exam, Dr. Fall asked Maimouna questions. "*Soxna si* ["Madame" in Wolof]," he said, "how long have you been bleeding? What color was the blood? Are you in pain?" The two midwives on call chimed in with responses from their earlier questioning of the patient. Maimouna had reported taking a *décoction*, or herbal infusion, to relieve a headache after a disagreement with her husband. She immediately began to bleed heavily, after not seeing her period for nearly two months, and suffered severe abdominal pain. Three days later, she sought help at a primary health care facility in a neighboring health district, at which point the nurse immediately referred her to the hospital.

Several hours later, as they performed uterine evacuation with a plastic manual vacuum aspiration (MVA) syringe and administered antibiotics, medical providers continued to question Maimouna. What exactly was the décoction that she swallowed? She replied that she had taken the same décoction before to relieve headaches. Why did she wait three days to seek medical care after she started bleeding? Maimouna replied that had she known she was pregnant, she would have sought medical attention sooner. Why had her husband not accompanied her to the hospital? She said she had not seen him since their argument several days earlier.

I stood in my own white coat at the edge of the group of medical providers surrounding Maimouna during her exam. I donned this coat in my capacity as an ethnographic researcher of the daily practice of *les soins après avortement,* or post-abortion care (PAC)—the treatment of abortion complications, followed by family planning services—at this district hospital in a sprawling *quartier populaire* or working-class neighborhood in a Senegalese city. At this particular moment, health workers were questioning Maimouna, or, in their own words, conducting *l'interrogation*. These were not idle questions, nor, pointedly, were all of them relevant to delivering quality obstetric care to the patient. Health workers interrogated her to determine whether the pregnancy loss she reported as spontaneous had instead been induced. In Senegal, the law forbids induced abortion under any circumstance and punishes practitioners with imprisonment, fines, and revocation of professional certification. Yet, clandestine abortion is not uncommon: between a third and a quarter of women in Senegalese prisons have been convicted of infanticide or abortion, with sentences ranging from several months to years (Iaccino, 2014; Moseson, Ouedraogo, Diallo, and Sakho, 2019). Maimouna's responses to health workers' questions, and the absence of her husband or other family members, made them suspicious that she had procured an illegal abortion. Nevertheless, they released her several days later and recorded her in the hospital's PAC register simply as a case of incomplete abortion. In other words, Maimouna appeared in the hospital record as a case of miscarriage.

In addition to observing PAC services and reviewing PAC records at this hospital and two others, I reviewed cases of illegal abortion prosecuted by the tribunal court of the region of Dakar between 1987 and 2010. These legal records reveal that some women may face not only interrogation by health workers but also arrest by the police when they receive PAC in Senegalese hospitals. At 3 P.M. on March 13, 2009, police officers arrived at a district hospital in Dakar two hours after receiving an anonymous tip that a young woman was being treated for complications of abortion. There, they found the twenty-year-old patient, Khady Ndiaye, "on her bed, in the grip of intense pain." The next day, they requisitioned the physician on call to confirm whether the patient had illegally terminated a pregnancy. On March 24, the physician issued a report indicating she had conducted an ultrasound procedure that revealed a "non-evolutive" pregnancy of eighteen weeks and six days and an absence of amniotic fluid, which led her to conclude that Khady had procured an illegal abortion. Her report also revealed that the patient had been treated with *curage digitale*, or digital evacuation, a procedure that involves the insertion of the index (and if possible, the middle) finger into the uterine cavity to remove "placental fragments or blood clots following an abortion" (Médecins Sans Frontières [MSF] 2019, p. 175).[1] On March 26, 2009, Khady "presented" herself to the police and "confessed" to taking an "infusion" of leaves from a papaya tree, coffee, and Paracetamol[2] that she had received from her cousin. On April 3, 2009, the court sentenced Khady Ndiaye and her cousin to six months in prison.

The clinical encounters of Maimouna Diallo and Khady Ndiaye illuminate how women's intimate reproductive experiences are inextricably tied to social, economic, legal, and professional institutions and processes. This nexus between personal and political dimensions of reproduction has been demonstrated in studies of clandestine abortion around the world (Grimes et al., 2006; Guillaume, Rossier, and Reeve, 2018; S. Singh, Remez, Sedgh, Kwokand, and Onda, 2018). In Senegal, as in other sub-Saharan African countries, a highly restrictive colonial-era abortion law is accompanied by significant religious and public opposition to abortion (Blystad et al., 2019). Almost all (96%) of Senegal's population practices Islam (Central Intelligence Agency, 2020). Conservative Islamic organizations like Jamra have portrayed efforts to relax the abortion law as a dangerous form of Western (and feminist) meddling, and their members actively lobby parliamentarians to reject legal reform (Archer, Finden, and Pearson, 2018; Gaestel and Shryock, 2017). These legal and social barriers do not deter women from attempting to terminate unexpected or unwanted pregnancies, and if they are unsuccessful, infanticide (Moseson et al., 2019). Nearly a quarter of all pregnancies end in induced abortion, and the estimated incidence of abortion is 17 per 1,000 women (Guttmacher Institute, 2015).[3] With safe abortions conducted by health workers in the private sector costing up to $375 in Senegal (Turner, Senderowicz, and Marlow, 2016), low-income women frequently turn to lay individuals who provide procedures that are more affordable but also more likely to lead to complications or death. While some women are treated with unsafe surgical procedures, others may ingest harmful products that may lead to severe bleeding, pain, infection, and organ failure. In Senegal, an estimated two-thirds of abortions are considered to be unsafe, because they are performed either by untrained practitioners or by the women themselves (Guttmacher Institute, 2015).

Restrictive abortion laws disproportionately criminalize low-income and single women who lack the resources to procure discreet, safe abortions or to fend off charges of homicide after experiencing a miscarriage. Low-income and single women who seek care at public hospitals are more likely to be reported to the police by health workers or anonymous sources.[4] At the same time, Maimouna Diallo's case suggests that health workers do not systematically report suspected or confirmed cases of illegal abortion to the police. In places with restrictive abortion laws, health workers may misclassify cases of abortion in hospital records or omit them altogether, contributing to the difficulty of accurately measuring the epidemiological scope of induced abortion (Gerdts, Tunçalp, Johnston, and Ganatra, 2015).

In this book, I explore how women's abortion experiences and their encounters with PAC are shaped not only by Senegal's legal prohibition on abortion but also by global systems of regulating reproduction, or what social scientists have called reproductive governance: the "mechanisms through which different historical configurations of actors—such as state institutions, churches, donor agencies, and non-governmental organizations (NGOs)—use legislative controls, economic inducements, moral injunctions, direct coercion, and ethical incitements to produce, monitor, and control reproductive behaviors and practices" (Morgan and Roberts, 2012, p. 243). These mechanisms of reproductive governance determine the kinds (and costs) of obstetric services and technologies available to women like Maimouna and Khady in government hospitals. Health workers' PAC record-keeping practices, designed to protect themselves and their patients from criminalization, produce data about abortion that shape policy makers' claims about what PAC does in hospitals and the kinds of women the intervention treats. In turn, these data bolster policy makers' commitments to national and global strategies to reduce maternal death as a matter of human rights. Women's experiences with abortion and PAC, and their encounters with health workers and health systems, are deeply embedded in the global production and diffusion of obstetric interventions, technologies, and data that have composed multiple regimes of global reproductive governance since the mid-twentieth century.

PAC: A GLOBAL REPRODUCTIVE HEALTH INTERVENTION

Although both Khady Ndiaye and Maimouna Diallo received PAC services at state health facilities, the former was incarcerated while the latter was not. PAC is a global reproductive health intervention that entails emergency treatment of incomplete abortion followed by contraceptive counseling and services to delay pregnancy. Currently implemented in over sixty countries worldwide (PAC Consortium, 2016), the PAC model was developed by global reproductive health advocates during the early 1990s as a harm reduction approach to the global health problem of unsafe abortion, which accounts for nearly 15 percent of global maternal deaths (Faúndes and Shah, 2015). Harm reduction approaches in public health draw on principles of neutrality, humanism, and pragmatism to improve health outcomes by reducing risk related to behaviors that are legally restricted or morally unacceptable (Briozzo et al., 2006; Erdman, 2011; Hyman, Blanchard, Coeytaux, Grossman, and Teixeira, 2013). A well-known example of public health harm reduction is safe needle exchange, in which access to clean needles reduces the risk of HIV among intravenous drug users, and by extension, their sexual partners. As a form of harm reduction, PAC called on medical professionals to provide quality, confidential, and nondiscriminatory treatment regardless of the legal status of abortion (Corbett and Turner, 2003). Additionally, the PAC model championed surgical methods of uterine evacuation, such as the MVA syringe (see figure I.1) and its electrically powered counterpart, electric vacuum aspiration (EVA), that were safer, more affordable, and more amenable to use by midwives and nurses at lower levels of the health system than dilation and curettage (Greenslade, McKay, Wolf, and McLaurin, 1994).[5] During this procedure, the physician uses a metal curette to remove "retained placenta or blood clots after incomplete abortion" (MSF, 2019, p. 180).[6] Put differently, the global PAC model "medicalized" (Conrad, 1992) the problem of abortion complications in countries with restrictive abortion laws by framing them as a medical and public health matter, to be managed by health workers in hospitals (rather than by legal or religious authorities) through emergency obstetric care

FIGURE I.1. Manual vacuum aspiration. Reproduced from Figure P-36, "Evacuating the contents of the uterus," in *Managing complications in pregnancy and childbirth: A guide for midwives and doctors,* by the World Health Organization (WHO, 2007, P-67, p. 319), https://apps.who.int/iris/bitstream/handle/10665/43972/9241545879_eng.pdf.

(EmOC) and contraceptive services to avert not just mortality but also unwanted or unplanned pregnancy.

In 1994, delegates from 179 countries, including Senegal, signed the Platform of Action of the United Nations (UN) International Conference on Population and Development (ICPD) in Cairo, which for the first time defined reproductive health or well-being as a human right. Although the ICPD called on governments to offer quality reproductive health care services, it did not recommend legal abortion as part of its reproductive rights framework. In countries where abortion is legal, the ICPD required governments to ensure the safety of services. For countries with restrictive abortion laws, the ICPD urged governments to provide PAC as a public health strategy to reduce mortality related to unsafe abortion (United Nations Population Fund [UNFPA], 2014). The ICPD included PAC in response to the global Safe Motherhood Initiative (SMI), established in 1987 by a group of UN agencies and international NGOs, which called for greater attention to the preventable problem of maternal mortality and identified complications of unsafe abortion as one of the top five causes of global maternal death (Abou-Zahr, 2003). The ICPD thus codified PAC's "harm reduction" approach as a reproductive rights strategy for reducing maternal mortality.

Over twenty years after the formulation of the global PAC model and its inclusion in the ICPD, there remains an urgent need for these services. Abortion rates in the developing world have remained unchanged while those in the developed world have declined (Sedgh et al., 2016). Almost all (97%) unsafe abortion takes place in developing countries (Ganatra et al., 2017), where laws tend to be stricter. Although Latin America has a higher incidence of unsafe abortion than Africa, women in Africa face a risk of death from unsafe abortion that is fifteen times higher (Faúndes and Shah, 2015). As devastating as the numbers related to mortality may be, they represent the tip of the iceberg, as the epidemiological burden of morbidity is even greater. Every year, nearly 7 million women are admitted to hospitals with complications of unsafe abortion. This number does not include the estimated 40 percent of women who experience complications but do not receive care (S. Singh and Maddow-Zimet, 2016). Complications of unsafe abortion may also result in secondary infertility, which may in turn jeopardize women's marriage prospects and financial security (Kumar, Hessini, and Mitchell, 2009).

Introduced to Senegal's health system by le Ministère de la Santé et de l'Action Sociale (MSAS/Ministry of Health and Social Action) in the late 1990s through a series of pilot projects, PAC is now available in many primary health care facilities and district and regional hospitals around the country. In 2016, an estimated 18,806 Senegalese women received PAC in 856 health structures, and most (95%) were treated in government facilities (Lince-Deroche, Sène, Pliskin, Owolabi, and Bankole, 2020). The introduction of PAC has been accompanied by ongoing advocacy with government and religious leaders by one organization in particular, l'Association des Juristes Sénégalaises (AJS; Senegalese Association of Women Lawyers), to permit abortion if pregnancy threatens the woman's life or health and in cases of rape or incest (Archer et al., 2018; Moseson et al., 2019; Suh, 2014).

Despite these developments, the clinical encounters of Maimouna Diallo and Khady Ndiaye reveal profound tensions between the treatment ethic of the global PAC model, on the one hand, and the legal, professional, and technological context in which Senegalese health workers practice obstetric care, on the other. Health workers' "denouncing" of women suspected of illegal abortion to the police runs contrary to the treatment ethic of the global PAC model, which entitles women to quality, confidential care regardless of the kind of abortion they have experienced, and to national codes of professional ethics that obligate medical providers to protect patient confidentiality. Even if medical providers do not systematically denounce women to the police, some humiliate and harass them by interrogating them repeatedly about their personal lives throughout treatment and hospitalization.

Although the MSAS has championed MVA technology for uterine evacuation since the initial piloting of PAC in the late 1990s, Khady Ndiaye was treated in 2009 with digital evacuation, a method that, like dilation and curettage, is not recognized by the World Health Organization (WHO, 2012) as a safe method of abortion care. Both digital evacuation and dilation and curettage have been documented in maternity wards throughout sub-Saharan Africa as methods of treating abortion complications when MVA is unavailable or there is a lack of providers trained in MVA (Izugbara, Egesa, and Okelo, 2015; Kiemtoré et al., 2016; Prada, Mirembe, Ahmed, Nalwadda, and Kiggundu, 2005; Izugbara et al., 2019; Kagaha and Manderson, 2020). My fieldwork in three hospitals demonstrated that even in health facilities where MVA was available, medical workers continued to use digital evacuation to treat PAC patients.

Maimouna's and Khady's clinical encounters illustrate the remarkable geopolitical funding configurations of Senegal's national PAC program, which has been supported since its inception by the U.S. government through its Agency for International Development (USAID). Starting in 1973 with the Helms Amendment to the Foreign Assistance Act, which banned the use of foreign aid for the "performance of abortion as a form of family planning" (Barot, 2013, p, 9), and in a bizarre contradiction with its generous support for contraceptive research and programming since the late 1960s (Murphy, 2012; Takeshita, 2012), the United States has profoundly influenced the global landscape of reproductive health care through anti-abortion policies. The Mexico City Policy (derisively dubbed the "Global Gag Rule" by reproductive health advocates) is among the most notorious anti-abortion measures in the global terrain of reproductive health advocacy, research, and programming. First issued as an executive order by President Ronald Reagan in 1984, it extended the 1973 Helms Amendment by prohibiting foreign NGOs that receive U.S. family planning aid from using their own funds, or funds from other sources, to engage in abortion service delivery, referral to legal abortion services, abortion advocacy, or abortion research (Barot, 2017; Starrs, 2017; van der Meulen Rodgers, 2018). Activated by every Republican president since 1984, this executive order has been in place for eighteen out of the last thirty-three years.[7] Considering that the United States has accounted for over two-thirds of global funding for family planning since 2003 (Grollman et al., 2018), the Mexico City Policy exercises tremendous control over reproductive health through the threat of withholding family planning aid. Ironically, although the Mexico City Policy aims to *reduce* the incidence of abortion in developing countries, data from sub-Saharan Africa and Latin America show that the odds of having an abortion increased during periods when it was activated, thus revealing that it has had the opposite effect (van der Meulen Rodgers, 2018).

PAC was conceived in a global reproductive health landscape profoundly affected by the hostility of the Mexico City Policy toward abortion (B. Crane, 1994). Its inclusion in the ICPD represents a political compromise on abortion in global health and development frameworks that do not recognize safe abortion as a reproductive right. Because PAC treats complications of spontaneous or induced abortions that have already occurred, it is the only abortion-related intervention that is exempt from the Mexico City Policy and thus eligible for financial support from USAID. USAID has spent over $20 million on PAC in forty countries since 1994. In 2003, USAID launched a five-year global PAC initiative that selected seven countries—Bolivia, Cambodia, Haiti, Mexico, Nepal, Senegal, and Tanzania—to receive special funds to institutionalize PAC within reproductive health care through operations research and community-based initiatives (Curtis, 2007).

Beyond PAC's puzzling ties to USAID, a donor agency that has been influenced by anti-abortion policies since the early 1970s, there is little statistical evidence tying PAC to reductions in national estimates of maternal mortality. Experts agree that as part of EmOC, PAC contributes, in theory, to reductions in maternal mortality by preventing abortion-related deaths (Bullough et al., 2005; Campbell and Graham, 2006; Gerdts et al., 2015). Additionally, PAC improves care for patients by replacing dilation and curettage with safer, more effective uterine evacuation methods such as MVA or EVA. These methods are associated with reduced patient costs, shorter periods of hospitalization, and fewer complications such as infection and uterine perforation (Huber, Curtis, Irani, Pappa, and Arrington, 2016).

Despite these advantages, establishing statistical associations between PAC and reductions in maternal mortality is inextricably bound with problems inherent to measuring abortion-related mortality itself. In countries with restrictive abortion laws, abortion-related mortality and morbidity are notoriously difficult to measure because women obtain services outside the formal health system, are often reluctant to seek care if complications arise, and may not disclose the cause of complications to health workers or family members. To avoid being implicated in police investigations of illegal abortion, health workers may not wish to disclose abortion-related deaths or services (Gerdts, Vohra, and Ahern, 2013). Hospital records of PAC thus lack the precision needed to statistically calculate not only the kinds of abortions being treated but also the kinds of abortions responsible for obstetric deaths when they occur, and the extent to which PAC averts such deaths on a national scale. In other words, the social context of PAC data collection limits the capacity to determine whether the intervention works in a statistical sense, and, if we are to use such metrics as a measuring stick for how resources should be directed, whether financial resources directed to PAC are justified.

Although Senegal's maternal mortality ratio decreased from 434 to 392 deaths per 100,000 live births between 2005 and 2010/2011 (Agence National de la Statistique et de la Démographie [ANSD and ICF International], 2012; N'Diaye and Ayad, 2006), and declined again to 273 in 2017 (ANSD and ICF, 2018), an epidemiological study of abortion conducted in 2013 estimated that 42 percent of women with complications from unsafe abortion did not receive PAC, with low-income women and women in rural areas least likely to do so (Sedgh, Sylla, Philbin, Keogh, and Ndiaye, 2015). In 2016, the estimated national cost of providing PAC was nearly $500,000 (Linche-Deroche et al., 2020). At a time of deepening financial austerity among governments and aid donors, when statistics demonstrating impact and cost-effectiveness have never mattered more in the field of global health (V. Adams, 2016; Biehl and Petryna, 2013; Erikson, 2012; Pfeiffer, 2019; Pfeiffer and Nichter, 2008), what are we to make of PAC's persistence in national and global strategies for maternal mortality reduction, and how do we reconcile its inextricable connection to abortion with its exemption from the Mexico City Policy?

HOW PAC WORKS

In this book, I illustrate how PAC, despite a lack of rigorous statistical evidence that it reduces maternal mortality, or even that it is available to the women who need it most, remains in place through simultaneously contributing to and enacting global forms of reproductive governance. My primary argument is that reproductive governance is not limited to national abortion laws or donor funding policies like the Mexico City Policy, but also occurs "from below" (Harding, 2008), as medical workers, health officials, and personnel from NGOs produce selective facts about women and abortion through mundane practices of daily clinical care, utilization of obstetric technology, and epidemiological surveillance of maternal mortality. I anchor this argument in scholarship from the fields of anthropology, science and technology studies (STS), and sociology that illustrates how data are not simply neutral facts or figures but active participants in the process of governance through their carefully orchestrated depictions of reality (V. Adams, 2013, 2016; Biruk, 2018; Merry, 2016). By allowing scientists and policy makers to "see exactly what they intend to see" (Biruk, 2012, p. 348), numbers shape decisions about social policies, services, and interventions. While much has been written about the role of numbers in population governance (Greenhalgh, 2005; Kanaaneh, 2002; Kligman, 1998; Murphy, 2017), scholars have more recently focused on how specific indicators of maternal and reproductive health, such as contraceptive prevalence or the maternal mortality ratio, enact governance in national and global arenas (Brunson and Suh, 2020; Oni-Orisan, 2016; Storeng and Béhague 2014, 2017; Wendland, 2016).

I demonstrate in this book how national and global stakeholders enact reproductive governance as they assemble and convey evidence about the kinds of women who receive life-saving obstetric care in government hospitals, what PAC technologies accomplish in these facilities, and how PAC affects maternal mortality. Through the systematic misclassification of suspected induced abortion as miscarriage in hospital records, PAC generates epidemiological narratives of induced abortion as a rare occurrence, thereby reinforcing discriminatory attitudes and practices toward women who are suspected of having procured an illegal abortion, or what scholars of reproduction have termed "abortion stigma" (Kumar et al., 2009; Norris et al. 2011). Selective reporting practices elide the persistence of obstetric techniques such as digital evacuation in hospitals that compromise women's safety and comfort during treatment. Generalized metrics of hospital performance, which do not distinguish between miscarriage and induced abortion and offer limited insight into the quality of care experienced by women patients, have been accepted as evidence that PAC works in reducing maternal mortality.

The clinical encounter of Maimouna Diallo, who survived her injuries, is particularly powerful in illustrating how health professionals pragmatically deploy demographic and epidemiological data in ways that idealize certain kinds of reproductive behaviors, identities, technologies, techniques, and interventions and demonstrate commitment to national and global accords on maternal and reproductive health. Although health workers at l'Hôpital de Ville suspected that Maimouna had illegally terminated a pregnancy, they recorded her in the PAC register as a case of incomplete abortion, and by default, a miscarriage. Aggregated across multiple levels of the health information system, such data points are established as facts that come to stand in for the kinds of women—presumably expectant mothers—who receive PAC in government hospitals. A preponderance of miscarriages not only is of little interest to law enforcement authorities but also resonates with Senegal's commitment to global efforts to reduce maternal mortality, formalized in the 1987 SMI (Abou-Zahr, 2003). Although Maimouna was treated with MVA, a preferred PAC technology, I will show in chapter 2 how, like Khady Ndiaye, she could just as easily have been treated with digital evacuation, depending on the time and day of her arrival at l'Hôpital de Ville, where MVA treatment was limited to weekdays and performed only by physicians. When calculated into impressive indicators of the percentage of patients that receive MVA, her case obscures the reasons why women continue to be treated with less effective techniques. Finally, because Maimouna survived, health experts can draw on her case to champion PAC as an effective maternal mortality reduction intervention, even if the numeric fact of her survival says nothing about the physical suffering and social and psychological distress she experienced before, during, and after treatment.

This book locates claims about the kinds of interventions and technologies that measurably improve maternal and reproductive health outcomes, or that "work" (V. Adams, 2013), and the kinds of women who receive and are deserving of affordable care within a broader geopolitical landscape of global health governance logics and funding directives. Some of these governance practices—such as the growing influence of evidence-based medicine in the field of global health, where rigorous statistical data, ideally from randomized controlled trials (RCTs),[8] are required to demonstrate impact and cost-effectiveness (V. Adams, 2016)—dovetail neatly with increasingly econometric investments in the fields of health and development. Historian Michelle Murphy (2017) has referred to this trend, emerging during the mid-twentieth century, as the "economization of life," in which decisions about policies or interventions are made according to projections of future economic growth. In the field of maternal and reproductive health, hospital-based, professionally controlled, and pharmaceutical interventions are associated with averted births or maternal deaths, which are in turn associated with improvements in national metrics of economic growth such as gross domestic product. Such instrumentalist logics, and the anti-abortion stance of the world's most significant donor of global reproductive health aid, starkly contradict global commitments to reproductive rights, in which women are fundamentally entitled to reproductive well-being, autonomy, and bodily integrity (Corrêa and Petchesky, 1999).

By locating women's clinical encounters with PAC and health professionals' PAC practices in a global context, I illustrate not only how global reproductive governance has unfolded numerically in Senegal during the late twentieth and early twenty-first centuries, but also how PAC itself enacts reproductive governance globally. Situated within national and global policy frameworks for reproductive health that simultaneously reject safe abortion and claim to uphold women's reproductive health and rights, PAC reinforces gender, racial, and class inequalities through its definitions of not only the kinds of women in the global South who receive and are deserving of obstetric care, but also the kinds of obstetric care to which such women are entitled. By strategically obscuring information about the frequency of induced abortion and about what happens in gynecological wards, PAC data narrow the scope of bodies, experiences, and identities that matter enough to count in global reproductive policy making. While these numbers matter most in demonstrating commitments to global treaties on maternal and reproductive health, they foreclose opportunities to take steps toward measures that have historically improved women's health, such as access to safe, legal abortion and the availability of quality obstetric care throughout the health system. In the next section, I engage explicitly with imbrications of violence and care in PAC as a mechanism of global reproductive governance.

AT THE INTERSECTION OF CARE AND VIOLENCE

While the term "obstetric violence" has often referred to the hyper-medicalization of pregnancy and delivery, I explore how it unfolds more broadly in substandard and neglectful treatment of women, particularly low-income women and women of color, during *any* kind of reproductive health care. Obstetric violence is not just about individual medical workers who mistreat women, or a few bad apples. Instead, this concept links unnecessary and abusive treatment and neglect during reproductive health care to underlying systems of inequality related to gender, race or ethnicity, class, age, and geography (Davis, 2019; Freedman et al., 2014; Sadler et al., 2016; Zacher Dixon, 2015). In this sense, we can consider under-medicalized births as a form of obstetric violence when women are unable to access lifesaving drugs, blood supplies, or surgeries (Heller, 2019). We can also interpret restrictive abortion laws—which leave women, and low-income women in particular, to resort to unsafe procedures—as a form of obstetric violence (Faúndes and Shah, 2015; Grimes et al., 2006).

Throughout the book, I illustrate how PAC, conceived as a form of public health harm reduction in response to global anti-abortion funding mechanisms and restrictive national abortion laws, simultaneously ensures women's survival and subjects them to bodily and structural forms of violence. When suspected of illegal abortion, women often endure the humiliation of what is widely understood among Senegalese health workers as l'interrogation. If the police become involved, women may be arrested and incarcerated. Policies related to MVA utilization, exercised within health facilities that are frequently underequipped, expose women to poor-quality care in the form of dilation and curettage or digital evacuation. Women who can afford to seek treatment for abortion complications in the private health care sector will likely receive good-quality, discreet care. Those who can afford a safe abortion may not experience complications at all. Exposure to obstetric violence as part of PAC, thus, is deeply embedded in gender, age, and class inequalities.

Obstetric violence in PAC is enacted not only through discriminatory abortion laws and poor-quality care but also through strategic measurement practices that produce data that suggest most PAC patients have experienced miscarriage, most patients are treated with MVA, and PAC contributes to maternal mortality reduction. While PAC indicators convey compliance with national and global commitments to maternal and reproductive health, they obscure physical suffering and psychosocial distress related to clandestine abortion before, during, and after treatment. Through these metrics, PAC defines, and ultimately limits, the kinds of obstetric care to which Senegalese women are entitled to merely *survive* abortion complications. Finally, by normalizing survival of abortion complications as a state of reproductive well-being, PAC data foreclose opportunities for abortion law reform, which has been associated with declines in abortion-related mortality in high-, low-, and middle-income countries (Faúndes and Shah, 2015; Fathallah, 2019). Data suggesting that most PAC patients have had miscarriages and that PAC services effectively keep these women alive suppress political will to change the abortion law.

What are we to make of a harm reduction intervention that exposes the most vulnerable women to bodily and structural harm? Feminist scholars have drawn extensively on Michel Foucault's (1978) theory of biopower—the exercise of power through the "calculated management of life"—to explore the deployment of metrics, interventions, and technologies in the definition and resolution of population problems (Andaya, 2014; Greenhalgh, 1995, 2005; Morgan and Roberts, 2012; Takeshita, 2012; De Zordo, 2016). I argue that imbrications of obstetric violence and care in PAC demonstrate the need to consider reproductive governance in relation to Cameroonian philosopher Achille Mbeme's theory of "necropower," which refers to the exercise of power through death, terror, suffering, dehumanization, and disposability (Mbembe and Meintjes, 2003). If we think of it in terms of necropower, PAC represents a profoundly stratified system of global reproductive governance that withholds affordable obstetric care from low-income women in Senegal (and other countries where abortion is legally restricted) until after they have resorted to unsafe procedures, and then punishes them in hospitals for transgressing gendered expectations of motherhood with threats, humiliation, and poor-quality care. In the face of decades of evidence showing that legal abortion reduces abortion-related mortality (Fathalla, 2019; Faúndes and Shah, 2015) and that PAC poses a tremendous financial burden on health systems in developing countries (S. Singh and Maddow-Zimet, 2016; Vlassoff, Shearer, Walker, and Lucas, 2008), the intervention's staying power in global and national reproductive health policies illuminates the disposability of women's bodies in global forms of reproductive governance. In other words, it is politically preferable to control women through threats of criminalization, death, and injury related to unsafe abortion than to implement policies and services that have been proven to reduce maternal mortality and health system costs related to PAC.

At the same time that PAC holds women hostage to restrictive abortion laws, it presents considerable professional, technological, and financial opportunities to a variety of stakeholders. Engagement in PAC research, programming, and advocacy confers global recognition of a commitment to reproductive rights on health authorities and NGOs, which leads to more funding for PAC. It pays, quite literally, to keep women alive after they have resorted to unsafe abortion. Indicators showing that health workers are being trained in MVA and that women are being treated with this technology ensure the investment of additional funding to keep more women alive. Since launching the first operations research project on PAC in 1997, the Senegalese MSAS has worked with and received technical support from at least nine international NGOs in the area of PAC, often with the financial backing of USAID.

PAC's connection with family planning promises additional opportunities to gain professional prestige and new markets for pharmaceutical research and sales. PAC patients represent an important group of potential contraceptive "acceptors" who can contribute to reaching the goals articulated by global and regional family planning initiatives like the Family Planning 2020 Initiative (FP 2020) and the Ouagadougou Partnership, described in the next section. For pharmaceutical companies involved in these initiatives, actual and potential PAC patients represent an additional client population for long-acting reversible contraceptives (LARCs) and other contraceptive methods (Bendix, Foley, Hendrixson, and Schultz, 2019). The integration of misoprostol into the global PAC model has also generated lucrative new markets for manufacturers of a drug that, in many countries, until recently was registered only for the treatment of gastric ulcers (Fernandez, Coeytaux, Gomez Ponce de León, and Harrison, 2009; Morgan, 2019; Weeks, Fiala, and Safar, 2005). A booming underground abortion economy operates alongside PAC, as women and providers use misoprostol to initiate abortions in private and then turn to government hospitals to receive PAC if complications arise (Sherris et al., 2005). Drawing on the concept of necropower, we see how PAC renders women's bodies disposable in the achievement of national and global maternal and reproductive health targets and the enrichment of pharmaceutical companies. PAC indicators celebrate the capacity of health systems to keep women alive—and to offer modern contraception to these survivors—while obscuring the material reality of reproduction in which clandestine and frequently unsafe abortion remains an option for too many women.

THEORIZING REPRODUCTIVE GOVERNANCE

Morgan and Roberts (2012) describe reproductive governance as an "analytic tool for tracing the shifting political rationalities directed towards reproduction" (p. 241). We can observe how reproductive governance is exercised through laws that regulate reproductive behaviors and practices such as abortion and contraception. Implicit in such laws are the "moral regimes" or "privileged standards of morality" (p. 242) that incentivize or idealize some reproductive behaviors, practices, and identities and actively stigmatize others. Restrictive abortion laws, for example, privilege not only the "innocent unborn" but also the selfless, nurturing, and responsible mothers who carry their pregnancies to term (Kumar et al., 2009). Reproductive policies reflect a calculated ranking of bodies, subjectivities, and identities along a gendered, racialized, and classed spectrum of normative reproductive behavior. In the United States, the enduring trope in the public imagination of the Black welfare queen, a single woman who deliberately has children out of wedlock to receive government benefits on the taxpayer's dime, motivated an overhaul of the welfare system in 1996 that reduced the length of time during which adults could receive such assistance (Bensonsmith, 2005; Bridges, 2011; Roberts, 1997).

As an analytic tool, reproductive governance draws significantly on Foucault's concept of biopower: the surveillance and management of populations through scientific knowledge produced by professional disciplines such as demography and epidemiology to achieve the political and economic goals of the state (Foucault, 1978; Foucault and Ewald, 2003). Population planning requires the collection and synthesis of reproductive data. Measurements related to fertility, abortion, pregnancy, delivery, and infant and maternal mortality and morbidity must be standardized into indicators that facilitate comparison across a variety of variables such as age, class, and residence. In turn, policy makers draw on these indicators to establish policies, design services, and calculate demographic and epidemiological targets for the future.

Reproductive governance requires careful policing of reproductive bodies to meet biopolitical targets related to population size. In the Belgian Congo, colonial medical officers pressured pregnant women to give birth in hospitals, not because they were particularly concerned with the well-being of African women,[9] but because they wanted to ensure the healthy delivery of babies who would eventually enrich the colony as laborers in mines, battlefields, and plantations (Hunt, 1999). In postcolonial China, Nigeria, and India, policy makers exercised demographic theories about the relationship between fertility and economic growth by implementing population policies that calculated fertility reduction targets over time (Connelly, 2006; Greenhalgh, 2008; Robinson, 2012). In Romania, the Ceaușescu regime perceived declining fertility rates as a threat to economic growth and modernization of the socialist state. To increase fertility, the government not only outlawed contraception and abortion but also mandated annual (or in some places, trimesterly) gynecological exams for women of reproductive age who attended or worked for state institutions such as schools or factories (Kligman, 1998).

National population statistics exert great influence as objective representations or facts of reproduction (such as total fertility rates, modern contraceptive prevalence, or maternal mortality ratios) that must be acted on through interventions such as family planning or obstetric services (V. Adams, 2005; Wendland, 2016). Decisions about population indicators or targets are thus political in the sense that they frame how population problems are defined and addressed. The power of numbers is evident not only in who does the counting (often "technocrats" with specialized statistical training in demography or economics) but also in what or who such experts decide matters enough to count (Merry, 2016).

While perceived as standardized, objective facts, population indicators may obscure the material conditions in which people make decisions about pregnancy, delivery, contraception, and abortion. The maternal mortality ratio, for example, offers little insight into the quality of maternal health care available to pregnant women (Wendland, 2016). Additionally, it says nothing about morbidity or "near miss events," which are often greater in number in developing countries (Storeng and Béhague, 2017; Storeng, Murray, Akoum, Ouattara, and Filippi, 2010). Indicators such as modern contraceptive prevalence, which measures the percentage of women using technological forms of birth control, overlook the importance of periodic abstinence in certain societies (Johnson-Hanks, 2002a). The demographic concept of birth spacing, in which contraception facilitates longer intervals between births to improve maternal and infant health, has been promoted by reproductive health advocates in developing countries as a form of empowering women. Yet, this concept obscures the social and economic contexts in which women accept or reject contraception (Duclos et al., 2019). In the Gambia, for example, women used contraception between births to maximize rather than limit family size (Bledsoe, Banja, and Hill, 1998).

In large part because women's bodies have been disproportionately (bio) medicalized for the purposes of fertility regulation (Clarke, Shim, Mamo, Fosket, and Fishman, 2003; Conrad, 1992; Daniels, 2009; Oudshoorn, 2003), women also bear the brunt of population policies that aspire to meet demographic targets and ideals. These embodied consequences are particularly dire when population targets fail to recognize the social and material conditions of reproduction. In Romania, prohibitions on abortion and contraception not only failed to increase birth rates but also led to staggering levels of mortality and morbidity related to clandestine abortion (Kligman, 1998). In China, fertility reduction targets were achieved through closely monitored, mandatory contraceptive practices such as sterilizing couples (usually women) who had reached the allowed number of children or requiring women who had exceeded this number to have abortions (Greenhalgh, 1994). The architects of South Africa's restrictive abortion law in 1975 turned a blind eye to disproportionately high rates of abortion-related mortality among Black women. During the era of apartheid, some viewed such mortality as an indirect method of curbing fertility in the Black population (Klausen, 2016). In sub-Saharan Africa, discourses urging women to "plan" their families stand in stark contradiction to social norms that encourage high parity within marriage and, among the poorest quintiles of society, the continuing threat of infant mortality (Foley, 2007; Renne, 2016). A recent study from a de-identified country in sub-Saharan Africa revealed how, in an effort to reach highly publicized family planning targets, health workers may subject women to coercive practices such as pressuring them to adopt or refusing to remove LARCs (Senderowicz, 2019).

Reproductive governance is not limited to individual countries, but since the mid-twentieth century has operated transnationally through UN agencies, philanthropic foundations, bilateral donors of aid, and national and international NGOs. The term "population control" describes the global response to the social, political, economic, and environmental consequences of the perceived problem of "overpopulation" (Bhatia et al., 2019). Grounded in demographic transition theory, in which fertility reduction leads to economic development and modernization (Greenhalgh, 1996; Murphy, 2017), population control promoted the use of modern contraception (with coercion, if necessary [Berelson and Lieberson, 1979]) to foster economic development and stave off the social and political unrest related to excessive human numbers (Connelly, 2008; Hartmann, 1995).

Although the first two World Population Conferences organized by the UN in 1954 (Rome) [10] and 1965 (Belgrade)[11] were primarily attended by population experts to share fertility data and discuss population planning, the 1974 conference in Bucharest was attended by delegates from 135 countries. The conference yielded a World Population Plan of Action that urged individual countries to adopt population policies with fertility reduction targets to achieve socioeconomic development. While the Plan of Action written during the 1984 International Conference on Population in Mexico City recognized the importance of human rights, health and well-being, and employment and education in the development process, the emphasis remained on creating population policies oriented around fertility reduction (Dixon-Mueller, 1993).[12]

In 1994, the ICPD in Cairo generated a Platform of Action that rejected earlier population control approaches to economic development that focused on establishing and meeting demographic targets through family planning. Instead, the ICPD framed women's reproductive health and rights as key components of the development process. It called on governments to not only ensure access to a broad range of safe and high-quality reproductive health services (including maternal health care) but also improve the social and economic conditions in which women and couples make decisions about fertility. In other words, the concept of reproductive rights was meaningless without the material conditions required to exercise reproductive autonomy (Corrêa and Petchesky, 1999; Lane, 1994). Although the ICPD did not articulate goals with respect to fertility reduction, it pledged to reduce 1990 levels of maternal mortality by three-quarters and to achieve universal access to reproductive health care services by 2015. These targets were adopted by the fifth Millennium Development Goal (MDG) to improve maternal health (WHO, 2015). In 2015, the third Sustainable Development Goal (SDG) "to ensure healthy lives and promote well-being at all ages" pledged to reduce the global maternal mortality ratio to fewer than 70 deaths per 100,000 live births and to achieve universal access to reproductive health care by 2030 (UN, 2018).

Some scholars have argued that far from truly dismantling population control, the ICPD simply rebranded fertility reduction efforts in the feminist language of reproductive rights (Hodgson and Watkins, 1997; Murphy, 2012; Petchesky, 1995). More recently, feminist scholars have raised concerns that the global health community has quite boldly returned to the demographic targets rejected by the 1994 ICPD. In 2012, a Family Planning Summit was organized by the United Kingdom Department for International Development, UNFPA, USAID, and the Bill & Melinda Gates Foundation in London to revitalize political commitments to increase modern contraceptive prevalence and reduce unmet contraceptive need. Pointing to other areas of global health, such as child health, that have experienced dramatic achievements through the establishment of measurable goals, the organizers called for similar metrics in family planning to serve as a "rallying point" for mobilizing resources and galvanizing action among governments, donors, and NGOs (Brown et al., 2014, p. 75). The summit resulted in the articulation of a global family planning target, dubbed "120 by 20," that aimed to have 120 million new family planning users in sixty-nine of the world's poorest countries by the year 2020. FP 2020 works with individual countries to establish and monitor family planning targets, supports research on new contraceptive technologies, and provides technical assistance in scaling up access to contraceptive methods through public and private outlets (Bendix et al., 2019). Additionally, FP 2020 has catalyzed regional initiatives such as the Ouagadougou Partnership, in which nine Francophone African countries pledged to have 2.2 million additional women on contraception by 2020 (Partenariat de Ouagadougou, 2015).

Reproductive governance thus unfolds globally through the collective establishment of demographic and epidemiological priorities, goals, and indicators by government bodies and nongovernment actors. Governments demonstrate power, expertise, and commitment to the global polity by participating in global conferences and initiatives, by signing accords, and by developing policies and programs that adhere to global benchmarks (Andaya, 2014; Bendix et al., 2019; Boyle, Longhofer, and Kim, 2015; Robinson, 2017). At the same time, nonstate actors exercise "soft" (Merry, 2016, p. 11) power or govern "at a distance" (Erikson, 2012, p. 372) through evaluating countries' progress on meeting indicators. Published rankings of countries' performance on indicators may bolster governments' reputations, at home and within the global community, as competent stewards of population health, or may embarrass them into efforts toward improvement (Merry, 2016). In Morocco, for example, a "political brouhaha" (p.268) was set in motion when an international NGO released a maternal mortality ratio that was significantly higher than the official government estimate, prompting the political opposition to question the current administration's ability to properly care for pregnant women (Storeng and Béhague, 2014). Nonstate actors reward governments for achieving or making progress toward targets through distributing resources in the form of financial and technical support for services, programs, research, and infrastructure (Erikson, 2012; Oni-Orisan, 2016; Sullivan, 2017; Wendland, 2016).

Undoubtedly, global reproductive policies like the Mexico City Policy directly infringe on the public health sovereignty of countries that receive U.S. family planning aid, especially where there are legal provisions for safe abortion (Cohen, 2000; B. Crane and Dusenberry, 2004; Starrs, 2017). At the same time, social scientists argue that evidence-based forms of global health governance, which rely on statistical data to measure associations between health interventions and outcomes, are increasingly challenging the nation-state's authority to regulate population health (V. Adams, 2016). Since the late 1970s, despite the global community's commitment to universal access to primary health care articulated in the 1978 Alma-Ata Declaration, global health decision-making has been increasingly governed by neoliberal logics of cost-effectiveness and privatization (Biehl and Petryna, 2013; Erikson, 2012; Pfeiffer and Chapman, 2010). Donors are more likely to invest in magic bullets, medication or interventions that yield the best health outcomes at minimal cost, at times with inadequate recognition of the conditions in which these technologies are used (or not) in daily medical and public health practice (Biehl, 2007; Cueto, 2013; Packard, 2007, 2016). Within a global health landscape that increasingly prioritizes statistical evidence of cost-effectiveness and impact (V. Adams, 2013, 2016; Storeng and Béhague, 2014, 2017), magic bullets come to stand in for the "staff, stuff, space, and systems" (Farmer, 2014, pp. 38–39) that compose the public health sector in which people seek and experience care. As governments in developing countries have withdrawn from the provision of health care following neoliberal economic reform (Thomson, Kentikelenis, and Stubbs, 2017), private actors such as NGOs have played an increasingly important role in health care delivery (Packard, 2016; Pfeiffer, 2019).[13] Additionally, the demand for better numbers has created new markets for health care consulting firms and agencies that specialize in the collection and analysis of health data (V. Adams, 2013; Erikson, 2012).

These neoliberal counting technologies of governance are vividly illustrated in the field of global maternal and reproductive health. Pharmaceutical technologies such as misoprostol (for preventing and treating postpartum hemorrhage [PPH]) or magnesium sulfate (for treating pre-eclampsia and eclampsia) that can be tested through RCTs are increasingly preferred over longer-term solutions that focus more broadly on strengthening health systems and reducing inequalities in access to health services (Storeng and Béhague, 2014). LARCs have been heavily promoted by FP 2020 as ideal technologies that offer the most bang for the buck in reducing fertility because method reliability is not compromised by user error (Bendix et al., 2019). Private actors such as ICF,[14] the University of Aberdeen's Initiative for Maternal Mortality Programme Assessment, and the University of Washington's Institute for Health Metrics and Evaluation (IHME)[15] receive lucrative contracts from donors to collect demographic data and to evaluate maternal health interventions in developing countries (DHS, 2008; Storeng and Béhague, 2017).

Numeric mechanisms of reproductive governance reinscribe hierarchies of race, gender, class, and geography in defining and measuring problems and finding solutions related to reproduction. Since the early twentieth century, neo-Malthusian[16] demographic theories about the relationship between fertility and the economy have problematized the reproduction of nonwhite populations in the global South as threats to the health, security, and environmental sustainability of wealthy populations in the developed world (Hartmann, 1995; Kuumba, 1999; Sasser, 2018). Preventing excess births in developing countries was widely understood as key to securing "the abundant life" in the West (Murphy, 2017). Although social scientists and feminist activists have offered powerful critiques of Eurocentric demographic theories of the relationship among fertility, economic development, and environmental degradation (Greenhalgh, 1995; Hartmann, 1995; Mamdani, 1972; Watkins, 1987, 1990, 1993),[17] population control remained the dominant global population paradigm from the late 1960s until the 1994 ICPD, funded in large part by USAID as a matter of national security. High levels of fertility (and maternal mortality and morbidity) in the global South continue to be understood as natural, objective facts related to the insufficiently modern reproductive behavior of nonwhite populations (Bhatia et al., 2019; Heller, 2019; McCann, 2017). Neo-Malthusian theories conveniently overlook how structural inequalities in the global distribution of resources related to the neoliberal restructuring of economies as part of the techno-scientific "development" of post-colonial countries have contributed to adverse health and environmental out-comes (Hartmann, 1995; Sasser, 2018; Storeng and Béhague, 2017).

Decision-making and resource allocation related to global reproductive governance remain concentrated in the hands of donor agencies, philanthropic foundations, pharmaceutical companies, and NGOs in the global North. Start-ing in the late 1960s, population control advocates worked closely with pharma-ceutical companies to test, market, and distribute contraceptive technologies to women in the global South (Kuumba, 1999; Murphy, 2012; Takeshita, 2012). More recently, FP 2020 has opened up vast new markets for LARCs in sub-Saharan Africa by negotiating the purchase of contraceptives with pharmaceuti-cal companies. For example, in addition to committing over $1 billion to FP 2020 in 2012 (FP 2020, 2013), the Bill & Melinda Gates Foundation negotiated a special price for Sayana Press (a self-administered injectable LARC)[18] in FP 2020 countries (Bendix et al., 2019). Rather than providing direct support to national epidemiological surveillance systems in developing countries, donors contract with private actors to gather health data and evaluate interventions (Storeng and Béhague, 2017). Not surprisingly, local professionals are usually tasked with the highly time-consuming yet less prestigious and lower-salaried work of conducting surveys or reviewing records "in the field" (Biruk, 2018).[19]

Global regimes of reproductive governance reinforce gender, race, and class inequalities by idealizing certain reproductive subjectivities, identities, and bodies while deeming others in need of intervention. According to mid-twentieth-century demographers in favor of population control, the dangers of overpopu-lation were driven by the traditional, "backward" fertility practices of women in the "Third World." In contrast, women in the West demonstrated responsible, rational, and modern behaviors by delaying marriage and childbearing (McCann, 2017). While feminist architects of the 1994 ICPD Platform of Action portrayed women as reproductive rights-bearing citizens, contemporary climate change advocates urge women in the global South to be "sexual stewards" of the envi-ronment by making rational, responsible decisions about contraceptive use and family size (Sasser, 2018). Global initiatives to "invest in girls," organized by international feminist NGOs and financed by for-profit corporations, highlight the potential of (contraceptively responsible) young women to advance "the good life" for their families and communities, thereby contributing to economic growth (Bhatia et al., 2019; Murphy, 2017). Campaigns to reduce maternal mortality and morbidity call on governments and donors to improve maternal health care to protect selfless, nurturing mothers. The global SMI has been careful not to advocate for legal abortion precisely because pregnancy termination violates gendered expectations of women's acceptance of and desire for motherhood, rendering women who have abortions less deserving of care and protection (Abou-Zahr, 2003; Kumar et al., 2009; Rance, 1997; Suh, 2018).

PAC IN GLOBAL REGIMES OF REPRODUCTIVE GOVERNANCE

To understand how PAC simultaneously contributes to and enacts global reproductive governance, we must situate the intervention within several familiar regimes of population governance since the mid-twentieth century, including population control, safe motherhood, and the ICPD platform of reproductive rights. Although advocates of maternal and reproductive health and environmental sustainability are eager to bracket population control as a relic of the Cold War era, a great deal of continuity exists between the mechanisms of reproductive governance—national and global institutions, policies, indicators, discourses, technologies, and subjectivities—associated with those regimes. Feminist scholars use the term "populationism" to signal contemporary strategies, logics, and approaches that accept as scientific fact the negative impact of human numbers on the environment. Although populationism calls for achieving environmental sustainability through voluntary access to contraception, its emphasis on averting births among nonwhite and poor populations in the global South, and in sub-Saharan Africa in particular, illustrates the endurance of racial hierarchies in the calculation of lives worth living (Bhatia et al., 2019; Murphy, 2017; Sasser, 2018). Despite a commitment to reproductive rights, populationist approaches prioritize target-driven, technical fixes to reduce excess births (Bendix et al., 2019).

Established in 1987 and 1994, respectively, the global SMI and the ICPD Platform of Action rejected population control's narrow focus on fertility reduction through family planning and called for maternal and reproductive health care grounded in reproductive rights. Nevertheless, both regimes of reproductive governance are increasingly oriented toward number-driven, magic bullet approaches. While the SMI initially called for multisectoral, system-wide approaches to reduce maternal mortality, donors are increasingly favoring pharmaceutical, hospital-based interventions (Storeng and Béhague, 2014). By counting the number of maternal deaths averted through contraceptive use, maternal health advocates emphasize the role of family planning in reducing women's exposure to maternal death (Ahmed, Li, Liu, and Tsui, 2012; Brunson, 2020). Reductions in the maternal mortality ratio, despite considerable debate over this indicator's capacity to accurately capture the state of maternal health care in a given country, remain an important marker of good maternal health governance (Oni-Orisan, 2016; Wendland, 2016). Although the 1994 ICPD omitted specific fertility reduction targets, calling instead for "universal access" to reproductive health care, FP 2020's "120 by 20" goal illustrates the resurgence of numeric family planning targets in global reproductive health governance (Bendix et al., 2019).

Conceptualized during the early 1990s, PAC represents a remarkable hybrid of the populationist logics of all three regimes. While PAC pragmatically situates abortion care under the politically acceptable umbrella of EmOC for mothers, the intervention's contraceptive component, which endeavors to prevent "repeat" abortion, resonates with efforts to avert excess births. PAC promises to improve the organization and quality of EmOC through the deployment of uterine aspiration technologies such as MVA and EVA, and more recently, the uterotonic misoprostol. The utilization of these technologies in obstetric care can be quantified in ways that demonstrate commitment to reproductive rights. Through PAC indicators, reproductive health advocates may demonstrate the achievement of goals related to maternal health and family planning without violating national laws restricting abortion or jeopardizing USAID funding for family planning under the Mexico City Policy.

In this book, I explore clinical activities, technologies, and measurement practices related to PAC, an intervention at the intersection of multiple regimes of global reproductive governance. At a time when global reproductive health stakeholders are increasingly concerned with establishing accurate measures of impact and cost-effectiveness, and in a region where rates of fertility and maternal mortality are among the highest in the world, this approach allows us to trace empirically how reproductive governance has unfolded in sub-Saharan Africa during the late twentieth and early twenty-first centuries. As a reproductive health intervention funded by USAID, tested and implemented in collaboration with international NGOs, and grounded in global treaties on reproductive rights, PAC represents an important *mechanism* of global reproductive governance. At the same time, I illustrate how PAC practitioners contribute to reproductive governance through the selective production and deployment of data about what PAC technologies accomplish in government hospitals, the kinds of women who receive obstetric care in these facilities, and the intervention's contribution to reductions in maternal mortality. These data *enact* reproductive governance by shaping perceptions of the kinds of obstetric care to which women are entitled, ultimately limiting possibilities for revision of a discriminatory and harmful abortion law.

TOWARD REPRODUCTIVE JUSTICE

As a feminist scholar, how do I justify a critical analysis of PAC at a time when access to abortion remains restricted across much of the developing world and is under renewed attack in wealthy countries like the United States? What purpose is served, theoretically or practically, by highlighting the necropolitical elements of the only abortion-related intervention exempt from the Mexico City Policy, reinstated by President Trump on his third day in office in January 2017? Global reproductive health advocates include PAC in multipronged strategies to reduce maternal mortality because the intervention can save women's lives in countries with restrictive abortion laws. In chapter 2, I demonstrate how PAC can facilitate the introduction of safe abortion technologies like MVA (and more recently, misoprostol) into health systems and services. Without a doubt, the political and programmatic accomplishments of establishing PAC services in countries with restrictive abortion laws, often with support from USAID, deserve recognition not only for improving the quality of care but also for catalyzing national conversations about unsafe abortion as a maternal health problem.

Since the early 1990s, women of color activists and scholars have understood reproductive justice as a framework for research, theory, and practice that highlights how inequalities related to gender, race, class, and ability constrain people's capacity to lead healthy reproductive lives (Luna and Luker, 2013; Ross and Solinger, 2017). Feminist scholars have a responsibility to critique mechanisms of global reproductive governance when they harm women. In this book, I show how Senegal's PAC program was introduced and practiced at the intersection of population control, reproductive rights, and safe motherhood regimes. I highlight the grave professional and political challenges faced by health professionals in the management of PAC technologies and the provision of services. I demonstrate how PAC knowledge production has been key to establishing the political legitimacy of the intervention and conveying stakeholders' accountability to global accords on maternal and reproductive health. Most importantly, I illustrate how women are simultaneously kept alive while subjected to harm by what PAC does and does not do in health facilities, health systems, and policy arenas.

PAC perpetuates reproductive injustice. Through careful attention to how PAC works within and contributes to national and global regimes of reproductive governance, I highlight concrete possibilities for advancing reproductive justice not only by revising harmful colonial-era abortion laws but also by making women-centered investments in health systems that improve access to safe and respectful reproductive health care for all.

ORGANIZATION OF THE BOOK

I began this chapter by illuminating the global significance of women's clinical encounters with PAC in Senegal, and traced the emergence of the global PAC model within a broader geopolitical history of global reproductive health governance, from the population control policies of the Cold War era to the rights-based agenda of the 1994 ICPD. In chapter 1, I highlight some of the ethical and methodological challenges of conducting PAC research and describe how this global ethnography (Browner and Sargent, 2011; Burawoy, Blum, George, Gille, and Thayer, 2000) of PAC emerged from my work experience as a public health professional with an international NGO in Senegal during the mid-2000s.[20] Chapter 1 situates Senegal's PAC program within a brief history of sexual and reproductive policies and programs from the colonial era until the present and describes how the intervention was tested, introduced, and scaled up throughout the country. I end by describing the clinical, technological, and organizational terrains of obstetric care in the three government hospitals where I observed PAC.

In chapter 2, I explore how MVA, a device that can both terminate pregnancy and treat complications of incomplete abortion, became the preferred PAC technology in Senegal. I illustrate how policies designed to limit MVA utilization to PAC have compromised quality of and access to care for low-income and rural women in particular. In chapter 3, I demonstrate how PAC transforms potentially criminal women into mothers deserving of obstetric care through a contradictory process in which health workers rigorously search their patients' bodies and behavior for signs of illegal abortion, and then mask suspected cases of induced abortion as miscarriage in hospital records. These practices of seeking out and hiding abortion generate a sanitized, uncontroversial account of PAC as a safe motherhood intervention that is unworthy of police scrutiny.

In chapter 4, I explore how PAC introduced new indicators that rendered abortion complications legible as a safe motherhood issue to national and global stakeholders, thereby displacing previous efforts to measure the incidence and fatality of induced abortion. I demonstrate how health professionals strategically mobilize and interpret PAC data to make claims about PAC technologies and patients and the intervention's impact on maternal mortality. In the conclusion, I discuss evolutions in PAC policies and practices since the end of my fieldwork in 2011. I juxtapose interpretations of PAC's effectiveness with a review of national and global evidence related to the cost of PAC and the relationship between maternal mortality and the legal status of abortion. I end with a reflection on achieving reproductive justice within transnational systems of reproductive governance.

1 · A "TRANSFORMATIVE" INTERVENTION

When I first arrived in Dakar in January 2005, I knew that PAC was part of what global maternal health experts had labeled EmOC, but had little understanding of its place in the global landscape of reproductive health politics. As a newly minted master of public health and a University of Michigan Population Fellow,[1] I had been assigned to the Senegal office of Management Sciences for Health (MSH), a global health NGO with headquarters in Medford, Massachusetts, that was contracted by USAID to support the Senegalese MSAS in reducing maternal death and increasing contraceptive prevalence. During this fellowship, my Senegalese colleagues tasked me with piloting a natural form of contraception known as the Standard Days Method (SDM)[2] in USAID's five regions of intervention. Although USAID supported various hormonal and barrier contraceptive methods in Senegal, the promotion of natural family planning in a setting with what global health experts considered "high" fertility (Senegal's total fertility rate [TFR] was estimated at 5.3 in the 2005 DHS [N'Diaye and Ayad, 2006]) offered an initial clue into the contradictory global reproductive politics at play. Around the same time the U.S. government implemented the Mexico City Policy in 1984, USAID began to support research and development of natural family planning methods (Dixon-Mueller, 1993).

The influence of the Mexico City Policy, reinstated by President George W. Bush in 2001, became even clearer when my Senegalese colleagues enlisted my help in monitoring and evaluating its PAC program. In 2003, USAID selected Senegal, along with six other countries, to receive special funding to "institutionalize" the agency's global PAC approach (Curtis, 2007). As USAID's contracting agency for maternal and reproductive health since the early 2000s, MSH supported the MSAS in training and supervising health workers in PAC and tracking the progress of services in USAID's regions of intervention. We documented our PAC activities in a paper published by MSH (Thiam, Suh, and Moreira, 2006). During our supervision and training activities, my colleagues spoke with health workers about treating abortion complications, but never about the kinds of abortions being treated, or the possibility that part of their PAC caseload was related to illegally terminated pregnancy. When I floated the idea of conducting a small, qualitative study that would entail interviewing health workers about what it meant to treat complications of abortion in a country with a restrictive abortion law, my colleagues declined. Some were rather annoyed by my failure, as an American, to grasp how such a study might jeopardize their compliance with USAID's funding restrictions on abortion-related activities. To protect their USAID funding at a time when the Mexico City Policy and the Helms Amendment were active, they were reluctant to engage in any kind of research or advocacy that did not directly relate to the clinical aspects of PAC.

It is precisely this "gagging" around abortion that motivated me to return to Senegal several years later as a PhD student to investigate the questions I could not while working with MSH. By the time I returned to Senegal in 2009 to conduct preliminary fieldwork, President Barack Obama had rescinded the Mexico City Policy. Yet, the 1973 Helms Amendment (which prohibits foreign assistance from being used for "the performance of abortion as a method of family planning" [Barot, 2013, p. 9]) remained in place, and, as I would learn through my research, compromised the quality of obstetric care in a country where USAID purportedly supported PAC.

In this chapter, I locate my research project and methods in the longer history of colonial and neocolonial reproductive policies and programs in which PAC was conceived. My research methods are inextricably tied to my work experience with MSH, during which I participated in one of the largest operations research projects on PAC in Senegal, described later in this chapter and throughout the book. The professional relationships I developed during this time with individuals in the Division de la Santé de la Reproduction (DSR/Division of Reproductive Health) of the MSAS and with national and international NGOs and donor agencies facilitated my entry into the hospitals where I observed PAC and interviewed health workers. I draw on these health professionals' perspectives to illustrate what it means to provide PAC services and manage a national PAC program within a complex and contradictory geopolitical landscape of global maternal and reproductive health.

A GLOBAL ETHNOGRAPHY OF PAC

This book is not (only) about the practice of illegal abortion and PAC in Senegal. Several ethnographers have documented health workers' and women's abortion practices and experiences in African countries with restrictive abortion laws (Bleek, 1981; Johnson-Hanks, 2002b; Rossier, 2007; Schuster, 2005). Since the early 1990s, studies have illustrated how PAC has improved access to, as well as the quality and organization of, obstetric care in sub-Saharan Africa and other regions (Huber, Curtis, Irani, Pappa, and Arrington, 2016). While I draw on these rich traditions of ethnographic and public health research, I adopt a somewhat different approach to studying abortion and PAC. By exploring how PAC service delivery and program management unfold at the intersection of national and global abortion policies, and how PAC data and technologies circulate across and acquire meaning through clinical, programmatic, and policy arenas, I offer a "global ethnography" (Burawoy, Blum, George, Gille, and Thayer, 2000) of abortion governance. PAC serves as an entry point into studying abortion that, in the words of anthropologists Ginsburg and Rapp (1991), "synthesizes these two perspectives—the local and the global—by examining the multiple levels on which reproductive practices, policies, and politics so often depend" (p. 313).

PAC facilitates analysis of a "global assemblage" (Ong and Collier, 2005) of clinical and programmatic practices, technologies, epidemiological and demographic data, institutions, and patients that simultaneously undergird and complicate processes and mechanisms of reproductive governance (Browner and Sargent, 2011; Morgan and Roberts, 2012). PAC is not merely a model of obstetric care, but rather is composed of clinical protocols that recommend certain uterine evacuation technologies (MVA, EVA, misoprostol) over others (dilation and curettage, digital evacuation) that in turn have been produced by and circulated among international reproductive health NGOs, bi- and multilateral aid agencies, and national ministries of health. These organizations have supported the piloting, implementation, and scale-up of PAC services in over sixty countries worldwide. Health workers in these countries have been trained to use PAC technology, and through daily obstetric care and record keeping in contexts with restrictive abortion laws, they generate data that national and global stakeholders draw on to make claims about how PAC "works" (V. Adams, 2013) in reducing maternal mortality and morbidity, thereby supporting the reproductive rights agenda articulated in global accords on health and development since the 1994 ICPD.

As the global, public, and scientific "face" of abortion, PAC is thus a theoretically and methodologically important object of study. In this book, I illuminate the meaning and location of abortion within medical and public health practice in settings with restrictive abortion laws by examining clinical, programmatic, and policy practices related to PAC, and in particular, the strategies deployed by stakeholders to separate PAC from induced abortion, demonstrate the intervention's impact on maternal mortality, and convey commitment to national and global accords on maternal and reproductive health. I excavate the inner workings of this public health intervention in Senegal—the various forms of work enacted by stakeholders to treat patients, develop and implement clinical norms and protocols, plan and monitor activities, collect and interpret data, and circulate and use technology. I connect stakeholders' work and discourses to the social, political, and legal context of PAC, in which medical and public health practices unfold at the intersection of national and global abortion politics.

Through this global, public, and scientific face of abortion, PAC offers an ethically feasible mechanism of studying politics and practices related to abortion in settings with restrictive abortion laws. Precisely because PAC has been widely accepted as a legitimate form of obstetric care, it offers a less threatening forum for research participants to discuss perceptions and experiences regarding induced abortion. It does not require participants to disclose personal and possibly illegal abortion practices. Instead, participants can explain how they think PAC works (or does not work), how it contributes to maternal mortality reduction, and how it relates to national and global abortion policies.

Global ethnographies of reproduction not only meld the local and the global but also complicate spatial and temporal dimensions of reproductive practices, discourses, experiences, policies, technologies, and subjects (Browner and Sargent, 2011). This study traces PAC throughout multiple terrains of intervention and practice in Senegal, including the earliest waves of operations research, the decentralization of services from national and regional hospitals to district health facilities, the daily provision of obstetric care in gynecological wards, the integration of global accords on reproductive health and rights into national protocols for reproductive health, and the negotiation of PAC with USAID's anti-abortion funding policies and the national prohibition on abortion. I illuminate how epidemiological, clinical, and demographic accounts of PAC patients and devices, created in gynecological wards, travel through multiple scales of the health information system, find their way into national and global reports and evaluations of PAC, and then circulate back into reproductive policies and discourses that regulate the kinds of care available to women in government health facilities and the kinds of women entitled to care.

My ethnography of Senegal's PAC program is anchored in temporally discrete but conceptually overlapping logics and strategies of global reproductive governance, from the period of French colonization that gave rise to Senegal's current abortion law, to the neocolonial period of population control during which the Senegalese government crafted a population policy under the influence of USAID, UNFPA, the World Bank, and other global entities, to the ICPD era of reproductive rights in which the PAC model was born. My encounters with Senegal's PAC program as a researcher unfolded during two distinct moments of global reproductive governance. My interest in what it meant to conduct PAC in a country with a restrictive abortion law was kindled while working with MSH to scale up PAC during the mid-2000s when the Mexico City Policy was in place. When I returned to Senegal in 2010 to investigate this question, the Mexico City Policy had been rescinded but the Helms Amendment remained active. In this study, I locate Senegal's PAC program in multiple regimes of global reproductive governance from the nineteenth century to the twenty-first, drawing on continuities and disruptions in practices, policies, and meanings related to abortion, obstetric care, and reproductive health over time.

A global ethnography of PAC required careful triangulation of multiple sources of data. I draw on five methods of data collection, conducted concurrently between November 2010 and December 2011. First, I directly observed PAC services in delivery rooms and separate MVA rooms at three hospitals (Hôpital Senghor, Hôpital Médina, and Hôpital de Ville) in three administrative regions of the country. Second, I reviewed PAC registers from hospital maternity wards and annual reports of obstetric care from administrative units at these hospitals. Third, I conducted in-depth interviews with eighty-nine PAC practitioners and key informants, including health providers, MSAS officials, employees of national and international NGOs and donor agencies, and members of legal and medical professional associations. Fourth, I conducted an archival review of forty-two cases of illegal abortion prosecuted by the regional tribunal of Dakar between 1987 and 2010 and cases reported by the Senegalese press. Last, I reviewed national and global literature on PAC and abortion from the 1980s until the present.

Senegal's PAC story is not entirely unique. The PAC practices, experiences, policies, and discourses documented in the Senegalese context may be extrapolated to PAC programs in other countries with restrictive abortion laws and where USAID has historically played an influential role in crafting population policy and promoting family planning. Although countries with PAC programs have unique histories of reproductive politics, each has had to negotiate PAC's contradictory geopolitical origins—in which national and global health experts recognized the contribution of unsafe abortion to maternal mortality but were gagged from advocating for safe, legal abortion by the Mexico City Policy and the Helms Amendment—with national abortion regulations. Throughout the book, I highlight parallels between Senegal and other countries with restrictive abortion laws in the challenges related to the clinical provision of PAC, the distribution of PAC technology, and the interpretation of PAC data. I hope that Senegal's story, as one of few global ethnographies of PAC in West Africa, is instructive in demonstrating the complex ways in which global reproductive health interventions unfold and inadvertently exacerbate inequalities in women's health outcomes and experiences.

RESEARCHING PAC

Since starting this project in 2009, I have been confronted with many provocative questions about my research by audience members during conference presentations, academic peer reviewers, colleagues, NGO representatives, students, and friends. Some have challenged my decision to conduct ethnographic research on PAC without interviewing women who have had abortions. Others have questioned the generalizability of my findings given that most of my research was conducted at large urban hospitals rather than primary health care facilities in rural areas. People have expressed concern that my research may inadvertently expose practices that lead to criminalization of health providers or women patients. For some people, my focus on obstetric violence in PAC threatens to contribute to long-standing Western discourses of incompetent African professionals (J. Crane, 2010; Iliffe, 1998; Jewkes, Abrahams, and Mvo, 1998). Others have taken issue with the practical and political implications of critiquing PAC, when it may be the only legitimate form of abortion care available to Senegalese women who cannot afford safe abortions.

A detailed description of my research methods appears in appendix A. Here, I grapple with the ethical, methodological, and epistemological conundrums that arise in the conduct of ethnographic research on illegal abortion and PAC in Senegal. More specifically, I reflect on what it means, as a feminist scholar, to study a global reproductive health intervention at the intersection of obstetric violence and care. I consider how multiple facets of my identity—Black woman, American, PhD student, and public health professional—simultaneously facilitated and foreclosed avenues of research. I explain how I negotiated ethical commitments to protect the confidentiality of research participants during and after fieldwork. I reflect on how the collection and analysis of data, and the subsequent portrayal of research participants' behaviors and practices, contributes to the production of knowledge regarding maternal and reproductive health in Senegal. These kinds of problems forced me to reckon with power imbalances inseparable from the research process, and the partial knowledges produced by what I want or am able to "see" (Collins 1989; Haraway 1998; Harding 1992).

In Senegal, two-thirds of healthcare provision occurs in primary health care facilities, administered by male and female nurses (Duclos, Ndoye, Faye, Diallo, and Penn-Kekana, 2019). Yet, my observations of PAC took place in three hospitals (two district hospitals and one regional hospital). Among the thirty-seven health workers I interviewed, only three were nurses.[3] The selection of interviewees and observation sites is directly related to the organization of PAC within the health system, in which many PAC cases end up being referred to district or regional hospitals, where they are treated by midwives or physicians. I selected l'Hôpital Senghor, l'Hôpital Médina, and l'Hôpital de Ville because they offered large caseloads of PAC patients for observation, offered a variety of health workers to interview, and were each located in a region where the MSAS received support from a different donor agency or NGO in implementing and evaluating reproductive health care. Additionally, l'Hôpital Senghor and l'Hôpital de Ville offered rich institutional PAC memories. Both had been among the first sites in their respective regions to pilot PAC and continue to serve as PAC training sites for physicians. One of the study hospitals had briefly served as the focal point for distributing the national supply of MVA kits.

PAC was available around the clock at the three study hospitals, where I observed health workers administer PAC in the delivery room, and at l'Hôpital Senghor and l'Hôpital de Ville, in special rooms for EVA and MVA. I attended early-morning meetings with gynecologists and midwives at l'Hôpital Senghor and l'Hôpital de Ville, during which the head gynecologist reviewed cases from the day before and gave instructions for further care if necessary. During my fieldwork at l'Hôpital Senghor, I lodged at the hospital and was able to observe PAC during night and day shifts in the gynecological ward. In between observation of services and review of records, I shared meals with health workers in the hospital cafeteria and tea in the break room of the maternity ward. It was often during these informal moments, gossiping over tea and watching Nigerian music videos and Indian soap operas, that people revealed sensitive information or shared alternative versions of events that had been articulated in formal interviews. For example, a female janitor at l'Hôpital Senghor explained, in contrast to what several midwives had told me, that the hospital had "denounced" a patient suspected of illegal abortion to the police several weeks before the beginning of my fieldwork. During a rare moment when we were alone in the MVA room at l'Hôpital de Ville, a nursing assistant revealed that a physician had taught her how to use the MVA syringe, a device that was restricted to physicians at this facility.

My previous work experience and my status as a doctoral student opened several important doorways to conducting research. Through my relationships with former colleagues from MSH, I established contact with important stakeholders and potential study participants in the MSAS, professional medical and legal associations, and national and international NGOs. At the same time, my status as a foreign researcher may have led some health professionals and patients to decline to participate in the study. Although my presence in the maternity wards was greatly facilitated by wearing a white coat,[4] this marker of belonging did not always translate into successful recruitment of participants. At each study hospital, at least one midwife refused to allow me to observe her administering PAC, engage with me in informal conversation, or participate in a formal interview. One day during fieldwork at l'Hôpital de Ville, a midwife who had declined to be interviewed called loudly to me as I was in the delivery room. She asked me what I was writing in my notebook. When I explained I was jotting down observations and questions to ask health providers later, she replied that I was not the first foreigner at the hospital "to write things down in a notebook" and that there had been others before me who had written things that "made the hospital look bad." When I asked her to explain what she meant, she declined to discuss further, waving me away as she continued to work.

For some individuals, the research topic itself likely rendered me problematic, if not downright suspicious. Although a representative of USAID's global PAC program in Washington, DC, declined to be interviewed, the individual emailed me articles and reports detailing the organization's stance and practices related to PAC. During a formal interview with a police commissioner, a police officer in the room interrupted to ask if I was recording the conversation.

When I replied that I had a digital recorder in my bag but was not using it, the officer demanded to see it. I took out the recorder and showed that the red recording button was in "off" mode. Although I left the inactive recorder on the commissioner's desk, the officer kept a watchful eye on my research assistant and me for the remainder of the interview.

Such moments, while somewhat dramatic, were quite rare during my fieldwork. For the most part, health professionals and other stakeholders were willing to participate in the study and did not demand to see my credentials as a researcher, and my status as a foreign researcher may have extended privileges that were incommensurate with my professional training and with my research protocol. For example, I was invited by several health professionals at the study hospitals to conduct family planning counseling sessions with PAC patients. After several weeks of observing MVA procedures, some health workers playfully asked if I wished to try one myself. On several occasions when patients declined to be observed during PAC, health workers chastised the women, telling them that they should stop being "difficult." Although I left the room as soon as a woman refused to be observed, it would not have been difficult to circumvent (and violate) the consent procedures approved by the MSAS.[5]

My research protocol was approved by ethics committees at Columbia University and the Senegalese MSAS before I started fieldwork. Still, some decisions regarding confidentiality were not made until I was actively conducting research on PAC in hospitals. To avoid drawing further attention to PAC patients, and to women suspected of illegal abortion in particular, I decided to restrict interviews in hospitals to health workers. I made this decision a week into my fieldwork at l'Hôpital Senghor during an early-morning meeting with the head gynecologist and several midwives who had just finished the night shift. Over the course of the meeting, the midwives brought to the physician's attention three PAC cases from the night shift in which the circumstances under which the abortions had occurred were unclear. For each case, the physician looked pointedly at me while instructing the midwives to "re-interrogate" these patients. It is possible that he wished to demonstrate to me, a foreign researcher who had just begun research on PAC at his hospital, his diligence in handling possible cases of illegal abortion. Whatever his reasons, I declined to interview PAC patients directly, choosing instead to explore women's clinical encounters through conversations and interviews with health workers during which I asked them to describe their patients and how they came to suspect some women and not others of illegal abortion.

I triangulate health workers' observations of their patients with a review of various kinds of accounts of abortion and PAC, including PAC registers at the three study hospitals, court records of illegal abortion prosecuted by the state, and cases of illegal abortion described by the Senegalese press. These data offer insight into the circumstances under which women arrive at hospitals with complications of abortion and how they are managed by medical workers and, at times, law enforcement officers. In chapter 3, I discuss information from twenty-six de-identified PAC patients (displayed in table B.1 in appendix B) at the study hospitals who may have been suspected of illegal abortion, and describe how health workers interpreted and acted on these data. In the few cases of induced abortion that appeared in the registers, I asked health workers to recall and discuss the details of the case. When they brought to my attention recent cases of confirmed or suspected induced abortion that had involved the police, I searched the registers to verify how they were recorded.

For an ethnographer interested in medical record keeping as a way of maintaining professional authority (Berg and Bowker, 1997; Jaffré, 2012), silences in the record are incredibly illuminating. For example, at l'Hôpital Senghor, a few midwives described a case of induced abortion investigated by the police in December 2010, a month before I began fieldwork at the hospital. When I could not find the case in the 2010 PAC register, midwives suggested looking in the delivery register since it was a "late" abortion. Although I searched the 2010 delivery register, my failure to identify the case raises the possibility that it may have been recorded as something else altogether in records that feed into the hospital's annual reports, and in turn, district and regional reports to the MSAS.

For health professionals attempting to measure the epidemiological scope of abortion, however, such omissions and reclassifications may complicate the production of robust numbers. In turn, the absence of rigorous statistics may hamper advocacy for improving interventions or changing policies (Gerdts, Vohra, and Ahern, 2013; Graham and Campbell, 1992; Storeng and Béhague, 2017). My purpose in sharing women's clinical encounters in the absence of direct interviews, therefore, is not limited to supporting my theoretical claims about how reproductive governance occurs through the recording and interpretation of data. As a feminist scholar committed to reproductive justice, I include these data to render visible women's embodied reproductive experiences and practices that are frequently obscured in settings with restrictive abortion laws.

Protecting the confidentiality of health workers was also of vital importance, especially for those who revealed involvement in the practice of abortion. For example, one study participant had been implicated in a case of illegal abortion I found in the legal archives. Although the individual denied involvement in this particular case of illegal abortion, they explained that they referred women to physicians who offered safe procedures. During my preliminary fieldwork project in 2009, the individual revealed that they had used MVA syringes to conduct safe but clandestine abortions. Another participant indicated that they regularly referred women with unwanted pregnancies to colleagues they knew who were able to perform safe abortions. To protect the confidentiality of study participants, I have de-identified the names and locations of the study hospitals and use pseudonyms.

Ethical commitments to research participants are not limited to protecting confidentiality, but also extend to their portrayal in the long afterlife of data following the completion of fieldwork. Concerns that PAC research will expose health workers to criminalization or reinforce racist perceptions of African health workers as incompetent, while understandable, may underestimate the complexity of health workers' experiences and perspectives related to abortion care. In this book, I strive to situate health workers' practices within the broader geopolitical context of maternal and reproductive health care, a complex terrain in which health professionals are obligated to respect their patients' reproductive rights and observe the national abortion law and the Mexico City Policy, all the while working within a health system deeply impacted by decades of neoliberal restructuring (Foley, 2009; Pfeiffer, 2019; Pfeiffer and Chapman, 2010; Sommer, Shandra, Restivo, and Reed, 2019). It is necessary to illustrate the political, technological, clinical, and professional conditions in which health professionals may simultaneously enact obstetric violence against their patients and protect them from the police.

It is troubling to imagine that Senegalese stakeholders are oblivious to what happens in hospitals and worry that I, as a foreign researcher, will expose practices that might be understood as complicity in illegal abortion. Such logic not only is incredibly condescending but also suggests that PAC is "good enough" for Senegalese women and that the transnational programmatic and funding mechanisms that support the intervention should remain in place. When I shared preliminary findings with research participants in the study hospitals and the MSAS, they were well aware of the complicated nature of PAC and eager to discuss how my research could lead to improvements in quality of and access to obstetric care. Similarly, global advocates of reproductive health can use PAC research to demand better forms of reproductive health care by illustrating, with great precision, how the intervention is experienced by health workers and women patients.

POPULATION POLICY IN SENEGAL:
FROM POPULATION CONTROL TO PAC

Although European colonial administrators and medical professionals enacted various strategies to regulate sexuality, fertility, and reproduction among their African subjects (Hunt, 1999; Ray, 2015; Stoler, 2002; Thomas, 2003), scholars of reproduction emphasize the interplay between internal and external forces in the development, implementation, and evaluation of twentieth-century population policies (Connelly, 2006; Greenhalgh, 2008, 2010; Hartmann, 1995; Robinson, 2016). Undoubtedly, Senegal's PAC program is anchored in a long history of French colonial prohibitions on contraception and abortion, followed by post–World War II population control efforts framed as "development" that were spearheaded primarily by USAID and global financial institutions like the International Monetary Fund (IMF) and the World Bank. At the same time, Senegalese health professionals, scientists, and population experts have played a significant role in defining population health policies and related programs like PAC and adapting them to make them palatable to the Senegalese people. Senegalese stakeholders have at once embraced and resisted policies related to fertility reduction and abortion and specific interventions like PAC. Their critiques and endorsements of donor, NGO, and government policies and strategies are explored throughout each chapter of this book.

Article 305 of Senegal's penal code prohibits abortion under any circumstance. Those who procure or attempt to procure an abortion, including the pregnant woman, health practitioners, or other accomplices, risk imprisonment, fines, and loss of professional license. Senegal's abortion law replicates the language that appeared in Article 317 of France's penal code in 1939 (Knoppers, Brault, and Sloss, 1990). Although the code of medical ethics permits physicians to conduct abortions in the case of fetal malformation or if the pregnant woman's life is at risk, the penal code does not recognize these exceptions. Additionally, therapeutic abortions must be approved by two other physicians, one of whom is recognized by the court as a medico-legal expert (Center for Reproductive Law and Policy [CRLP], 2001). A report of reproductive rights published in 2001 found "no record" of health worker convictions (CRLP, 2001). In contrast, my review of archives in the regional tribunal of Dakar found that between 1987 and 2011, nineteen "practitioners" of abortion were convicted. Almost all of these individuals were paramedical or unskilled practitioners: nine were practicing or retired nurses, and seven were nursing assistants, janitors, or *matrons* (traditional birthing assistants). Only in one case, in 2008, were two health professionals prosecuted: a midwife and a physician.

Population planning began in earnest in sub-Saharan Africa during the late 1970s and early 1980s, the same period that ushered in several decades of structural adjustment, or the neoliberal reorganizing of economies under the guidance of the IMF and the World Bank to increase competitiveness and attract foreign investment (Dembele, 2012). As prominent American and European economists and demographers framed averted births in terms of economic gain (Connelly, 2008; Greenhalgh, 1996; Murphy, 2017), fertility reduction was adopted as a critical component of economic restructuring to catalyze development. The U.S. government exercised both hard and soft power approaches to enacting population control in developing countries. During the mid-1960s, President Lyndon B. Johnson insisted on personally signing off on shipments of food aid to India during a period of famine to force the government to "deal with" its own "population problem" (Connelly, 2008, p. 221). This approach was known as "the short leash" (p. 213). With USAID providing half of all global population aid between the 1960s and 1980s (Donaldson, 1990), aid in exchange for the implementation of

population control measures was funneled through less coercive, but no less per-
suasive forms. Between 1973 and 1993, USAID provided more funding to countries with population policies. Such countries could gain up to $1.7 million by
having a population policy (Barrett and Tsui, 1999). During the 1980s and 1990s,
USAID was the primary provider of low-cost contraceptives in sub-Saharan Africa
(Robinson, 2016).

Starting in the early 1980s, USAID funded Futures Group, a healthcare consulting firm, to develop the Resources for the Awareness of Population Impact
on Development (RAPID) program, which entailed country-specific presentations that used statistical modeling to dramatically demonstrate the social and
economic consequences of overpopulation (Robinson, 2017). During the 1980s
and 1990s, two-thirds of sub-Saharan African countries adopted population policies (Robinson, 2015). Some African countries, such as Nigeria and Kenya, explicitly articulated fertility reduction targets (Chimbwete, Watkins, and Zulu, 2005;
Robinson, 2012), while others, like Malawi and Senegal, framed population policies in terms of birth spacing and maternal health (Robinson, 2017). Although
the engagement of African policy makers in population planning signaled their
desire to participate in the global polity (Chimbwete et al., 2005; Robinson, 2017),
the relationship between resources and the articulation of population policies is
difficult to ignore: higher levels of structural adjustment debt to the World Bank
and the IMF are statistically associated with the presence of population policies
in sub-Saharan African countries (Robinson, 2015).

During the 1974 World Population Conference in Bucharest, many developing countries rejected population control approaches promoted by USAID as
the solution to economic development, arguing instead that "development is the
best contraceptive" (Hodgson and Watkins, 1997, p. 489). Nevertheless, family
planning efforts in Senegal had already begun. Senegal's largest family planning
NGO, L'Association Sénégalaise pour le Bien-Être Familial (ASBEF/Senegalese
Association for Familial Well-Being), was established in 1968 and became an
affiliate of the International Planned Parenthood Federation (IPPF) in 1975.
Concerned about rising fertility rates during the late 1970s, the Senegalese government established a commission to develop a population policy with support
from Pathfinder International, USAID, and UNFPA. In 1980, the same year that
Senegal became the first sub-Saharan African country to receive a structural
adjustment loan from the World Bank and the IMF, the government repealed
the prohibition on contraception (Robinson, 2017). However, the ban on abortion
remained in place, and the government added an article to the penal code that
criminalized public discourse on abortion and public and private advertisement
or distribution of abortion services and methods (Center for Reproductive Rights
[CRR], 2003). In 1982, Futures Group conducted RAPID presentations with Senegalese policy makers. USAID funded a delegation of Senegalese officials to Zaire
(now the Democratic Republic of Congo) to learn about family planning under

the political regime of President Mobutu Sese Seko, who had been in power since 1965 (Hartmann, 1995). By 1985, over thirty national NGOs in Senegal were conducting family planning and reproductive health activities throughout the country (Robinson, 2017).

Senegal's population policy, issued in 1988, identified population as a natural arena of government intervention and management, no different from other areas of government responsibility, such as agriculture and fishing (Robinson, 2016). The policy aimed to decrease fertility, reduce mortality in all its forms, and geographically redistribute the population to improve quality of life (CRR, 2003). The absence of numeric targets related to fertility reduction reflected resistance among Senegalese policy makers to equate population planning with family planning. For these stakeholders, population was a resource, rather than a problem, that could be carefully managed and harnessed toward the achievement of economic growth. Fertility reduction could not simply boil down to top-down family planning programs, which would be out of step with cultural and religious expectations related to family and childbearing, but should entail more comprehensive efforts to protect maternal and child health through child spacing. Nevertheless, external actors continued to exercise considerable influence over this process. The 1988 population policy was released at least in part due to pressure from the World Bank, which stipulated the articulation of a formal population policy as a precondition for releasing the country's third structural adjustment loan (Robinson, 2017).

Along with 178 other countries, Senegal endorsed the 1994 Platform of Action of the ICPD. With its recognition of maternal health as a component of reproductive rights (Abou-Zahr, 2003), the ICPD broadened the scope of global population efforts beyond family planning to include obstetric and neonatal care. In 1997, as part of ongoing efforts to integrate ICPD principles into the national health care system, the Senegalese government formed the National Reproductive Health Project, which aimed to reduce maternal and child mortality and morbidity by increasing access to pre- and postnatal care, family planning, and treatment and prevention services for sexually transmitted infections (CRR, 2003).

The need for PAC emerged at the intersection of a continuing emphasis on family planning and a new focus on the role of obstetric care in reducing maternal death. During the late 1990s, Senegal was one of several African countries included in the piloting, implementation, and evaluation of EmOC, a hospital-based maternal health intervention spearheaded by Averting Maternal Death and Disability (AMDD) at Columbia University in New York and funded by the Gates Foundation (Paxton, Maine, Freedman, Fry, and Lobis, 2005).[6] EmOC includes uterine evacuation, which is a signal function of PAC. Additionally, epidemiological research on abortion conducted by Senegalese scientists during the early 1990s, discussed in chapter 4, inspired calls for improvements in the management of abortion complications in government hospitals. Consequently, the National Reproductive Health Project called for a 50 percent reduction in the rate of induced and spontaneous abortion (CRR, 2003). The Ministry of the Family's Plan of Action for Women (1997–2001) explicitly addressed mortality related to unsafe abortion, urging increased awareness of the dangers of clandestine abortion, improved medical care and psychosocial support for women with abortion complications, and additional studies of the socioeconomic consequences of unsafe abortion (CRLP, 2001). In response to the results of the first operations research project on PAC, described in the following section, the MSAS integrated PAC into national norms and protocols for maternal and reproductive health in 1998.

USAID has supported PAC activities in Senegal since the late 1990s through contracting health NGOs such as the Population Council,[7] Johns Hopkins Program for International Education in Gynecology and Obstetrics (JHPIEGO),[8] EngenderHealth,[9] Intrahealth,[10] Child Fund,[11] and MSH. PAC remains part of USAID's portfolio for reproductive health aid in Senegal. In 2018, USAID (2019) allocated $7.8 million to reproductive health care, $9.8 million to family planning, and $400,000 to "population policy and administrative management."

The 1994 ICPD is one of numerous regional and global treaties on human rights ratified by the Senegalese government, including the 1981 Convention on the Elimination of all Forms of Discrimination Against Women (CEDAW), the MDGs, the 2003 Protocol to the African Charter on Human and People's Rights on the Rights of Women in Africa (Maputo Protocol), and the 2015 SDGs. Unlike the ICPD, the Maputo Protocol explicitly calls on governments to provide safe abortion in the case of rape or incest or if the pregnancy threatens the health or life of the pregnant woman (African Commission on Human and People's Rights, 2003). Organizations such as l'AJS have invoked the language of the Maputo Protocol in their advocacy for "medicalized abortion" under these circumstances. A 2005 law on reproductive health recognized PAC, but not abortion, as a reproductive health service to which all citizens are entitled. In 2013, the DSR organized a multidisciplinary task force, spearheaded by l'AJS, to address the problem of unsafe abortion through research and advocacy with religious leaders, parliamentarians, the media, and the public (Moseson, Ouedraogo, Diallo, and Sakho, 2019). In 2014, the task force drafted a bill on safe abortion that used the language of the Maputo Protocol. Although the bill was delivered to the MSAS and to the Committee for the Reform of the Criminal Code, to date the abortion law remains unchanged (Archer, Finden, and Pearson, 2018).

The lack of harmonization between the penal code and human rights treaties is not unique to Senegal. Globally, women's participation in government is more likely to result in abortion law reform than ratification of reproductive rights treaties like the ICPD. Additionally, abortion law reform tends to follow the adoption of a public health harm reduction approach to abortion (Boyle, Longhofer, and

Kim, 2015). The experiences of Rwanda, Mozambique, and Ethiopia appear to support this model. The governments of Mozambique and Ethiopia relaxed abortion laws in response to epidemiological data demonstrating the contribution of unsafe abortion to maternal mortality (Durr, 2015; Guttmacher Institute, 2012; Holcombe, Berhe, and Cherie, 2015). With 61 percent of the national Parliament and half of its cabinet seats occupied by women, Rwanda demonstrates a significant amount of female leadership in government (Ssuunal, 2018). In 2012, Rwanda relaxed the law to permit abortion in the case of rape, incest, forced marriage, and fetal impairment. The government is currently considering eliminating the involvement of the court in determining a woman's eligibility for abortion (Rwirahira, 2018).

BUILDING AN EVIDENCE BASE FOR PAC, 1997 TO 2009

Having identified complications of abortion as a major public health problem by the mid-1990s, the MSAS started a series of operations research projects to test the feasibility of launching the PAC model endorsed by the ICPD. The first PAC pilot project was implemented in three large hospitals, including the national university hospital, Centre Hospitalier Universitaire (CHU) Le Dantec, in Dakar between 1997 and 1998. The MSAS partnered with two reproductive health NGOs contracted by USAID: the Population Council and JHPIEGO. As part of the intervention, midwives were trained to use MVA technology to treat complications and to provide contraceptive counseling during and after treatment. By the end of the first pilot project, a little over half of PAC patients[12] had been treated with MVA, and the use of less effective methods such as digital evacuation and dilation and curettage had decreased by approximately half. Additional improvements included a decline in the length of hospitalization from 3 to 1.6 days and the cost of treatment from 35,800 to 26,700 CFA francs ($70 to $50). The project was less successful, however, with respect to family planning: nearly two-thirds of patients did not receive family planning counseling (CEFOREP, 1998a).

The next operations research project, conducted in collaboration with UNFPA in 1999, aimed to test the feasibility of implementing PAC in two regional hospitals and a district hospital in the regions of Diourbel and Kaolack. Regional and district hospitals generally have fewer medical specialists and less equipment than tertiary-level hospitals in Dakar. Still, the second project yielded results similar to the first: the acceptability of MVA as a method of uterine evacuation among midwives, an increase in the percentage of patients treated with MVA, and reductions in the cost of treatment and the duration of hospitalization (Thiam et al., 2006).

The third project, conducted between 2001 and 2003 in collaboration with EngenderHealth, tested the provision of PAC at six district hospitals and twelve primary health care facilities in the regions of Kaolack and Fatick.[13] By the end of the project, these hospitals had treated over half (57%) of PAC cases with MVA. The average length of hospitalization decreased from 1.3 days to approximately 9.6 hours. The percentage of patients who received family planning counseling increased from 38 percent to 70 percent, and 20 percent of all PAC patients accepted a contraceptive method (EngenderHealth, 2003).

In 2002, to further explore the feasibility of PAC at the level of primary care, the MSAS, in collaboration with Intrahealth, implemented PAC in a district in the region of Fatick. In addition to training medical providers in PAC, the project sensitized communities with respect to recognizing danger signs during pregnancy and the importance of immediately transporting women with such symptoms to health facilities. Some of the communities involved in the project established emergency funds and transportation systems to refer women with obstetric emergencies to the nearest health facility (Thiam et al., 2006).

The fifth operations research project, conducted between 2003 and 2006, was implemented in five regions of the country in collaboration with MSH. In my capacity as a University of Michigan Population Fellow with MSH between 2004 and 2006, I participated in the evaluation of the MSAS's largest PAC project to date. The project trained over 500 physicians, midwives, and nurses and introduced PAC equipment to twenty-three district hospitals. Over this three-year period, the percentage of facilities with adequate space, supplies, and equipment for PAC increased from 29 percent to 95 percent. The percentage of district hospitals with at least one provider trained in PAC increased from 39 percent to 100 percent, and the number of women admitted for PAC in these facilities more than doubled from 1,178 in 2003 to 2,530 in 2005. The percentage of patients treated with MVA nearly doubled from 27 to 54 percent. The percentage of patients who received family planning counseling increased from 36 to 78 percent, and the percentage of patients who received a method increased from 15 to 56 percent (Thiam et al., 2006).

Clinical and operations research on PAC continued into the late 2000s. In 2008, the MSAS entered into a partnership with Ipas, an international reproductive rights NGO,[14] to train midwives in PAC in the regions of Dakar and Diourbel. In 2010, the DSR collaborated with Ipas and WHO to conduct a situational analysis of unwanted pregnancy and unsafe abortion.[15] At the time of my fieldwork in 2010 and 2011, the DSR was collaborating with Child Fund on a community-based approach to PAC in three regions of the country. Child Fund agents worked with community representatives to sensitize people on referring women with abortion complications to the nearest hospital. The terminology used to describe abortion complications, however, was quite innovative. A midwife who worked with Child Fund explained that using the term "abortion" was too provocative because it immediately evoked clandestine abortion. "The question of abortion is quite delicate," she said. "You can't just discuss it anywhere or anyhow." She and her colleagues therefore developed the phrase "preventing hemorrhage during the first trimester of pregnancy" to communicate the urgency of obstetric conditions in a culturally acceptable manner without specifying whether the hemorrhage was related to spontaneous or induced abortion.[16]

In 2009, Gynuity Health Projects, a reproductive health research NGO,[17] enrolled a large hospital in Dakar in a multicountry study on the use of misoprostol for the treatment of incomplete abortion (Shochet et al., 2012). Also known by the brand name Cytotec, misoprostol was until recently registered only for the treatment of gastric ulcers. Since being placed on the national List of Essential Medications (LEM) in 2013, it can now be used for PAC, for labor induction, and to manage PPH (but not pregnancy termination) (Reiss et al., 2017). Between 2011 and 2012, Gynuity Health Projects tested the feasibility of providing misoprostol at the community level for the treatment of incomplete abortion. During the study, 481 women seeking PAC at eleven primary health care facilities received misoprostol. Nearly all patients (99.4%) were successfully treated without the need for additional intervention (Gaye, Diop, Shochet, and Winikoff, 2014).[18]

PAC: A "TRANSFORMATIVE" INTERVENTION

When I returned to Senegal to conduct research on PAC as a doctoral student, I was equipped with thinking tools from the fields of medical sociology and anthropology. Although I drew on my identity and knowledge as a public health professional to gain access to my research sites and to develop rapport with my interlocutors, some of whom I had worked with as a Population Fellow with MSH, I began to think about what people were saying to me about PAC and what I was observing in hospitals as a social scientist. One of the recurring themes from my conversations with MSAS officials, NGO personnel, and health workers that struck me the most was the perception that PAC had not only improved but essentially "transformed" the treatment of abortion complications in Senegal. These narratives of transformation illustrate what sociologist Peter Conrad (1992) called "conceptual" and "institutional" forms of medicalization, in which treating abortion complications was defined as a medical affair, rather than a legal or moral affair, to be managed by trained professionals in health facilities. My interlocutors' descriptions of PAC aligned closely with early conceptualizations of the global PAC model that framed the intervention as a form of public health harm reduction (Erdman, 2011), in which the availability of quality services and effective technology throughout the health system would avert mortality and morbidity related to complications of unsafe abortion.

Health professionals outlined four primary ways in which PAC had transformed the treatment of abortion complications in Senegal. First, PAC training improved health workers' clinical skills so that they could treat women immediately, rather than referring them to other health facilities. M. (abbreviation of Monsieur) Gueye, a demographer who worked with a reproductive health research NGO, described how failure to recognize complications of abortion could lead to delays in care:

> Health personnel often weren't instructed on the signs of abortion, so the emergency of the situation wasn't well perceived. We saw, for example, and this was something really remarkable, with the studies we did with UNFPA, we realized that women could visit more than three health facilities, nearly eighty hours after the first sign of abortion, they go to the facilities . . . and they didn't see the obvious signs . . . so the pregnant woman, she's bleeding, they'll think you're supposed to stop the bleeding, give her a product to stop the bleeding, when the abortion is already taking place, and there's a reaction that's giving rise to this hemorrhaging. So the woman continued to go to the facilities, where they continued to try to stop the bleeding, and there were no results, so they went to another facility, and another, until someone did a uterine evacuation.

Mme (abbreviation of Madame) Sankharé, a DSR official and a midwife, agreed, shaking her head as she described how "for a long time, women were wasting their time with the treatment of incomplete abortions." PAC "speeded up" the treatment, so women no longer had to "go to the hospital and come back" repeatedly.

Second, the replacement of dilation and curettage with MVA reduced the cost of obstetric care and the hospitalization period for patients, thereby making care more efficient in hospitals. Dr. Dème, a DSR official and a gynecologist, described how MVA streamlined services for women in one hospital and allowed a faster turnover of hospital beds:

> Perhaps you didn't experience this, but I did. In 1987, I went to the maternity ward at Le Dantec Hospital. I was in a rural zone prior to this. I came to work on my specialty. When I arrived . . . we saw beds with pathological pregnancies, that is, pregnancies with problems. Three-quarters of the beds in the ward were occupied by women who presented with incomplete abortions who were waiting for us to do their checkup, to insert the laminaria.[19] . . . These women, we gave them appointments, then they did the checkup somewhere else, then they came back and we hospitalized them. These appointments, this back and forth, there were some who just never came back. When we introduced MVA, we saw that they didn't need to do the checkup, the problem was there, we were able to treat the problem. She won't have to occupy the beds that should be occupied by patients with more serious conditions. So things really changed.

Third, the decentralization of PAC from national and regional hospitals to district hospitals significantly increased access to lifesaving services for women in rural areas. Dr. Dème explained that before the introduction of PAC, health workers in district hospitals without an operating theater would have to refer patients to the nearest hospital with one: "Take the case of a woman in Popenguine district hospital, where there is no operating block, who has an incomplete abortion. She has to go all the way to Mbour. Now we can treat her at Popenguine. At the district hospital in Saint-Louis, they don't have to refer, or the district hospital at Dagana, they don't have to refer her, they can treat her there instead of evacuating her to Ndioum. In Matam it's the same thing, in Kanel, in Ranérou, in Fatick, in Guinguineo they no longer have to refer cases." Dr. Dème indicated that he was "very satisfied" with this reorganization of services, which for him represented a series of "significant advances" in clinical care.

Fourth, PAC transformed the ethic of care for abortion complications from one that singled out women suspected of illegal, induced abortion to one in which the kind of abortion the patient had experienced did not matter. The global PAC model, grounded in the ICPD's vocabulary of reproductive rights, obligated health workers to provide quality obstetric care to all patients regardless of the origins of the abortion. PAC training emphasized health workers' ethical duties to not only treat patients but also respect their patients' privacy. MSAS officials and NGO personnel recalled how the introduction of PAC dramatically improved health workers' bedside manner when it came to women suspected of illegal abortion. Both Mme Mbow, a midwife who worked for an international health NGO, and Mme Ngom, a midwife and a regional MSAS official, recalled instances where women suspected of abortion had been poorly treated. "I remember when I was a student," Mme Mbow said, "a woman came and had an abortion, and she was cornered and seen as guilty." Mme Ngom described how she had once witnessed health workers threatening to withhold care from a patient suspected of abortion.

My interlocutors acknowledged that treating abortion was perceived as a legal matter, fraught with tension, and that health workers often crossed the line into work typically reserved for law enforcement agents. "Before, it was like the police," said Mme Mbow. M. Gueye agreed, noting how this orientation led to discrimination against women: "The health agent positioned himself more like, how would I say, a judge, an inquisitor, than a health agent. Women suspected of induced abortion were rejected. Cases of induced abortion were very poorly received. . . . The problem was that, from a strictly human and ethical point of view, there was negligence because the duty of health personnel is not to assume the role of judge. They have to first treat people, treat them and then try to prevent the same event from happening, especially induced abortions, by offering contraceptive methods. So I think that the reception of women posed a problem."

In contrast, the new PAC model liberated health workers from attending to the legal aspects of a suspected case of illegal abortion. "Now, you have to treat the emergency before continuing with the interview to learn more," Mme Mbow said. "Even when there are doubts, you have to properly welcome the woman." M. Gueye highlighted the "novelty" of this new approach, in which health workers were not supposed to judge women who had experienced illegal abortions, but rather counsel them in contraception to prevent unwanted pregnancies in the future. "With the introduction of the PAC model, the first thing was to abolish this tendency, to say that you must first treat a patient, someone who is in need," he explained. "You have the means to treat her, so first treat her and then help her prevent the same thing from happening if it's an induced abortion."

As direct practitioners of PAC, health workers at the three study hospitals echoed the imperative to treat articulated by MSAS officials and NGO personnel. "The role of the doctor is to treat the patient," explained Dr. Diatta, the head gynecologist at l'Hôpital Senghor. "Even if she has had an induced abortion, the doctor must care for her." Dr. Ly at l'Hôpital Senghor agreed, arguing that "doctors just want to do their work, and that is to treat." Furthermore, in their understanding of PAC, health workers grounded the obligation to treat as no different from other maternal and reproductive health services. "PAC is a service like the rest—delivery, family planning," insisted Mme Kouyaté, a midwife at a primary health care facility in the first study region. "We have to care for the woman." According to Mme Bâ, a midwife at l'Hôpital Médina, health workers saw "no difference" between induced and spontaneous abortion. "Above all, we are concerned with the health of the woman," she explained. "We treat and ask questions later. We don't stand there and cross our arms and refuse to treat if it's a case of induced abortion."

THE STUDY HOSPITALS

Senegalese health workers are not alone in their perception that PAC is a regular feature of reproductive health care. Studies show that throughout sub-Saharan Africa, medical professionals frequently confront abortion-related obstetric emergencies. Retrospective reviews of hospital records at Kenyatta National Hospital in Nairobi, Kenya, estimated that 60 percent of emergency gynecological admissions were related to abortion complications (Gebreselassie, Gallo, Monyo, and Johnson, 2005). Between 2002 and 2004, abortion complications accounted for 12 percent of general hospital admissions, and approximately 60 percent of gynecological admissions at a hospital in Ethiopia (Gessessew, 2010). Even in South Africa, where abortion upon request has been legal during the first trimester of pregnancy since 1996, nearly 50,000 women were admitted to public hospitals in 2000 with complications of unsafe abortion (Jewkes, Rees, Dickson, Brown, and Levin, 2005). In Burkina Faso, approximately 23,000 women received care

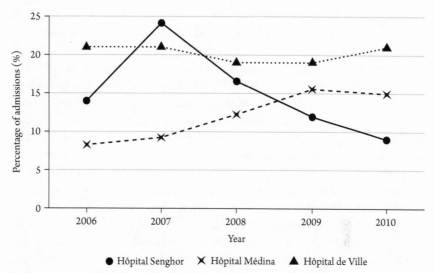

FIGURE 1.1. Abortion as a percentage of admissions to the maternity ward in three hospitals, 2006–2010.

for abortion complications in 2008 (Bankole et al., 2013). In 2016, an estimated 37,870 women in Kinshasa, the capital city of the Democratic Republic of Congo, received PAC (Lince-Deroche et al., 2019).

In 2016, 18,806 women received PAC in Senegalese health facilities. Almost all (77%) of these patients were treated in district hospitals and primary health care facilities. While incomplete abortion accounted for 70 percent of cases treated at all facilities, higher-level facilities were more likely to treat severe complications such as shock, lacerations, or perforations. In a 2016 study of PAC at forty-one health facilities, midwives on average spent more time providing PAC on each patient than physicians (22.2 minutes and 9.6 minutes, respectively) (Lince-Deroche, Sène, Pliskin, Owolabi, and Bankole, 2020).

Drawing on hospital records at the three hospitals where I conducted field-work, I calculated abortion as a percentage of total admissions to the maternity ward between 2006 and 2010 (see figure 1.1). At all three sites, where at least one form of uterine evacuation (MVA, EVA, digital evacuation, or dilation and curettage) was available around the clock, PAC was a significant component of health providers' work in gynecological wards. As a Population Fellow with MSH, I had participated in PAC supervision visits at one of these hospitals and thus was already aware of the burden posed by PAC on maternity wards. From a sociological perspective, however, these data raised other important questions about the provision, organization, and quality of PAC (and PAC record keeping) that merited consideration in light of the legal context of abortion in Senegal, which

I explore throughout the next three chapters. Here, I briefly describe how health workers treated abortion complications and the challenging technical environment in which they administered care.

The first hospital where I conducted research (Hôpital Senghor) was a tertiary facility located in a coastal city with a population of 176,000, where fishing and tourism are the primary sources of income. Midwives at this hospital treated most PAC patients and managed PAC records. Between 2009 and 2010, they treated an average of thirty-two cases of incomplete abortion per month. Midwives administered uterine evacuation services in the delivery room, with a separate room for MVA and EVA. After treatment, women rested in one of several recovery rooms in the maternity ward. In 2010, PAC accounted for 9 percent of gynecological admissions, down from 24 percent in 2007.

At the second study facility (Hôpital Médina), health workers treated an average of thirty-five PAC cases per month between 2009 and 2010. L'Hôpital Médina was a district facility in a coastal town with a population of approximately 230,000, located about seventy-four kilometers from the regional capital. Like their counterparts at l'Hôpital Senghor, midwives at l'Hôpital Médina performed most PAC treatment and record-keeping procedures. However, midwives at l'Hôpital Médina conducted all PAC procedures, including MVA, in the three-bed delivery room, displayed in figure 1.2. In 2010, PAC accounted for 15 percent of admissions to the maternity ward at l'Hôpital Médina.

The third study facility (Hôpital de Ville) was a district hospital in a coastal town with a population of 330,000, located approximately nineteen kilometers from the regional capital. Between 2009 and 2010, medical workers here treated an average of 107 PAC cases each month. L'Hôpital de Ville differed from the other two hospitals in that its physicians conducted the lion's share of PAC. Physicians performed MVA in a separate room in the maternity ward, and EVA and dilation and curettage in an operating block. Midwives conducted digital evacuation in the main delivery room. PAC accounted for up to 21 percent of gynecological admissions at this hospital in 2010.

At all three hospitals, health workers triaged women according to their clinical state upon arrival at the facility. Those who arrived in a state of shock received uterine evacuation services immediately. Some women required treatment of infection or a blood transfusion for hemorrhage. If providers determined that a patient was stable, they conducted l'interrogation to establish a standard medical history to manage the case. They performed a vaginal exam with the use of a speculum and, if necessary, an ultrasound to determine the status of the fetus and to measure the size and shape of the uterus. After the vaginal exam and the ultrasound, the patient received uterine evacuation services and, depending on the type of treatment or the severity of complications, was hospitalized. Upon completion of uterine aspiration, providers in the maternity ward recorded each case in a special PAC register. They counseled the woman, during or after treat-

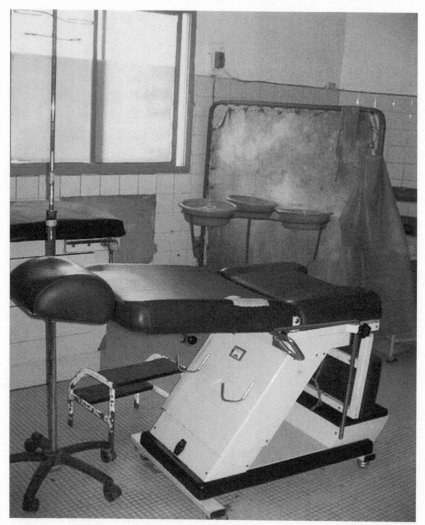

FIGURE 1.2. Delivery room at l'Hôpital Médina.

ment, to use contraception to delay her next pregnancy. Unless health workers confirmed that a pregnancy termination had occurred and notified the police, or the police learned about the case from a source outside the hospital, the woman left the hospital as soon as she was able.

Although the PAC model promotes separate treatment rooms for patients (Billings and Benson, 2005; Johnson, Ndhlovu, Farr, and Chipato, 2002; Wood, Ottolenghi, and Marin, 2007), at all three study hospitals providers conducted the initial examination and interrogation and performed digital evacuation in the delivery room. Dr. Ly lamented the state of PAC infrastructure at l'Hôpital

Senghor: "PAC patients need a certain measure of confidentiality, which we don't have here. All patients are together in the delivery room. Especially for cases of induced abortion. Anyone can find you here in the delivery room, even your neighbor. What if you're not married? These are special cases and they need privacy."

Dr. Sylla—the head gynecologist at l'Hôpital Médina, where midwives managed both abortion complications and deliveries in the delivery room (sometimes at the same time)—echoed the need for a separate PAC room. Her efforts to designate a PAC room in the maternity ward, however, were blocked by the district health planning committee, which declined to release funds to make the required infrastructural changes.

The incongruence I observed between health professionals' working conditions and the clinical and infrastructural requirements of the global PAC model was hardly unusual. In 1987, African Ministers of Health enacted the Bamako Initiative, which decentralized health care decision-making to local health committees. Although the Bamako Initiative aimed to improve rural populations' access to primary health care, it was part of a broader pattern of neoliberal economic restructuring that gutted financing for health systems, ultimately impeding health workers' ability to provide quality services to their patients (Foley, 2009; Kanji, 1989; McPake, Hanson, and Mills, 1993; Ridde, 2003). Some studies show that structural adjustment policies have worsened maternal and child health outcomes in sub-Saharan Africa (Sommer et al., 2019; Thomson, Kentikelenis, and Stubbs, 2017). Health facilities often face stockouts of drugs and other medical supplies and equipment despite the initiative's goal to locate such products in hospitals rather than private pharmacies (Lange, Kanhonou, Goufodji, Ronsmans, and Filippi, 2016; Paganini, 2004; Uzochukwu, Onwujekwe, and Akpala, 2002). Infrastructural constraints may range from a lack of hospital beds to frequent shortages in running water and electricity (Beninguisse and De Brouwere, 2004; Foley 2009; Geurts, 2001; Maimbolwa, Yamba, Diwan, and Ransjö-Arvidson, 2003). A participant in a community evaluation of primary health care facilities in Tanzania aptly captured the dire situation faced by government facilities: "It is like a dance hall in there because there is no equipment" (Gilson, Alilio, and Heggenhougen, 1994, p. 771).

In addition to decentralizing authority to local decision-makers, the Bamako Initiative instituted user fees at government health facilities. A 2016 study of PAC in forty-one health facilities found that direct patient costs, including medication, laboratory tests, and equipment, ranged from $8.31 in primary health care facilities to $34.44 in district hospitals (Lince-Deroche et al., 2020). During my fieldwork, I observed PAC patients and their families purchasing a variety of materials, including Betadine (an antiseptic), Xylocaine (a locally applied anesthetic), the latex gloves that providers would use during treatment, and bottles of bleach to sterilize MVA material. Sometimes, health workers may take advantage of patients' involvement in the procurement of hospital supplies. In Benin, for example, delivery patients complained bitterly about having to purchase an entire bottle of bleach, knowing that health workers would use whatever remained after their treatment for themselves or other patients (Lange et al., 2016). Other opportunities for extortion may arise when health workers "volunteer" to facilitate payment on behalf of patients at the hospital cashier. For example, during a tea break in the staff room at l'Hôpital Médina, a community health worker told me that some midwives deliberately misinformed patients about the price of services and pocketed the difference.

Throughout this book, I document instances of obstetric violence because, as elsewhere in both developed and developing countries (Castro and Savage, 2019; Davis, 2018, 2019; d'Oliveira, Diniz, and Schraiber, 2002; Heller, 2019; Jewkes et al., 1998; Zacher Dixon, 2015), it was a regular feature of obstetric care. At all three hospitals, I observed midwives, and some physicians, perform a procedure known as "abdominal expression" (Heller, 2019), in which the health worker presses on the pregnant woman's abdomen to expulse the baby from the uterus. Health workers raised their voices at women, and at times smacked them on their legs or roughly pushed their legs apart, when they did not comply with instructions to push or submit to an examination or other procedure. Sometimes, health workers verbally shamed women for defecating during delivery. One afternoon at l'Hôpital de Ville, a woman in labor began to defecate while lying on an observation bed in the delivery room. The physicians were seated at a table in the center of the room, reviewing files and completing paperwork. One of them glanced in the woman's direction, loudly announced that she was defecating, and yelled at her to go to the toilet. Slowly, she got off the bed and shuffled toward the toilet. As she passed by the doctors sitting at the table, she accidentally brushed against Dr. Thiam, who angrily yelled at her to stay away from him. On another occasion, a female doctor shouted at and slapped a woman who had begun to defecate during delivery, calling her "undisciplined" and "crazy."

PAC patients were also subjected to obstetric violence when they demonstrated what health workers viewed as "difficult" behavior. At l'Hôpital de Ville, in the MVA room, Mme Sow (a nursing assistant) yelled at a patient who was anxious about the procedure and would not let the physician insert the speculum. Mme Sow told the patient that she was "wasting their time" and that if she did not want to be treated she should leave. Eventually the woman climbed back onto the examination bed and permitted the doctor to proceed with MVA. When her treatment was completed, Mme Sow began to clean up the room in preparation for the next patient. At one point, she threw a crumpled piece of paper toward the trash can next to the examination bed. Instead, the paper hit the woman's exposed buttocks as she lay on the table, and fell to the floor.

Even seemingly compliant patients were subjected to neglectful care. At l'Hôpital de Ville, a research assistant and I observed a physician, Dr. Thiam, who did not systematically administer the Xylocaine injection. On one occasion, he administered the numbing injection *after* he had already begun the procedure. When I asked him why, he said he had forgotten to do so earlier. About a month later, we saw him administer the injection on the first two MVA patients, but not the third. When we asked him why, Dr. Thiam said he found that some women could "handle the pain" without anesthesia.

These instances of neglect, abuse, and substandard care appear throughout the book not to pathologize Senegalese health workers but to situate violent obstetric practices within a broader geopolitical landscape of health care in which government health providers often lack the political and economic power to lobby for improved working conditions, including salary and benefits. Public sector health professionals in sub-Saharan Africa have been particularly vulnerable to cuts in wages and employment as governments strive to meet the "wage bill ceilings" imposed by structural adjustment programs (Thomson, Kentikelenis, and Stubbs, 2017). Reductions in government spending on medical supplies and equipment compromise health workers' capacity to provide quality care for their patients. For example, midwives and nurses in a study of obstetric services in South Africa reported that their working environment constantly undermined their efforts to ensure good clinical outcomes for patients. Moreover, they often felt unfairly blamed by the community for structural problems beyond their control (Jewkes, Abrahams, and Mvo, 1998). In some cases, health workers attempt to force the government's hand. At the time of my fieldwork in Senegal in 2011, providers belonging to two national health worker unions had been on strike since July 2010 to improve working conditions and equalize the distribution of health resources throughout the country. Although they continued to provide health services (some on a limited basis), they withheld patient data from the MSAS (Tichenor, 2016).

Despite these ongoing attempts to improve their working conditions, health workers often resigned themselves to "making do." "We'd like to have separate rooms for more privacy," Dr. Ly at l'Hôpital Senghor told me. "But you've seen the delivery room. . . . You see how we keep the women crammed together like sheep." He then shrugged and said, "But that's how it is in Africa." In a health system gutted by decades of development strategies like the Bamako Initiative, health workers did what they could to care for their patients while contending with low salaries, inadequate medical equipment and infrastructure, low confidence in their abilities in the eyes of the community, and burnout (Foley, 2009; Heller, 2019; Jaffré, 2012; Jaffré and Olivier de Sardan, 2003). Such working environments left plenty of room for obstetric violence to not just occur but become a mundane part of obstetric care.

In the chapters that follow, I interrogate the extent to which the global PAC model has "transformed" the treatment of abortion complications from the perspectives of health officials, medical workers, and NGO personnel. I illustrate how the medicalization of abortion care in the form of harm reduction not only facilitates neglectful and discriminatory treatment of women but also entrenches reproductive health inequalities through selective portrayals of what happens in hospitals and the kinds of women who receive care.

2 · A TROUBLESOME TECHNOLOGY

The Multiple Lives of MVA in Senegal

At l'Hôpital de Ville, physicians conducted MVA in *la chambre d'AMIU* (the MVA room), displayed in figure 2.1. Located across the courtyard of the maternity ward from the delivery room, the MVA room consisted of two small rooms: one with an examination bed where doctors conducted MVA, and an adjoining room with two single beds where women could rest after the procedure. As the designated manager of the MVA room, Mme Sow assembled the syringe before each procedure and disassembled and sterilized it in the electric autoclave for the next patient. She stored spare MVA syringes and cannulas in a cabinet across from the examination bed, and locked the door to the MVA room when service hours ended.

The securing of MVA under lock and key was not unusual in a facility offering PAC. The device's capacity to terminate pregnancy has engendered similar practices in other Senegalese health facilities (Population Council, 2007) and other African countries with restrictive abortion laws (Cook, de Kok, and Odland, 2016; Mutua, Manderson, Musenge, and Achia, 2018; Ndembi, Mekuí, Pheterson, and Alblas 2019; Odland et al., 2014; Paul, Gemzell-Danielsson, Kiggundu, Namugenyi, and Klingberg-Allvin, 2014; Tagoe-Darko, 2013). At l'Hôpital de Ville, not only was the device secured in a cabinet in the MVA room, but MVA services were restricted to certain hours during the weekday and performed only by physicians. Given these attempts to keep the device "in the hands of trustworthy men," in the words of Dr. Ndao, a district health official, I was somewhat puzzled to learn that Mme Sow, the MVA room manager, was a paramedical provider—a nursing assistant. Although she stated that she had not been formally trained, informal chats with Mme Sow and observations in the MVA room revealed her familiarity with the device. For example, my research assistant and I observed her instructing a physician, Dr. Sarr, to stop using the syringe shortly after he had started treating a patient. *"C'est bon"* [that's enough], she told him,

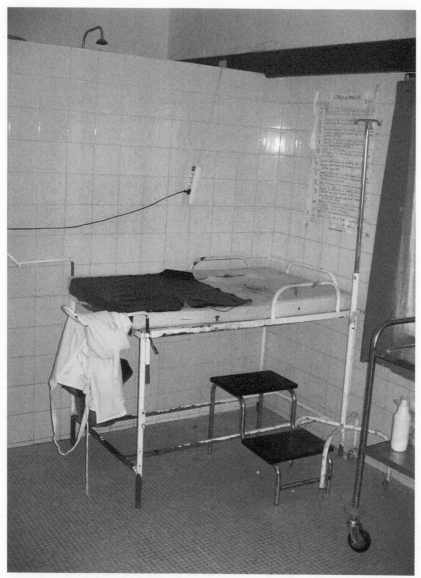

FIGURE 2.1. MVA room at l'Hôpital de Ville.

rather curtly. One morning, while another physician, Dr. Thiam, was conducting MVA on a patient, he asked her for a cannula of a different size. She shook her head, explaining that the one he wanted was being sterilized. Then she handed him a different cannula, saying, "It's practically the same thing." After Dr. Thiam left the room, she told my research assistant and me that he often did not use the syringe correctly. When we asked her if she had ever used the syringe, she revealed that a physician had "once" supervised her while she conducted the procedure on a patient.

That a paramedical provider had seemingly unfettered access to an abortion device represents one of many striking contradictions between MVA policies and discourses that aimed to prevent the misuse of an abortifacient technology and what happened in daily obstetric practice in Senegalese hospitals. Mme Sow's proximity to MVA—and the questions it raises about who can use the device, for what, and where—is part of a much longer, complicated story this chapter tells of MVA as a globally circulating abortion technology. MVA is a tool of reproductive governance with origins in vacuum suction devices developed by European and American doctors in the late nineteenth century that transformed into a PAC device in countries with restrictive abortion laws such as Bolivia, Mexico, Honduras, Niger, Mali, Burkina Faso, and Senegal a century later.

STS scholars offer important theoretical tools for tracing how technologies shape and are shaped by social, political, organizational, professional, and economic relations. Technologies can lead multiple "lives" (Carpenter and Casper, 2009; Casper and Morrison, 2010; Mol and Berg, 1994; Timmermans and Berg, 2003; Whyte, van der Geest, and Hardon, 2002) as scientists, patients, consumers, pharmaceutical companies, government institutions, manufacturing companies, and others with lay or professional claims to or interests in these devices negotiate what they are designed to do and how they are deployed to accomplish particular goals. Those who are "active around" (Clarke and Montini, 1993) the technology participate a great deal in fashioning it into "the right tool for the job" (Clarke and Fujimura, 1992).

For example, the Pap smear remains the most widely used cervical cancer screening tool in the United States since its introduction in the 1940s, despite its limited capacity to accurately detect and classify cancerous cells. This device became the "right tool" because it served the political goals of newly emerging national cancer organizations and the professional interests of physicians who wished to integrate cancer screening into routine gynecological practice (Clarke and Montini, 1993). Takeshita's (2012) history of the intrauterine device (IUD) shows how the "jobs" that reproductive technologies are designed to accomplish reflect demographic and epidemiological goals of those "active around" the devices, including global population and development experts and U.S. medical professionals. During the late 1960s and throughout the 1970s, at the height of the era of population control (Connelly, 2008; McCann, 2017; Murphy, 2012), the IUD was the ideal tool for "blocking" the wombs of insufficiently modern, overabundantly fertile (Black and brown) women in the global South. By the mid-2000s, this device had been refashioned into a reliable method for contraception and menstrual suppression for modern, educated middle-class (white) women in the global North (Takeshita, 2012). Similarly, as I illustrate in this chapter, MVA has at once been the "right tool" for the job of abortion within the reproductive regime of population control and a device for PAC in countries with restrictive abortion laws that are signatories of the 1994 ICPD.

When it comes to technologies designed for women, STS scholars have grappled with what makes technologies feminist. Although feminist technologies do not necessarily have to be designed by women, technologies can be understood as feminist if they "benefit and empower women" (Layne, 2010). Of course, technologies in and of themselves cannot be feminist (or anything else). Rather, the social, political, and economic relations in which they are designed and used determine how and whether they improve women's lives and health (Layne, Vostral, and Boyer, 2010). In this chapter, I show how uterine aspiration devices have been designed simultaneously for the purposes of population control and women's reproductive autonomy (Murphy 2012). Additionally, I illustrate how the political context of PAC in Senegal limits MVA's capacity to improve women's reproductive health.

The sociological concept of "boundary work" describes the strategies enacted by professionals to protect jurisdiction over tasks, techniques, and technologies (Abbott, 1988, 1995a, 1995b; Gieryn, 1999; Lamont and Molnár, 2002). It facilitates analysis of how local and global actors, including Senegalese health workers, health officials, and personnel from national and international NGOs, have endeavored to define MVA as the right tool for the job of PAC since its introduction to the health system during the late 1990s. In this chapter I demonstrate how, in a country where abortion is altogether prohibited, MVA's dual capacity to terminate pregnancy and treat abortion complications required stakeholders to establish the device's clinical and political legitimacy as a PAC device during the period of pilot research in regional and district hospitals and the formulation of policies regarding where it could be used and by whom. Additionally, I illustrate how the struggle to restrict MVA to the practice of PAC amplified tensions over power, resources, and professional prestige between physicians and midlevel providers like nurses and midwives, who provide the bulk of reproductive health care in government health facilities, and between practitioners and decision-makers at central and peripheral levels of the national health system.

Equally important to tracing the multiple lives of MVA in Senegal is attention to what it does *not* do and the ways in which, despite being established as the preferred technology for PAC, it has been only partially integrated into regular obstetric practice in government hospitals precisely because of its vexatious connection to the illegitimate "job" of induced abortion. In the previous chapter, I illustrated how the global PAC model "transformed" the treatment of abortion complications in Senegal because of MVA—a handheld plastic syringe that could be used by midlevel providers in low-resource clinical settings. Here, I disrupt this triumphal narrative of MVA as a magic bullet for the public health problem of unsafe abortion by showing how policies designed to prevent the (mis)use of the device for illegal abortion constrain health workers' capacity to use it effectively in daily obstetric practice. Gaps in MVA training for nurses and midwives, inadequate MVA supplies, and restrictions over who can use it (and when and where) give rise to delays in care and costly referrals between primary health care facilities and district and regional hospitals that are absorbed by women patients.

These factors increase the likelihood that health workers will treat women with methods not recognized by the WHO (2012) as safe techniques of abortion care—dilation and curettage and digital evacuation. The latter procedure has been documented in Senegal and other African countries in health facilities with no MVA equipment or where there is no provider trained in MVA, or in situations where gestational age exceeds fourteen weeks (Izugbara, Wekesah, et al., 2019; Izugbara, Egesa, and Okelo, 2015; Kiemtoré et al., 2016; Prada, Mirembe, Ahmed, Nalwadda, and Kiggundu, 2005). While clinical protocols for digital evacuation in Senegal call for the use of gloves and pain medication, these materials are not systematically used. In some facilities, matrons (traditional birth attendants who may or may not have received biomedical training) rather than nurses or midwives conduct the procedure (Population Council, 2007).

The persistence of less safe and less effective uterine evacuation techniques suggests that within the Senegalese health system, MVA is not always the right tool for the job. By tracing the multiple lives of MVA as a tool of reproductive governance, I highlight troubling disparities between national and global PAC narratives of what this device does and how it "works" in treating abortion complications, and illustrate the organizational, clinical, and professional conditions that give rise to obstetric violence in the application of the device to or its withholding from women's bodies in daily obstetric care in government health facilities.

A GLOBALLY CIRCULATING DEVICE

From the start, this syringe device has been both inextricably linked to and painstakingly distinguished from the "job" of abortion. A Scottish physician, Sir James Young Simpson, was the first to report using a syringe device to "induce menstruation" in 1863. In turn, Dr. Simpson had been inspired by Dr. Frederick Hollick's description in 1849 of applying an airtight cup against the abdomen to "bring on the menstrual flow" (Tunc, 2008, p. 356). American physicians also experimented with suction devices, "littering" the U.S. Patent Office with their inventions during the nineteenth century (Murphy, 2012). By the early twentieth century in the United States, when abortion was largely restricted to therapeutic purposes in hospitals, physicians were using manual aspiration devices to diagnose uterine pathologies and to "treat" conditions like amenorrhea and dysmenorrhea, which were likely euphemisms for abortion (Tunc, 2008).

In countries with less restrictive abortion laws, physicians had greater freedom to publish research on abortion technology. During the 1920s, Russian physician S. G. Bykov described openly in international medical literature how manual vacuum aspiration devices could be used effectively to terminate pregnancy (Joffe, 1996; Tunc, 2008). Starting in the late 1950s, as part of China's birth control program, Chinese physicians experimented with various abortion technologies, including manual suction devices that could be used in rural settings because they did not require electricity (Murphy, 2012). In the United States, by the early 1930s, physicians were experimenting with motorized, electric pumps to conduct aspiration to treat complications of incomplete abortion and to perform endometrial biopsies. Although Chinese and Russian physicians continued to improve EVA devices throughout the 1950s and 1960s, dilation and curettage remained the most frequently used method in the United States for practicing therapeutic abortions and treating abortion complications (Joffe, 1996; Tunc, 2008).

It was not until the late 1960s that EVA technology was formally introduced to American gynecologists (Tunc, 2008). At a 1968 conference sponsored by the Association for the Study of Abortion (a group of American physicians involved in advocacy to decriminalize abortion), Yugoslavian physician Franc Novac demonstrated the latest iteration of vacuum aspiration technology. He delivered a powerful technological rationale for replacing dilation and curettage with vacuum aspiration: "When the gynecologist who knows only the conventional dilation and curettage (D&C) method first sees the apparatus in action, he is impressed by the cleanness, apparent bloodlessness, speed, and simplicity of the operation. While a D&C gives the impression of rude artisan's work, an abortion performed with suction gives the impression of a simple mechanical procedure" (Joffe, 1996, p. 43). By the early 1970s, this technological innovation had replaced dilation and curettage for conducting therapeutic abortions in the United States. The state-by-state decriminalization of abortion in the early 1970s, coupled with the uptake of the technology by aspirator manufacturers around the country, led to the mainstreaming of EVA into American medicine (Tunc, 2008). In contrast, dilation and curettage in the United Kingdom did not begin to decline significantly until the early 1990s, when the Royal College of Obstetricians and Gynecologists stopped recommending it for women under forty (Seamark, 1998).

Despite the growing popularity of EVA among American physicians, its manual predecessor had not entirely disappeared. Interest in MVA technology was likely rekindled by Harvey Karman, a nonphysician who infamously practiced illegal abortion in California during the 1950s. After serving two years in prison following the death of one of his "patients" (Goldberg, 2009), Karman was eager to develop better abortion technologies. During the early 1960s, he fashioned a bendable plastic cannula that differed notably from the metal, plastic, and glass curettes that physicians were using with both electric and manual aspiration devices.

Soft and flexible, Karman's cannula reduced the risk of uterine perforation, was easily attached to or removed from the electric aspirator or syringe, and could be used with local or no anesthesia. Karman demonstrated that his device could be used safely by nonphysicians in nonhospital settings. By the early 1970s, several prominent gynecologists were promoting Karman's device in their advocacy to improve abortion technology and to liberalize abortion laws (Joffe, 1996; Murphy, 2012). Other gynecologists were less enthusiastic about Karman's cannula precisely because it threatened physicians' control over the practice of abortion.

Radical feminist health groups had been practicing abortions using MVA procedures and technologies gleaned from Chinese medical journals since the late 1960s (Murphy, 2012). At a time when physicians still maintained a monopoly over the practice of legal therapeutic abortions in hospitals, these groups were dedicated to facilitating women's access to safe, albeit clandestine, abortion by placing technologies in the hands of lay practitioners. After attending a demonstration by Karman in 1971, abortion activist Lorraine Rothman patented a model known as the Del-Em Menstrual Extraction device. Described in the patent as "an apparatus whereby substantially all of the menstrual fluid incident to a normal monthly 'period' may be removed" (Murphy, 2012, p. 159), Rothman's device distinguished itself from other aspiration devices employed by feminist health groups as abortive methods. Instead, Rothman defined Del-Em as a home health device to allow women to "regain control over their reproductive lives" (Murphy, 2012, p. 158). Women could assemble the device themselves, using materials available at hardware stores, and then perform menstrual extraction in nonmedical settings. Designed and used by women to regulate reproduction, Del-Em was the quintessential "feminist" technology (Layne et al., 2010).

Karman's plastic cannula also caught the interest of Reimert Ravenholt, director of USAID's Office of Population at a time when the U.S. government perceived fertility regulation in newly decolonized nations in the global South as a matter of national security. Demographers identified contraceptive unmet need (the gap between women's desire to space or limit births and the nonuse of modern contraception) as a significant driver of high fertility in the developing world. By the late 1960s, Ravenholt had launched an "inundation strategy" to flood developing countries with cheap contraceptives (primarily IUDs and oral contraceptive pills) to reduce this unmet need (Murphy, 2012, p. 163). Between 1968 and 1972, 80 percent of all global assistance for family planning came from USAID (Takeshita, 2012).

Karman's cannula offered a useful opportunity to integrate abortion into USAID's contraceptive "inundation strategy" in the form of "menstrual regulation" (Murphy, 2012). USAID contracted Burnett Instruments to develop a manual aspiration device using Karman's bendable plastic cannula. Pathfinder Fund, a nonprofit organization that began family planning programs in Africa, Asia, and Latin America during the 1950s (now known as Pathfinder International), was contracted to develop utilization protocols for the menstrual regulation kit. In contrast to what radical feminist health groups were calling menstrual extraction, menstrual regulation was defined as evacuating "the uterine contents from a woman who is at risk of being pregnant, before she can be declared 'obviously pregnant' by clinical examination and other diagnostic measures" (Murphy, 2012, p. 151). Like the feminist health groups, however, Ravenholt perceived the benefits of making this abortion technology available for use by nonphysicians or in places with limited medical infrastructure. In addition to contracting other organizations to produce and test the menstrual regulation kit, including the International Pregnancy Advisory Committee (now known as Ipas) and the International Fertility Research Program, USAID purchased and distributed thousands of kits to health professionals and family planning programs in Vietnam, Korea, Bangladesh, Pakistan, Indonesia, Singapore, and Thailand. In Bangladesh, Pathfinder Fund trained female community health agents known as "lady health workers" to use these kits to administer menstrual regulation (Murphy, 2012). Bangladesh integrated menstrual regulation into its family planning program in 1979. These services are available in government health facilities despite the fact that the penal code permits abortion only for therapeutic purposes (P. Adams, 2018).

In 1972, USAID invited 300 practitioners and policy makers from fifty countries to a meeting on menstrual regulation in Hawaii. A supply of 10,000 kits had been ordered for distribution at the meeting. A physician who attended the meeting later reflected: "It was about abortion technology in the Third World. USAID had literally rooms full of these kits! The kits consisted of the 50cc syringe, a variety of cannulas and instructions on how to do abortions. This was an international meeting. People came from the Pacific Basin, from all over Latin America. It's incredible to think of AID spending this kind of money now on that!" (Joffe, 1996, p. 45).

Ravenholt's menstrual regulation program was cut short by the Helms Amendment to the Foreign Assistance Act of 1973, which prohibited the use of federal funds "for the performance of abortion as a method of family planning or to motivate or coerce any person to practice abortions" (Barot, 2013, p. 9). No longer able to directly procure or distribute the menstrual regulation kits, Ravenholt delegated the program to organizations such as IPPF, Ipas, and Pathfinder International. By 1978, these organizations had distributed approximately 175,000 kits despite the Helms Amendment (Murphy, 2012). Although the Helms Amendment brought USAID's involvement in abortion in developing countries to a halt, it did not curtail USAID's support for family planning. USAID became the largest distributor of oral contraceptive pills in the world, selling 780 million cycles by 1979 (Takeshita, 2012) through family planning programs supported by such organizations as the Population Council, IPPF, and Pathfinder International.

In the early 1980s, the Reagan administration began introducing anti-abortion policies that restricted funding for biomedical research on abortion or training of medical providers in abortion techniques (Dixon-Mueller, 1993).[1] In 1987, three years after the Mexico City Policy had virtually silenced global conversation about abortion, the SMI recognized complications of unsafe abortion as one of the top five direct causes of global maternal death. WHO recommended uterine aspiration, both manual and electric, as the preferred technology for the treatment of abortion complications, defined as PAC in 1991 by Ipas. In 1993, Ipas established the Post-abortion Care Consortium, including EngenderHealth (known until 2001 as the Association for Voluntary Surgical Contraception), IPPF, JHPIEGO, and Pathfinder International, to promote PAC as an effective public health strategy to reduce abortion-related mortality and morbidity. The PAC Consortium urged health authorities in developing countries, where abortion complications were frequently treated with dilation and curettage in hospitals with operating theaters, to integrate MVA into maternal health care (Corbett and Turner, 2003; Greenslade, McKay, Wolf, and McLaurin, 1994). The qualities of MVA that had rendered it "the right tool for the job" for abortion in developing countries faced with the threat of overpopulation—safe, easy to use by physicians *and* midlevel professionals, and amenable to rural facilities lacking electricity—could just as easily be applied toward treating complications of unsafe abortion in developing countries with restrictive abortion laws. By 1993, MVA had been introduced to over one hundred countries through the PAC Consortium (P. Adams, 2018).[2]

For some members of the PAC Consortium, PAC offered a pragmatic means through which to distribute an abortifacient technology in countries with restrictive abortion laws and within the anti-abortion funding constraints imposed by the 1973 Helms Amendment and the 1984 Mexico City Policy. During an interview conducted in 2011 with Dr. Perez, a senior member of a reproductive health NGO, she explained:

> The private sector is providing comprehensive services including induced abortion services. Of course, public sector providers are also private sector providers. So part of our strategy ... part of the beauty, in some ways, of the PAC concept is that it allows you to train on any uterine evacuation procedure, and public providers will and do provide abortion services privately. So it's always been our approach in highly restrictive settings to train on PAC ... knowing that there will be private provision. ... It definitely gave us cover, to put it bluntly, to do a lot of training in a lot of places, especially in Latin America. Abortion laws there are so severely restricted that that was the only way. And we knew and still know that in Latin America providers are doing private provision of induced services. We have not been able to document the extent to which providers are doing that privately. ... I mean, it's illegal, they're not going to tell us what they're doing. So we haven't been able to document it, but we know that that's the case.

In the same way that menstrual regulation provided a "cover" for USAID to disseminate abortion technologies in developing countries before the 1973 Helms Amendment, Dr. Perez suggests that under the "cover" of PAC, NGOs could introduce MVA and train health workers to use the device to treat abortion complications in public facilities as part of the national maternal mortality reduction strategy. In private, however, these providers could use the very same device to practice safe, albeit clandestine, abortions. Put differently, MVA could meet the goals of global safe abortion advocates and national health officials eager to reduce maternal mortality without explicitly engaging in abortion law reform or jeopardizing USAID funding for family planning under the Mexico City Policy.

In 1994, while the authors of the ICPD's Platform of Action omitted safe abortion from the document's definition of reproductive health, they identified the Consortium's PAC model as a public health solution to reduce mortality related to unsafe abortion in countries with restrictive abortion laws. MVA became the device of choice for administering PAC. USAID began to support PAC in 1994, spending over $20 million in forty countries by 2001. With the Helms Amendment still in place, USAID could not purchase MVA kits, but channeled funds to NGOs implementing PAC programs to support "policy and advocacy, operations research, training, service delivery, and health communication" (Curtis, 2007, p. 371) related to PAC. In 2012, an estimated twenty-eight African countries had active PAC programs, many of which received funding from USAID (PAC Consortium, 2012). In 2017, Ipas issued the license to produce MVA kits previously held by Woman Care Global to another NGO, DKT International (PRWEB, 2017).[3] In 2018, DKT International (2018) sold 180,658 aspirators and 1,698,434 cannulas worldwide.

MVA TROUBLES AROUND THE WORLD

Despite the integration of MVA into the global PAC model, PAC advocates and stakeholders—known as "catalyzers" in some Latin American countries (Billings, Crane, Benson, Solo, and Fetters, 2007) and "champions" in Francophone West Africa—have struggled to introduce this device into clinical practice. In many of these countries, NGOs like Ipas donated initial supplies of MVA kits to health workers during PAC training or as part of PAC operations research projects. Since then, hospital managers and Ministry of Health officials have faced significant barriers to incorporating MVA into national systems for procuring and distributing medical supplies. Despite the clinical and cost-saving benefits of using MVA rather than dilation and curettage, the device's capacity to terminate pregnancy has complicated MVA's integration into obstetric practice.

In Guatemala, for example, the Ministry of Health tested the feasibility of introducing PAC in twenty-two out of thirty-three district hospitals across the country between 2003 and 2004. After the creation of special zones within the hospitals for MVA procedures, the percentage of patients treated with MVA increased from 38 to 68 percent in the study facilities. Despite this success, PAC catalyzers carefully framed the intervention as a maternal mortality reduction strategy because of concerns that the availability of MVA would "promote" illegal abortion in government hospitals. At the end of the study, hospitals had to procure MVA kits using their own funds (Kestler, Valencia, Valle, and Silva, 2006).

While catalyzers in Mexico used the term "PAC" to pressure the government to scale up services beyond the pilot research sites, their counterparts in Bolivia changed the name to *atención a las hemorragias de la primera mitad del embarazo* (care for hemorrhage during the first half of pregnancy). Like their Guatemalan counterparts, Bolivian PAC catalyzers were eager to situate the intervention in existing discourses related to safe motherhood. They focused the intervention on "saving women's lives" to ensure political commitment from the Ministry of Health and to fend off perceptions that the technology encouraged clandestine abortion in government hospitals (Billings et al., 2007). Bolivian physicians referred to MVA as a "saving women" device to distance their work from pregnancy termination (Rance, 2005). In both countries, catalyzers described the procurement and institutionalization of MVA as the greatest challenge to implementing PAC because of the device's proximity to induced abortion. Although MVA is "officially registered" in both countries, the device has not been integrated into national supply systems, leaving individual hospitals to purchase MVA directly from local distributors of medical supplies (Billings et al., 2007).

In Honduras, the Ministry of Health and the Honduran National Society of Obstetrics and Gynecology (SGOH) had worked with Ipas since the mid-1990s to pilot and extend PAC. In response to a 2010 study that revealed how difficulties in acquiring MVA contributed to low rates of MVA use in hospitals, the International Federation of Gynecology and Obstetrics (FIGO) gave the SGOH emergency funding in 2012 to purchase 250 kits that were distributed to twenty-five hospitals. FIGO and Ipas provided additional support for training health workers in MVA. Even after this intervention, however, MVA remained outside regular channels for procuring medical equipment (Chinchilla, Flores, Morales, and de Gil, 2014).

Similar challenges to institutionalizing MVA procurement and utilization have been observed throughout sub-Saharan Africa. In Malawi, MVA was first tested at a large hospital in 1994 and extended to district hospitals by the early 2000s. Recent studies suggest, however, that MVA utilization is declining at government hospitals (Cook et al., 2016; Odland et al., 2014). Following initial donations of MVA by Ipas, the syringe remains outside formal medical supply systems. Once such projects come to an end, a health worker in Malawi observed, "there's no supply of equipment, so it naturally goes to extinction" (Cook et al., 2016, p. 308).

Throughout much of Francophone West Africa, MVA was introduced to and implemented in clinical settings through a variety of strategies that reflect similar anxieties on the part of PAC champions about the device's capacity to terminate pregnancy. NGOs donated MVA material during health worker training conducted from the late 1990s into the early 2000s in Burkina Faso, Guinea, Mali, Niger, and Senegal. In a 2008 review of PAC in the region financed by USAID, the Centre Régionale de Formation, de Recherche, et de Plaidoyer en Santé de la Reproduction (CEFOREP/Regional Center for Training, Research, and Advocacy in Reproductive Health) noted that although all five countries had integrated PAC into national guidelines and protocols for reproductive health care, none had integrated MVA into national medical supply systems. In Niger, for example, the sole syringe in use at the national teaching hospital at the time of the review had been purchased by a midwife during a professional trip to Dakar; she was later reimbursed for the expense. In Burkina Faso, hospitals in the capital city of Ouagadougou purchased MVA from a local distributor of medical supplies. In Guinea, the government placed MVA on the LEM for EmOC, but the device was not available through the national pharmacy system (Dieng, Diadhiou, Diop, and Faye, 2008).

THE "RIGHT TOOL" BUT FOR WHAT "JOB"?

In Senegal, PAC champions included officials in the DSR, demographers from CEFOREP, and personnel from NGOs such as the Population Council, JHPIEGO, EngenderHealth, and MSH. Senior members of the faculty of medicine in the Clinique Gynécologique et Obstétricale (Gynecological and Obstetric Clinic) of CHU Le Dantec played a particularly influential role in the testing, introduction, and extension of PAC because of their national prominence as maternal health scientists. By the early 1990s, some of these scientists were generating epidemiological estimates of the contribution of unsafe abortion to maternal mortality in large hospitals in Dakar and calling for improvements in the treatment of abortion complications on a national scale as a strategy for reducing maternal mortality (CEFOREP, 1998b; F. Diadhiou, Faye, Sangaré, and Diouf, 1995).

In a political context hostile to abortion, however, translating these recommendations beyond the research context posed a significant challenge. "The philosophy of PAC presents problems because of the easy access to abortion," Dr. Ndao, a district health official and early PAC champion, explained to me. "That's a problem in a context where induced abortion is not authorized. It would be an open door to do abortion in this country." At the root of this "problem" was the MVA syringe, a device that could facilitate the clandestine provision of abortion in government hospitals. "That was the danger with implementing MVA," Dr. Ndao said, "because there was just one person who could do everything, and they could do it anywhere. All you needed was a gynecological table and some antiseptic products, Xylocaine, and the syringe to do something else besides PAC."

In Senegal, the perceived "ease" with which MVA could be used to conduct illegal abortions in government hospitals raised troubling questions about the difference—or lack thereof—between PAC and pregnancy termination.[4] According to Dr. Diallo, a physician who worked with a multilateral reproductive health agency, during early conversations between PAC champions and high-ranking MSAS officials, "the Director of Health Services himself" threatened to block the testing of PAC altogether "because the line between using the syringe to treat a difficult abortion and doing an induced abortion is thin." Other PAC champions recalled similar concerns expressed by high-ranking officials about what PAC entailed and how it might facilitate illegal abortion in hospitals. "At the beginning, there was a lot of suspicion," Dr. Mané, a Senegalese physician who worked with a multilateral health organization, told me. "There were really a lot of problems involved with introducing PAC because people thought PAC was services for inducing abortion." The availability of MVA syringes raised the risk of PAC devolving into an abortion free-for-all in government hospitals. According to M. Gueye, a demographer and PAC champion who worked with a reproductive health research NGO, there were concerns that "if we introduce the syringe, c'est fini [that's it], everyone will do abortions!"

Senior gynecologists at CHU Le Dantec took the lead in demonstrating that PAC was *not* equivalent to pregnancy termination and could therefore be integrated into existing obstetric care services in government hospitals. As maternal health experts, these physicians perceived themselves as independent from political interference from the government. "The professors said," M. Gueye told me, "since we're at the university, we're going to do research. The government cannot stop us, so we'll go through the university. That's how it happened." In collaboration with CEFOREP, the Population Council, and JHPIEGO, these physicians conducted a pilot project that introduced PAC to three hospitals in Dakar between 1997 and 1998. "We used operations research as a doorway to advocacy," explained Dr. Dème, one of the investigators and a DSR official, "because if you recall, at the beginning, people confused PAC and the MVA syringe." The operations research project "facilitated" advocacy by placing the stamp of scientific and moral credibility on PAC. Through the conduct of objective scientific research, these champions generated statistical data that showed that using MVA was a safer and more cost-effective form of uterine evacuation than dilation and curettage or digital evacuation, the methods in use at most regional and district hospitals to treat abortion complications. Most importantly, according to Dr. Dème, since the champions could show that the results were yielded from the treatment of complications related to abortions "that had already happened," the MSAS could no longer justify "blockages" of PAC.

Despite the rigorous statistical data on clinical safety and savings in cost and time yielded by these highly pragmatic boundary work strategies, PAC champions could not entirely erase the taint of abortion associated with the intervention. Dr. Mané explained that even with these "concrete results," some health officials did not want to "hear talk of the term post-abortion care." The term does not appear in the title of the findings report that was circulated to MSAS officials and other stakeholders: "Introduction des Soins Obstétricaux d'Urgence et de la Planification Familiale pour les Patientes Présentant des Complications Liées à un Avortement Incomplet" (Introduction of emergency obstetric care and family planning for patients presenting with complications of incomplete abortion) (CEFOREP, 1998a). This careful selection of language to describe PAC services and technologies echoes the PAC experience in Bolivia, where PAC catalyzers described PAC as care for hemorrhage during the first half of pregnancy (Billings et al., 2007), and where physicians have referred to MVA as the "saving women" device (Rance, 2005).

According to Dr. Mané, "to make sure that PAC was accepted" in Senegal, PAC champions pragmatically framed the intervention in terms of two pre-existing maternal health interventions: EmOC and family planning. The government had supported family planning since 1981, when it revised the colonial-era prohibition on contraception and established a population policy as part of the conditions related to structural adjustment loans from the World Bank (Robinson, 2015, 2016, 2017). Starting in the late 1990s, Senegal was one of several testing sites for the introduction of EmOC, a hospital-based intervention designed by AMDD, an NGO based at Columbia University in New York (Paxton, Maine, Freedman, Fry, and Lobis, 2005).

To a certain degree, this strategy worked. In 1998, the MSAS integrated PAC into national norms and protocols for reproductive health. The following year, the MSAS authorized the next phase of operations research to test the feasibility of extending these services beyond Dakar to tertiary hospitals in regional capital cities. With support from UNFPA and JHPIEGO, PAC was introduced to four tertiary hospitals in the regions of Diourbel, St. Louis, Kaolack, and Ziguinchor and a district hospital in the region of Fatick (Dieng et al., 2008). Even with the support of high-level MSAS officials, however, PAC champions remained concerned about how the introduction of MVA to regional facilities would be perceived. According to M. Gueye, the selection of study sites for the extension phase ended up being "a personal affair" rather than a randomly determined process: "We didn't do it systematically. We chose facilities that were headed by reliable people, reliable gynecologists. We said, we know someone in Diourbel who is trustworthy, we know someone trustworthy in Kaolack. That means someone who is not known as someone who does induced abortion, someone who is responsible. There were even facilities in Dakar that we skipped because we didn't trust the people there. If you leave them with the material, who knows what could happen! [*laughter*]."

Others confirmed M. Gueye's description of the selection of study sites for the second phase of PAC pilot research. M. Niasse, a demographer who worked for an international family planning NGO, recalled: "I remember that when we were introducing PAC, it was a big problem. The first people who started to roll out the program were handpicked." Dr. Ndao, who was involved in the very first PAC pilot project in three hospitals in Dakar, described how the moral character of health workers loomed large in the selection of PAC testing sites: "We had to secure MVA and put it in the hands of trustworthy people," he explained. "We said that we will put it in the hands of trustworthy men, men whom we know will not be potential abortionists."

In addition to ensuring the MSAS that pilot sites would be selected with caution (if not randomly), PAC champions used statistical data to demonstrate the need to extend PAC services beyond tertiary regional hospitals to lower levels of the health system. For example, a review of abortion statistics from 1995 found that 68 percent of cases had originated from district hospitals and primary health care facilities (EngenderHealth, 2003). In response, the MSAS authorized a pilot study of PAC, with support from EngenderHealth, at six district hospitals and twelve primary health care clinics in two regions between 2001 and 2003. While MVA training was limited to health workers in district hospitals, health workers in primary health care facilities received training in contraceptive counseling. Between 2003 and 2006, the MSAS worked with MSH to introduce PAC to 23 district hospitals and 300 primary health care clinics in five regions. Nurses in primary health care facilities received training in contraceptive counseling, referral, and digital evacuation (Thiam, Suh, and Moreira, 2006).

A 2008 evaluation of PAC in West Africa, published by CEFOREP and the Population Council, heralded Senegal as a PAC pioneer for its decentralized approach to introducing and scaling up these services (Dieng et al., 2008). Yet, at the time of my fieldwork between 2010 and 2011, over a decade after PAC had been incorporated into national protocols for maternal and reproductive health care, the MVA syringe continued to stoke disagreements among MSAS officials, NGO personnel, and health workers. MVA was neither on the LEM nor part of the Pharmacie Nationale d'Approvisionnement (PNA/National Pharmacy Supply). Additionally, the MSAS decided that the decentralization of MVA would not extend beyond its use by physicians and midwives in district hospitals. Midwives and nurses in primary health care facilities were not allowed to use the device. In what follows, I explain why the MSAS made these decisions and describe the impact of national MVA policies and informal MVA practices in hospitals on the provision and quality of PAC in regional, district, and primary health care facilities.

PROCURING MVA: AN "INCOHERENT" SYSTEM

During the piloting phase, Ipas donated MVA kits to newly trained providers. As the MSAS began to decentralize MVA from regional to district hospitals, the DSR desired a more sustainable approach to ensuring a national MVA supply given its exclusion from the PNA. One possibility included working with a private distributor of medical equipment to make MVA available to authorized health centers. Although PAC champions in Burkina Faso opted for this solution, their Senegalese counterparts were leery of this approach. "I wasn't comfortable with that," Dr. Dème explained, "because it meant that anybody could go and buy an MVA kit. We had to figure out how to make the supply system more secure."

Starting in 2006, the DSR identified a large referral hospital in the region of Dakar as the focal point for the procurement and distribution of MVA. The hospital had served as a study site for several PAC pilot projects, and its head gynecologist was a highly respected member of the medical community and a PAC champion. The hospital purchased MVA kits directly from Ipas. Health facilities that wished to purchase the device had to submit an order, pay for it up front in cash at the DSR headquarters in Dakar, and then travel to the hospital to pick it up. Problems soon arose as administrators at other health facilities began to complain about a lack of transparency in the process, arguing that the hospital was inflating the price (between 25,000 and 28,000 CFA francs, or $57 and $65 in 2008) to make a profit (Population Council, 2007).

By the time I began my fieldwork in 2010, the DSR had tasked CEFOREP with the procurement and distribution of MVA. The process, however, remained similar. Hospitals had to receive approval from DSR officials before they could purchase and pick up the syringe at CEFOREP headquarters in Dakar. Various PAC stakeholders, including MSAS officials and NGO and donor personnel, expressed dissatisfaction with this approach. "People have to go all the way to Dakar to buy the syringe," complained Mme Ngom, a regional reproductive health coordinator in the first study region. "The circuit is too long. Normally it should be available through the regional pharmacy." The burdensome process of having to travel all the way to Dakar to renew MVA kits led to the overuse of these devices in health facilities. While the average life span of the MVA syringe is between twenty-five and fifty procedures, with careful maintenance it can be used up to one hundred times (Hudgins and Abernathy, 2008). "Sometimes it's difficult to renew the syringes," Mme Mbow, who worked for an international health NGO, said. "When we go on supervision visits we see there are syringes with broken nozzles. . . . The supply system causes some problems." M. Gueye expressed similar concerns about the impact of the current distribution system on the quality of care. "It blocks the system," he said. "It pushes facilities to overuse the syringes, to use them beyond the authorized time period. You can see how that creates other problems that have to be resolved."

Beyond the potential to push syringes beyond their shelf life, PAC stakeholders pointed to the incongruence between the MVA procurement system and the fundamental goals of the PAC program to reduce maternal mortality. The centralized nature of this system, and its isolation from the PNA, lacked sustainability and created unnecessary barriers to access for patients and health professionals. "You can't want something and its opposite," argued Mme Sankharé, a midwife and DSR official. "This system, that requires people to go to CEFOREP, hinders accessibility. The MVA should be in the PNA, and that's that—it will be more accessible to people if it's integrated into the regular distribution system." M. Gueye pointed out that MVA was the only medical commodity with procurement protocols requiring health workers to travel all the way to Dakar. "It simply isn't sustainable," he said. "Health workers should be able to get it at the PNA, which has branches all over the country."

Dr. Gomis, a pharmacist who worked with an international health NGO, questioned the logic of the distribution system. As with the selection of study facilities for early PAC research, he suggested that the current procurement system was based on the personal preferences of influential PAC champions. "I wouldn't even say it's the choice of the DSR," he said. "It's the choice of one person, and that's Dr. X,[5] nothing else. It makes no sense. It's not necessary for the head doctor of a district to go all the way to Dakar and pay 30,000 CFA for an MVA kit." Dr. Sabaly, who worked with a bilateral donor agency, also found fault with the logic of the distribution system. "The system is too centralized, it's parallel to the regular system," he explained. "There is much more dangerous equipment that's part of the regular circulation system than MVA. When a doctor wants opium, he can get it because it's authorized." For Mme Sankharé, the system made little sense because it did nothing to stop the practice of clandestine abortion: "People who want to do illegal abortions will continue to do illegal abortions."

While stakeholders acknowledged the "sensitivity" of the material, they believed that solutions could be found to supervise its distribution through the PNA. "The PNA can still monitor the purchases and ensure that there are clear criteria for use," said Mme Sankharé. Dr. Sabaly agreed, and described a system in which the head physician of a region would give authorization to procure MVA from the PNA. "It doesn't have to be like aspirin," he joked, "but it can still be monitored!"

Even the head of the DSR, Dr. Ndiaye, expressed a great deal of frustration with the current distribution system, calling it "quite incoherent." He disliked having to validate MVA purchases for health workers before they picked up the material at CEFOREP headquarters. "It has nothing to do with me," he said. "It's a way for CEFOREP to manage the problem, to cover themselves with the institution of the DSR." Dr. Ndiaye found this practice unnecessary, arguing that as health professionals, CEFOREP staff had the expertise to manage the process without the involvement of the DSR. Additionally, he disagreed with the restriction of MVA to public providers, saying it made no sense "to create barriers" for the private sector when "modalities" could be established to grant access to private practitioners. "It's a question of individual responsibility," he argued, echoing Mme Sankharé's belief that MVA restrictions would not stop clandestine abortion practices.

As the head of the DSR, Dr. Ndiaye interfaced directly with representatives from donors such as UNFPA and USAID. Consequently, he was keenly aware of the constraints they faced in supporting PAC due to USAID's anti-abortion policies. For example, he described how he had asked UNFPA to incorporate donations of MVA into their annual safe motherhood plan of action. "Now, with the constraints the Americans put on them with respect to abortion," he said, referring to policies like the 1985 Kemp Kasten Amendment,[6] "I don't know." Dr. Ndiaye criticized USAID, suggesting that it made little sense for USAID to "support" PAC without assisting in the procurement of the technology. "In reality, they say they support the policies of the country," he said, "but when you supply MVA, you are in fact an actor with respect to abortion, and they don't want to go that far. They have to protect their own interests." Here, Dr. Ndiaye highlighted the Helms Amendment, still in place under the Obama administration despite the suspension of both the Mexico City Policy and the Kemp-Kasten Amendment at the time of my fieldwork in 2011.

"IN THE HANDS OF TRUSTWORTHY MEN"

In addition to isolating MVA from the regular distribution system of the PNA, the MSAS limited use of the device to physicians and midwives in regional and district hospitals. Midwives and nurses who worked in primary health care facilities were not allowed to use MVA. Instead, they were required to either refer women eligible for MVA to the nearest hospital or perform digital evacuation.

Some PAC stakeholders suggested that the restriction of MVA to regional and district hospitals was due to the limited technical environment of primary health care facilities. Specifically, these facilities frequently lacked the ultrasound machines and electric-powered autoclaves that are used in many district and regional hospitals to establish the state of the fetus, to determine the contents and shape of the uterus, and to sterilize MVA material. Since the decentralization of health decision-making from the MSAS to local health committees as part of the government's adoption of the 1987 Bamako Initiative, primary health care facilities often faced shortages of basic services like water and electricity (Foley, 2009). "We work without means," M. Sall, a head nurse from a primary health care facility located in the second region of study, said. "Our only means come from the health committees, or the revenue from the sale of medication and services. We pay for our own electricity—as a state facility!—our own water, and our own telephone." Under these circumstances, ultrasound machines and electric auto-claves were rarely found in primary health care facilities, leaving health workers limited in their capacity to follow PAC protocols.

Most of the health professionals I interviewed, however, believed that the MSAS's restrictions on MVA were ultimately grounded in concerns that the device would be misused at primary health care facilities. More specifically, they believed that MSAS officials were concerned that nurses, the supervisory clinical officers at these facilities (many of whom are men), would use the device to practice illegal abortion as a lucrative side business. "The Ministry didn't have a problem with the material in the hands of midwives," Dr. Diallo said. "It was when we wanted to extend further into the health system and involve the nurses in rural health clinics that we ran into difficulties with the Director of Health Services.... He trusted midwives but not nurses." Nurses could not be trusted *not* to use the material for "something else besides PAC."

Many of the health professionals I interviewed believed that MVA abuse was more likely at primary health care facilities precisely because they were located at the periphery of the health system and irregularly supervised by MSAS authori-ties. They felt strongly that nurses would be unable to resist the temptation to use MVA to practice safe, albeit illegal, abortion. "People will pay up to 300 or 400,000 CFA for an abortion," Dr. Diallo said. "That's twice the monthly salary of a nurse. If you put that material in his hands, he will use it to earn money." Dr. Sarr at l'Hôpital de Ville agreed that nurses could not be trusted with the syringe: "In the primary health care facility, the provider is alone. I don't want to say that I doubt their morality, but if you see the conditions in the districts . . . Sometimes they offer you enormous amounts of money. If you can't resist money you run the risk of doing illegal abortion. With MVA, it's so simple." Dr. Sylla, a gynecologist from l'Hôpital Médina, was more blunt in her evaluation of the likelihood of MVA being misused at primary health care facilities. "The nurses at primary health care facilities are men, and they are more likely than midwives to use the material to induce abortion," she said. "It's just my personal opinion."

While Dr. Sylla framed her assessment as a personal opinion, scholars of medi-cine have understood physicians' discourses about the immorality of midlevel and paramedical providers as a tactical form of professional boundary work. Physicians have questioned not only the technical skill but also the moral apti-tude of competing practitioners as a way of securing professional authority over healing technologies and techniques. In their efforts to protect professional jurisdiction, physicians have questioned the morality of *both* male and female providers. For example, American physicians portrayed midwives, and those from Black and immigrant communities in particular, as physically and morally unfit to supervise childbirth (Fraser, 1995; Wertz and Wertz, 2019). They conjured up images of incompetent, greedy male "abortionists" who would exploit desperate women to pressure state governments to grant them exclusive monopolies over the practice of therapeutic abortion (Joffe, 1996; Reagan, 1998). In postcolonial Uganda, physicians portrayed unscrupulous "traditional needle men" as a public health threat and urged health authorities to criminalize the sale of medication by unskilled practitioners (Iliffe, 1998).

Repeated narratives about the untrustworthiness of male nurses offer little concrete evidence that male nurses are more likely than any other health worker to conduct illegal abortions with MVA. They do, however, illustrate physicians' perceived lack of control over midlevel providers at peripheral levels of the health system. M. Sall highlighted how these perceptions of nurses served as a "cover story," a way of articulating things that cannot be said (Briggs, 2000; Lubiano, 1992), when he dismissed them as "fears that are based on nothing at all." Nurses at primary health care facilities observed the same professional ethics as physicians and were well aware that the law prohibits abortion. "There is no reason to fear that paramedical personnel will use MVA to practice induced abortion," M. Sall argued. "One could just as well do illegal abortions without the material." M. Badji, a nurse at a primary health care facility I visited with Child Fund community outreach workers in the second study region, similarly disagreed with stereotypes of male nurses as potential *avorteurs* (abortionists). He highlighted similarities in the accomplishment of clinical tasks between nurses and midwives as a way of questioning the MSAS's rationale in restricting the device from nurses. "Nurses," M. Badji told me, "are really *sage-femmes* [midwives]. We do deliveries all the time. We do everything: prenatal care, postnatal care, and childhood vaccinations. We are *hommes sage-femmes* [male midwives]."

By framing the moral failings of male nurses as a "fact," physicians are able to keep MVA technology under their supervision at regional and district hospitals, even when the device is frequently used by midwives in the daily practice of PAC at these facilities. For MSAS officials, this "fact" offers a convenient rationale for withholding MVA from peripheral levels of the health system. Put differently, the untrustworthiness of male nurses glosses over the institutional forms of disinvestment that limit the technical environment of primary health care facilities regardless of MVA, despite the fact that nurses regularly practice reproductive health care. It is precisely this failure to invest that motivated nurses like M. Sall to participate in the *rétention des données*, or data strike, that was taking place during my fieldwork, in which unionized health workers limited the provision of services and withheld data from the MSAS (Foley, 2009; Tichenor, 2016). "We work with great difficulty, and it saps our morale," M. Sall said. Some nurses, discouraged by working conditions and inadequate pay, simply "gave up" and went into the private sector or "emigrated to Europe." Others, like himself, "often went on strike" to demand improvements in working conditions. For nurses like

M. Sall, being able to provide basic health services, much less conducting illegal abortions with MVA, was challenging enough.

A DEVICE INSIDE/OUTSIDE OF PRACTICE

Gaps between global PAC protocols and MSAS policies extended into hospitals where supervisory health workers developed informal practices to manage the procurement, circulation, and utilization of MVA. My fieldwork at three hospitals illustrates how MSAS policies and informal practices at hospitals, designed to prevent the misuse of MVA, have limited its utilization despite its designation by the global PAC model as a preferred PAC technology. Taken together, these national policies and informal practices have profoundly compromised women's access to high-quality, affordable obstetric care throughout the health system.

By no means is the isolation of MVA from standard medical supply systems a situation unique to Senegal. Similar problems have been documented in countries with even longer periods of PAC programming than Senegal. In Malawi, for example, where PAC was piloted as early as 1994, declines in MVA were observed as dilation and curettage was on the rise (Cook et al., 2016; Odland et al., 2014). Declines in MVA use have also been documented in some hospitals in Honduras despite an injection of syringes into the health system with the support of FIGO and Ipas (Chinchilla et al., 2014). In Uganda, shortages of MVA material encouraged health workers to use dilation and curettage to treat abortion complications (Paul et al., 2014).

My review of PAC data from annual reports at three hospitals, illustrated in figure 2.2, revealed that the percentage of cases treated with MVA increased over time, whereas the use of dilation and curettage declined or disappeared altogether. At l'Hôpital Senghor, I did not find any cases of dilation and curettage in the PAC registers in the maternity ward or in the annual reports of obstetric care I obtained from the administration. At l'Hôpital Médina, dilation and curettage disappeared entirely, whereas at l'Hôpital de Ville, the practice declined but remained in use for a small percentage of cases. Dr. Fall and Mme Sène, supervisors at l'Hôpital de Ville, explained that dilation and curettage continued to be practiced because the facility served as a training site for physicians. At all three hospitals, however, digital evacuation (practiced by midwives) continued to account for a significant percentage of cases. While difficulties in procuring new MVA kits and resulting shortages in the material have contributed to the persistence of dilation and curettage in some hospitals in Malawi, Honduras, and Uganda, my fieldwork suggests that Senegalese health workers have turned to digital evacuation when unable to practice EVA or MVA.

In the remainder of this chapter, I show how digital evacuation persists while MVA, despite accounting for the greatest percentage of cases, is not used by

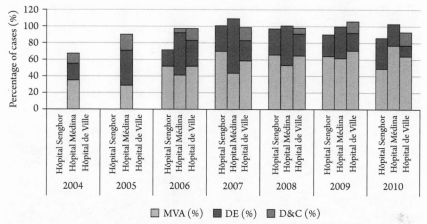

FIGURE 2.2. Percentage of PAC cases treated with MVA, digital evacuation (DE), and dilation and curettage (D&C) at three hospitals, 2004–2010. L'Hôpital Senghor routinely referred to and recorded EVA as MVA. At l'Hôpital Senghor and l'Hôpital de Ville, I was unable to retrieve PAC data between 2004 and 2005. Percentages exceeding 100 may be due to incomplete data on the number of abortions treated at the hospital. At l'Hôpital de Ville, starting in 2009, misoprostol was used as a PAC method, but these data are not displayed in this graph.

health workers as frequently as it could be. I argue that digital evacuation, a method that is not recognized by WHO as a safe technique of abortion care, remains part of the PAC tool kit as health workers endeavor to provide obstetric care while abiding by national policies on MVA training, authorization, and procurement and hospital-specific MVA policies. I juxtapose these practices alongside PAC and MVA practices in other countries to highlight how restrictive abortion laws constrain women's access to the high-quality care envisioned by the global PAC model.

At l'Hôpital Senghor, midwives practiced uterine aspiration around the clock. Although they recorded the procedure as MVA in the PAC register, they practiced EVA by attaching MVA cannulas to an electric aspirator in the maternity ward (Suh, 2015). Midwives complained vigorously about the state of the aspiration material. The cannulas were often broken or went missing "during sterilization." The aspirator itself, according to Mme Gassama, "often didn't work." Faced with shortages of or inadequate material, midwives likely used digital evacuation to treat some patients, even those eligible for uterine aspiration, to reduce their patient caseload. Although Mme Koulibaly, the midwife responsible for monitoring and evaluation, explained that the hospital renewed its MVA supply once or twice a year, the process of renewal itself revealed MVA's isolation from the PNA. For example, Mme Coly described how she was once asked to pick up a kit while on a personal trip to Dakar. Her experience is not unlike the midwife from

FIGURE 2.3. MVA kit at l'Hôpital Médina.

Niger who reportedly picked up a kit while on a professional trip to Dakar (Dieng et al., 2008).

Facility-specific restrictions on the circulation of MVA contributed to the overuse of MVA syringes and the persistence of digital evacuation at l'Hôpital Médina, where MVA was offered around the clock. Although Dr. Sylla, the head gynecologist at l'Hôpital Médina, showed me several MVA kits in her office cabinet that she had received as donations from the MSAS, she permitted only one kit to be circulated among several shifts of midwives in the maternity ward because "the material shouldn't be available to everyone." The midwives at l'Hôpital Médina complained bitterly about having to share one MVA kit, displayed in figure 2.3, arguing that it compromised the management and quality of the syringe. Mme Diop, the head midwife, believed that each midwife should have her own MVA kit and be responsible for sterilizing the material. "Now, there's just one kit in circulation. What is the condition of the material in that box?" she mused.

Another midwife, Mme Sakho, showed me how she placed vitamin E oil on the syringe to facilitate the movement of the plunger in and out of the barrel. Medical tape was wrapped around the head of the syringe to keep it in place. "We just have to make do," she told me. "It often doesn't work." The considerably high rates of digital evacuation at l'Hôpital Médina, as well as at l'Hôpital Senghor, suggest that midwives fell back on digital evacuation when the MVA syringe was being sterilized or was not working. Similarly, in Uganda, health workers observed that a lack of MVA equipment led to "overuse of the equipment and questionable safety of the procedure" (Paul et al., 2014, p. 6).

Locking up the MVA syringe to prevent abuse or—in the words of Mme Sène, the head midwife at l'Hôpital de Ville—to keep the syringe "secure" was not uncommon. Mme Koulibaly, the midwife responsible for monitoring and evaluation in the maternity ward at l'Hôpital Senghor, showed me an extra MVA kit and accompanying cannulas in her office cabinet. Included in her stash were old and broken cannulas. "It's not good to throw away old or broken material," she explained. "People can always use them for other purposes." Similarly, Mme Sow, the nursing assistant in charge of the MVA room at l'Hôpital de Ville, kept a supply of MVA syringes locked in a cabinet to which only she had the key. An evaluation of PAC by the Population Council conducted in 2007 found that in some facilities, MVA syringes were kept under lock and key to prevent abuse. Similar practices have been documented in Gabon (Ndembi et al., 2019) and Malawi (Cook et al., 2016). In addition to contributing to delays in care and the overuse of syringes in circulation, these practices may incentivize health workers to abandon MVA altogether and opt for practicing dilation and curettage or digital evacuation.

Other factors can lead to the displacement of MVA as a preferred PAC technology. A study in Pakistan showed that physicians in a public hospital perceived MVA as more expensive than dilation and curettage because the material requires replacement more frequently. Although MVA is more cost-effective for patients and hospitals in the long run, this logic resulted in a greater percentage of patients being treated with dilation and curettage than MVA and misoprostol combined (Zaidi et al., 2014). In Uganda, some health workers preferred dilation and curettage over MVA because the former can be used beyond the first trimester of pregnancy. Like their Pakistani counterparts, they expressed concerns about timely replacement of MVA material that was permanently damaged during sterilization (Kagaha and Manderson, 2020). In both contexts, health workers' perceptions of cost and effectiveness influenced decision-making about the technologies used to treat PAC patients.

Among the three hospitals where I observed PAC, l'Hôpital de Ville was the only one that restricted MVA services to weekdays from morning until late afternoon. Women who arrived at night on weekdays or during the weekend would be treated with dilation and curettage or EVA in the operating block or digital evacuation in the delivery room. During my fieldwork at this hospital, I had the opportunity to interview Dr. Ndao, the gynecologist who had enacted this policy in the early days of PAC at the facility. Dr. Ndao explained that the policy was designed to prevent the abuse of MVA during the night shift when senior gynecologists were not at the hospital. Describing the night shift as "uncontrolled," he argued that unsupervised interns could take the syringe into some "corner" of the hospital to practice illegal abortion. Dr. Ndao's primary concern was the security of the device, even if the strategies designed to prevent abuse subjected women to less effective and, in the case of dilation and curettage, more costly methods.

L'Hôpital de Ville differed from l'Hôpital Senghor and l'Hôpital Médina in its distribution of PAC tasks. Whereas midwives at l'Hôpital Senghor and l'Hôpital Médina treated most PAC cases, physicians at l'Hôpital de Ville treated the vast majority of PAC cases. My review of PAC registers at l'Hôpital de Ville, displayed in table 2.1, shows that in 2009 and 2010, physicians treated approximately 73 percent and 78 percent, respectively, of PAC cases.

Dr. Fall and Mme Sène, the senior gynecologist and midwife, respectively, at l'Hôpital de Ville, explained that the distribution of PAC tasks reflected the hospital's status as a training facility for physicians. Mme Sène added that midwives had their hands full "with the burden of work" in the delivery room and that "many" doctors were available to practice MVA. Some midwives, however, suggested that the distribution of PAC labor reflected concerns that midwives would abuse the syringe by practicing illegal abortion. Mme Ndir recalled that the former head gynecologist had said as much during a visit to the delivery room. "He said there were some midwives he trusted, and others he didn't." She disagreed with this position, saying, "I think he could have created a space in the delivery room to do MVA, so that if someone is doing it, everyone can see and it wouldn't be possible to use MVA clandestinely." What Mme Ndir described was

TABLE 2.1.   Treatment of PAC cases by type of provider at l'Hôpital de Ville, 2009–2010

Provider	2009		2010	
	N	%	N	%
Doctor	1,072	73.1	848	77.6
Midwife	241	16.4	179	16.4
Joint	23	1.6	4	0.3
No information on type of provider	131	8.9	60	5.4
Total PAC cases treated	1,467		1,091	

a designated MVA room or area. This space already existed at l'Hôpital de Ville and was managed by a nurse's assistant, Mme Sow, but only physicians were permitted to use the device here.

The absence of task shifting, coupled with a lack of MVA training among midwives,[7] further contributed to the persistence of dilation and curettage and digital evacuation and delays in care at l'Hôpital de Ville. "Many of the midwives in the delivery room are not trained in MVA," explained Mme Sène, the head midwife. The senior gynecologist, Dr. Fall, believed that women's access to MVA would be enhanced through a greater number of trained midwives. Although he told me that he planned to conduct on-site training with midwives, my fieldwork at this site ended before these activities began.

Despite these human resources limitations, women who arrived at l'Hôpital de Ville at night or on weekends still received treatment, even if this entailed dilation and curettage in the operating block (a small percentage of women were also treated with EVA here) or digital evacuation by a midwife in the delivery room. Ironically, delays in care at l'Hôpital de Ville occurred *during* authorized MVA hours, when doctors had multiple MVA procedures to conduct during a limited time period. "If we have eight patients for MVA, we may have to send one away, or tell her to come back the next day," explained Mme Mbodji, a midwife at l'Hôpital de Ville. Alternatively, depending on the dilation of her cervix, the patient may be treated with digital evacuation by midwives in the delivery room.

Three of the midwives I interviewed provided PAC at primary health care facilities in the first and second study regions. Two of them, Mme Kouyaté and Mme Diongue, had been trained in MVA but were prohibited from using the device while stationed at their facilities. All three complained about having to refer patients eligible for MVA to the nearest hospital. This policy led to delays in care and forced patients and their families to incur additional transportation costs. Mme Camara, a midwife and district health official in the second study region, explained that referrals discouraged women from seeking care: "They won't come because they don't have the means to travel." Furthermore, if informed that they have to travel all the way to the district or regional hospital, said Mme Camara, women "may wait two or three days before going, and that's plenty of time to become infected." The delays in care related to referrals, and the additional costs posed on patients and their families, greatly alarmed Mme Diongue, a midwife at a primary health care facility in the second study region. "This is an area that's very far away from the city, where people are very poor," she said. "Women come to the health facility in a state of emergency, without any money."

The midwives' observations are supported by a recent study estimating that up to 41 percent of low-income rural women and 32 percent of low-income urban women with abortion complications, for whom primary health care facilities are often the first point of contact with the health system, do not receive medical treatment (Sedgh, Sylla, Philbin, Keogh, and Ndiaye, 2015). A recent survey of primary health care facilities found that only 50 percent had a vehicle to transport women with complications to a referral hospital, and even fewer (30%) had the means to communicate with another referral facility (Owolabi, Biddlecom, and Whitehead, 2019). In addition to incurring transportation costs, women referred from primary health care facilities to the three study hospitals faced a good chance of encountering delays in care or being treated with digital evacuation precisely because of the facility-specific restrictions on MVA described above. Similar delays in care related to referrals have been observed in Kenya, where women may be sent to an advanced facility for an ultrasound before returning to the facility where they first sought care for MVA (Mutua et al., 2018).

MVA, PAC, AND OBSTETRIC VIOLENCE

A recent survey of PAC in ten developing countries found significant gaps in health systems' capacity to provide these services. In seven out of ten countries, less than 10 percent of primary health care facilities could provide basic PAC, which includes uterine evacuation, the provision of antibiotics, and referral. In eight out of ten countries, less than 40 percent of referral facilities could provide comprehensive PAC, which includes surgery (Owolabi et al., 2019). These gaps translate into poor quality of care for women patients, who must often wait for hours with inadequate pain medication or antibiotics. While low-quality care may be related to health system problems such as inadequate task shifting, an absence of providers trained in MVA, or stockouts in equipment or medication, it also represents a specific form of obstetric violence: neglectful or abusive treatment of women with complications of confirmed or suspected induced abortion. In Kenya, some PAC patients lose consciousness before they receive care (Mutua et al., 2018). At the Komfo Anokye Teaching Hospital in Kumasi, Ghana, an estimated 50 percent of PAC patients do not receive pain medication, even when requested (Tagoe-Darko, 2013). Midwives in Uganda observed some of their colleagues deliberately delaying care or withholding pain medication from women they suspected had illegally procured abortions (Cleeve, Nalwadda, Zadik, Sterner, and Allvin, 2019). In contexts with high levels of abortion stigma, such punitive treatment serves to separate "good" mothers who have experienced miscarriage from "bad" women who have procured abortions (Suh, 2014, 2018). Put differently, abortion stigma frequently translates into obstetric violence against PAC patients.

The following fieldwork observation from l'Hôpital Médina illuminates how obstetric violence is inextricably bound up with PAC, even when MVA is available, providers are trained, and patients are not necessarily suspected of illegal abortion. On a warm morning in May 2011, there was a lull in the three-bed delivery room. A woman who had just given birth watched anxiously as the midwife's assistant weighed her baby. The woman who prepared meals in the hospital cafeteria had dropped by the maternity ward to ask Mme Bâ, the midwife on call who had delivered her baby several weeks ago, to give her an exam. A young woman sat in the chair by Mme Bâ's desk right outside the delivery room, also waiting to be examined.

As the woman from the cafeteria climbed onto the examination bed, Mme Bâ teased her about how quickly she had become pregnant. I walked out of the delivery room and saw that the woman who had been waiting by the desk had slumped onto the floor, her skirt soaked with blood, her eyes rolled toward the back of her head. Immediately, I called Mme Bâ, who rushed out of the delivery room and, with the help of one of the hospital guards, lay the patient on the floor. As Mme Sidibé, a nurse, inserted an IV into the woman's arm, the assistant midwife removed the woman's skirt and conducted a vaginal exam with the guard lingering in the doorway. Mme Sidibé explained that the woman was experiencing *"une menace d'avortement"* (threat of abortion) and was in shock because she had lost a great deal of blood. Her cervix was open, and they would use MVA right away to treat the emergency.

A few minutes later, the guard had disappeared, so I helped the midwife's assistant and the nurse lift the woman and slowly walk her to a bed in the delivery room while Mme Bâ assembled the MVA syringe. The MVA procedure lasted about ten minutes, after which Mme Bâ took apart the syringe and explained that the woman was probably about two months along. "See how MVA saves lives?" she said to me. "Imagine what would have happened if I wasn't here. All the patients come here for MVA, from all the twenty-five health posts in the district."

Although this patient survived, her experience highlights multiple instances of obstetric violence. First, she experienced a delay in care, after having been referred from a primary health care facility and incurring the costs of transportation. This delay in treatment did not occur because Mme Bâ was tending to other patients who had arrived and been triaged earlier, but because she was examining a friend who had dropped by the maternity ward. Yannick Jaffré, a medical anthropologist who has studied maternal and infant health care throughout West Africa, describes how such delays are generated through the "relational ethics" of maternity care, in which "quality of care is exercised according to social ties between patient and provider, rather than standard norms and uniform skills" (Jaffré and Suh, 2016, p. 180). In this set of relationships, and against a backdrop of limited resources, "where one can't do everything for everyone, everything is done for a chosen few and nothing for others. Parents, friends, and acquaintances have priority, then the affluent who may be expected to pay and last of all everyone else" (p. 180). Not only did this patient have to enter into a state of shock to receive attention from Mme Bâ, but her vaginal exam, normally conducted in the delivery room, was conducted in an open room in the maternity ward with a male guard looking on. In a context where women value discretion in matters of pregnancy, delivery, and abortion (Foley 2007; Jaffré and de Sardan, 2003), such violations of modesty may contribute to women's reluctance to seek care at government hospitals. Although this woman was treated with MVA, her comfort, safety, dignity, and privacy received little priority in clinical efforts undertaken to ensure her survival.

CONCLUSION

Capable of accomplishing multiple "jobs," MVA has long troubled the boundaries between legitimate and illegitimate obstetric care. Within global and national regimes of reproductive governance, MVA has at once been an efficient abortifacient capable of carrying out the fertility reduction goals of population control, a feminist tool designed and used by women to achieve reproductive autonomy, and a safer, less costly method than dilation and curettage for conducting PAC in developing countries. PAC stakeholders in Senegal, like their counterparts in Bolivia, Burkina Faso, Guatemala, Honduras, Malawi, Mali, Mexico, and Niger, have worked carefully to establish MVA as the "right tool" for the legitimate "job" of PAC through carefully designed operations research and MVA procurement systems, along with restrictions regarding who can use the device, and where.

Efforts to prevent MVA abuse have limited health workers' capacity to effectively use the device as part of routine obstetric practice. In facilities authorized to use MVA, dilation and curettage and digital evacuation techniques persist, despite the risks of perforation and infection associated with these methods, because of shortages in human resources, inadequate supplies of MVA material, and informal policies designed to keep the device secure. Health workers in primary health care facilities, even if trained in MVA, must practice digital evacuation or refer PAC patients to regional and district hospitals. After referral, those eligible for MVA may wait hours or days to receive this care, or end up being treated with dilation and curettage or digital evacuation anyway. Local stories of MVA reveal how the broader landscape of obstetric care, including the U.S. Helms Amendment, the national prohibition on abortion, interprofessional politics, and limited health system resources, threatens MVA's celebrated identity as "the right tool for the job" of PAC.

That both national MVA policies and informal practices at hospitals have subordinated the quality of care for women—timely access to safe, effective, affordable, and functional uterine evacuation techniques—to the maintaining of the security of the device illustrates how MVA straddles the boundaries not only between legitimate and illegitimate abortion care but also between obstetric care and violence. These imbrications of violence and care occur at the intersection of global accords on reproductive rights that omit safe abortion and U.S. funding policies that champion MVA as a safe PAC technology while refusing to pay for it because the device is an abortifacient. While this chapter shows how delays in or withholding MVA enacts obstetric violence against women, the next illustrates how the application of MVA and other PAC techniques unfolds within a medico-legal context that significantly limits health workers' capacity to provide confidential, nondiscriminatory care. The provision of PAC and the application of its technologies raise troubling questions about the rights-based treatment ethic of this intervention and the extent to which it can be conceived as a form of harm reduction.

3 · "WE WEAR WHITE COATS, NOT UNIFORMS"

Abortion Surveillance in Hospitals

Over lunch in the cafeteria at l'Hôpital Médina one afternoon, M. Dia, the head nurse, repeated what many of his colleagues had already told me: most of the PAC cases they treated were related to miscarriage. Indeed, the preponderance of cases of spontaneous abortion that I noted in my review of the hospital's PAC records confirmed this claim. For example, over the course of twenty-four months between 2009 and 2010, health workers documented only three cases of induced abortion. M. Dia insisted that health workers did not care about the kind of abortion the patient had experienced. "We are not the police," he told me. "It's not up to us to manage delinquents. Our main concern is health. It's up to the criminal justice authorities to see if it's a case of induced abortion. When the patient comes, we have to treat her, and the rest is not our problem. We wear white coats, not uniforms."

This distinction between health workers and police officers, between the medical and legal management of abortion, echoes the treatment ethic of the global PAC model, in which the type of abortion experienced by the patient should not influence the health professional (Corbett and Turner, 2003; Curtis, 2007; Greenslade, McKay, Wolf, and McLaurin, 1994), whose duty is to offer high-quality, lifesaving obstetric care regardless of the legal status of abortion. Yet, my observations of PAC at l'Hôpital Senghor, l'Hôpital Médina, and l'Hôpital de Ville reveal profound contradictions between the global ethics of PAC treatment and the daily realities of obstetric care, in which health providers, because of the threat of police investigation into illegal abortion at the hospital, are *extremely* concerned about the kind of abortion the patient has experienced. Furthermore, suspected or confirmed cases of induced abortion may pass through the hospital more frequently than officially documented in the PAC register. Treating abortion complications thus requires navigating between competing sets of obligations, including professional duties to provide nondiscriminatory treatment, protect patient confidentiality, and cooperate with law enforcement authorities in the investigation of illegal abortion.

In this chapter, I argue that rather than being a mundane obstetric procedure, PAC entails a constellation of clinical, discursive, and textual practices in which potentially "delinquent" women are transformed into mothers deserving of quality obstetric care. This transformation occurs through a contradictory process in which health workers rigorously search their patients' bodies and behavior for signs of illegal abortion and then obscure suspected cases of abortion as miscarriage in the hospital record. Through this process of seeing, speaking, and writing the body (Atkinson, 1995; Good, 1994), health workers assemble a "reproductive subject" (Morgan and Roberts, 2012): an expectant mother who experienced the loss of a presumably desired pregnancy. Institutional records reinforce this identity by classifying most PAC patients as cases of miscarriage. The underlying claim is that the clinical management of such patients is unworthy of police scrutiny, thereby allowing health workers to maintain control over what happens in the gynecological ward.

Sociologists have described the steps taken by professions to protect their jurisdictional turf as "boundary work" that may involve obtaining legal monopolies over certain techniques and technologies (Gieryn, 1983) or expanding professional authority over tasks previously considered the jurisdiction of other occupations (Halpern, 1990). This work, however, also occurs through everyday practices at the job. Examples from the medical field include physicians' interpersonal and institutional subordination of practitioners of complementary and alternative medicine (Mizrachi, Shuval, and Gross, 2005), nurses' attempts to distinguish their tasks from those of auxiliary support workers (Allen, 2000), and pharmacists' regulation of patient access to controlled substances (Chiarello, 2013).

This chapter tells a story of jurisdictional skirmishes over abortion between medical providers and law enforcement authorities in Senegal. But that struggle is only part of the story. Health workers' boundary work over abortion also constitutes a broader set of processes and accountabilities (Sullivan, 2017) of global reproductive governance between national health and law enforcement authorities, international NGOs, and donors of health and development aid. I argue that it is precisely through health workers' daily practices of patient interviews, vaginal exams, ultrasounds, and record keeping that PAC patients become legible—"known" (Geissler, 2013), or recognized—within and beyond the hospital as expectant mothers. Medical providers deploy a particular ideal of motherhood as an interpretive lens through which they assess the likelihood that a patient procured an illegal abortion. Clinical abortion classification schemes mirror idealized notions of motherhood in which "normal" women welcome pregnancy even when it is unplanned or occurs beyond the boundaries of marriage (Kumar, Hessini, and Mitchell, 2009). Medical workers can thus reclassify even suspicious cases as instances of spontaneous abortion to create a sanitized, uncontroversial account of PAC that legitimates their work from the perspectives of law enforcement officials, national health authorities, and international NGOs and donor agencies.

DISCIPLINING WOMEN IN THE GYNECOLOGICAL WARD

Reproductive health care has long been recognized as a terrain, in both global North and South contexts, for the reinforcement of gender, class, race, and ethnic inequalities between women and health professionals. Medical workers assess women's capacity for motherhood according to their compliance with instructions for behavior during pregnancy and delivery (Davis-Floyd and Sargent, 1997). In the United States, women who refuse surgical interventions, and in particular low-income women and women of color, are perceived as unfit for motherhood. If their behavior during pregnancy and delivery is deemed harmful to the fetus, women may be subjected to arrest and imprisonment (Daniels, 2009; Paltrow and Flavin, 2013; Roberts, 1997). Anthropologists Dána-Ain Davis (2018, 2019) and Khiara Bridges (2011) remind us that regardless of socioeconomic status, obstetric racism places pregnant and birthing Black women in the United States at risk of neglectful, disrespectful, punitive treatment that may result in poor maternal and infant health outcomes.

In hospitals throughout sub-Saharan Africa, where midlevel providers like midwives often provide the bulk of reproductive health care (Berer, 2009), health workers enforce classed and gendered expectations of motherhood in a variety of ways. Midwives verbally abuse low-income pregnant women who arrive at the hospital without a personal supply of bed sheets and sanitary pads (Geurts, 2001; Jewkes, Abrahams, and Mvo, 1998). Women who express reluctance about using family planning, who wish to observe traditional practices during pregnancy and delivery, whose births are deemed to be inappropriately spaced, or who delay seeking antenatal care because they do not wish to reveal their pregnancy status may also be treated poorly by health workers (Beninguisse and De Brouwere, 2004; Chapman, 2006; Eades, Brace, Osei, and LaGuardia, 1993; Gilson, Alilio, and Heggenhougen, 1994; Maimbolwa, Yamba, Diwan, and Ransjö-Arvidson, 2003). Midwives may scold women who are perceived as too old or too young to be having children (Jaffré and Prual, 1994). Health workers may discourage women from vocally expressing pain during labor as silence during this time is perceived as a marker of appropriate and chaste motherhood. Women who express or demand relief from pain are perceived as overly entitled and may be subjected to sexualized insults such as "You liked it all right when it was time to give, so don't shout now" (d'Oliveira, Diniz, and Schraiber, 2002, p. 1682). During my observations at the three study hospitals, birthing women who cried or groaned too loudly were frequently instructed—gently or curtly—by midwives and other health workers to be quiet.

Sometimes, midwives punish women physically for inappropriate behavior. At a hospital in Niger, a midwife, frustrated by the duration of labor for a young primigravida, instructed her assistants to conduct an episiotomy and use forceps: "It's these lazy women who refuse to push. They like pleasure but not suffering. Tear her and use forceps as necessary" (Jaffré and de Sardan, 2003, p. 137). During a night shift at l'Hôpital Senghor, I observed a patient who was similarly punished for not submitting to the "suffering" of labor and delivery. The patient was on a delivery bed, crying loudly while surrounded by midwives and nurses. One of the nurses, when I asked her what was happening when she momentarily stepped away from the bedside, told me that the woman "didn't want to suffer, but you have to suffer to give birth." One of the senior midwives sternly instructed the woman to lie flat so she could examine her. Although she eventually complied, she continued to move around on the bed. Frustrated, the midwife smacked her legs and roughly pushed them apart. The woman, still moaning and crying, continued to writhe around on the bed. Infuriated, the midwife raised her voice in anger, lunging at the woman as if to strike her. Her colleagues stepped in immediately and pulled her away from the patient. Several moments later, the woman was surrounded by five or six health workers, pressing on her abdomen. The woman's head hung over the edge of the bed as she screamed in agony. Whether health workers disciplined women verbally or physically, their expectations of women's behavior during delivery reveal a great deal about the hospital as a site where the boundaries of appropriate femininity and motherhood are actively enforced.

Health workers' expectations of illness behavior reflect the power relations between patient and provider that characterize what sociologist Talcott Parsons called "the sick role." In return for treatment, and exemption from their regular responsibilities owing to their illness status, patients are supposed to comply with medical professionals' instructions (Parsons, 1951; Segall, 1976). The power differential is also evident in the ability of the provider to define, and possibly discredit, the patient's experience with and understanding of illness (Goffman, 1963). But providers' perceptions suggest a more neoliberal power dynamic is also at work here, in which patients themselves have a moral responsibility to monitor and optimize their own health through the timely seeking of biomedical health care (Clarke, Shim, Mamo, Fosket, and Fishman, 2003). In addition to eating nutritious food, sleeping under treated mosquito nets, and refraining from heavy labor that might increase the risk of miscarriage, women must comply with scheduled appointments for prenatal care and other services. During a night shift at l'Hôpital Senghor, I observed Dr. Ly scold a woman for arriving after her scheduled appointment for a cesarean section. She had arrived with her family members late at night and was extremely weak. As several hospital attendants carried her on a stretcher upstairs to the operating theater, Dr. Ly continued to yell at her about her "lack of discipline" and threatened to make her walk up the stairs.

In the United States, medical providers discipline women according to norms regarding the desirability of motherhood not only during pregnancy and delivery but also in events related to spontaneous and induced abortion. They may question a woman's fitness for motherhood if she fails to appropriately demonstrate grief over fetal loss (Fordyce, 2014). Physicians reinforce motherhood when they privilege medically indicated abortions over elective procedures or when they demonstrate more empathy to women who appear emotionally distressed about having an abortion (Kimport, Weitz, and Freedman, 2016). Even in places with very liberal abortion laws, like the Netherlands, women are expected to show a certain level of contrition during the abortion procedure (Løkeland, 2004).

When high fertility is socially desirable and induced abortion is legally restricted, a different calculus of women's fitness for motherhood becomes necessary. My observation of PAC at l'Hôpital Senghor, l'Hôpital Médina, and l'Hôpital de Ville suggests that health workers draw on gendered expectations of the linkages among women's sexuality, fertility, and marriage to assess the likelihood that patients have illegally terminated pregnancy. In Senegal, motherhood within marriage is an "obligatory" and highly respected social role for women. As heads of household, men are also obligated and take pride in their ability to provide financially for their dependents (Hernández-Carretero, 2015). Women are expected to wait until marriage to begin sexual relations and to demonstrate their fertility by becoming pregnant shortly thereafter (Foley, 2007). In 2017, women's median age at first marriage was 20 and 21.8 at first birth. The TFR is 4.6 children born per woman, with higher fertility rates among rural women (5.9) than urban women (3.4) (ANSD and ICF, 2018). Although men and women may have different expectations of family size (Bankole, 1995), the concept of an "unwanted" pregnancy within marriage falls beyond the boundaries of appropriate femininity, in which motherhood is a natural, desirable, and inevitable outcome of sexuality (Kumar et al., 2009). In 2017, Senegalese women's ideal number of children was 5.7, and 76 percent of women in union wanted another child (ANSD and ICF, 2018). In contexts where polygamy remains common, high parity is often the most logical reproductive strategy for women to maintain financial security (Foley, 2007). In 2017, 32 percent of Senegalese women reported being in a polygamous union (ANSD and ICF, 2018). The social significance of children as gendered markers of normal adulthood and forms of belonging in kinship networks and gift-giving collectivities promotes high fertility within marriage (Foley, 2007). In places where the state inadequately contributes to forms of social security for the elderly, children represent a crucial investment in the future (Dodoo and Frost, 2008).

Within this calculus of gendered expectations regarding sexuality, fertility, and kinship, the most plausible explanation for the presence of a married woman with abortion complications at the hospital becomes the miscarriage of a presumably desired pregnancy. Unmarried women with complications of abortion threaten to unravel the gendered logics binding women's sexuality and fertility to marriage. Some scholars argue that abortion may be *less* shameful than pregnancy outside marriage because it permits, even if risks to the woman's health are involved, a certain masking of inappropriate sexual relations that may yield children outside of or before marriage (Bleek, 1981; Johnson-Hanks, 2002b; Rossier, 2007). Knowledge of patients' marital status, therefore, is a critical component of health workers' surveillance over women's sexuality and reproduction in Senegalese hospitals.

ENCOUNTERING ILLEGAL ABORTION IN THE HOSPITAL

Despite the criminalization of abortion in the penal code, illegal abortion appeared in government hospitals in a variety of ways. Several midwives told me that women frequently approached them with requests for abortion, some even claiming that they received such requests at the hospital *presque tous les jours!"* [nearly every day!]. During an interview in the delivery room at l'Hôpital de Ville with Mme Dieng, a midwife, I observed one such request. A young woman approached Mme Dieng and quietly told her she was pregnant but could not have the child. She asked the midwife if she could "help her." Mme Dieng replied that she was not permitted by law to perform induced abortion but could provide her with prenatal care and family planning services following delivery. Although some providers indicated that they threatened to denounce such women to the police, others said they discouraged women from seeking abortion by explaining the risks of clandestine and unsafe procedures performed by avorteurs.

More regularly, health workers encountered patients with complications of possible or probable illegal abortion. When treating such cases, health workers found themselves in a precarious professional situation that required negotiating frequently contradictory sets of obligations and expectations. Despite jurisdictional claims over PAC as a set of clinical obstetric tasks, few professional guidelines existed for the legal and administrative management of suspected or confirmed cases of illegal abortion. Furthermore, law enforcement authorities expected health providers to cooperate with investigations of illegal abortion in a variety of ways, including notifying the police of patients who have had illegal abortions, cooperating with requisitions for medical information, and testifying during formal prosecutions of illegal abortion. The daily practice of PAC required navigating a significant gap between the treatment ethic of this global reproductive health intervention and the legal context of obstetric care. In turn, health workers' decisions held profound implications not only for the quality of obstetric care but also for the circumstances under which women became subject to investigation, arrest, and prosecution for illegal abortion.

Among the thirty-seven health workers I interviewed, only a third believed that abortion should be permitted in cases of rape or fetal malformation, or if the pregnancy threatened the health or life of the pregnant woman. Not a single provider was in favor of legal abortion upon request, and most described abortion provision as a morally and professionally discrediting practice. Many expressed concern that a relaxed abortion law would encourage "debauchery" among women (few mentioned men) who would now be free to have sexual relations without consequences. Despite their disapproval of abortion, health workers unanimously perceived PAC as an important public health intervention that effectively saved women's lives, especially with the decentralization of MVA to district hospitals. Mme Bâ, a midwife at l'Hôpital Médina, explained proudly, "Now women can come here for treatment and leave thirty minutes later." In Uganda, midwives expressed similar ambivalence toward liberalizing the abortion law at the same time that they strongly supported and took pride in their ability to provide PAC (Cleeve, Nalwadda, Zadik, Sterner, and Allvin, 2019).

Health workers insisted that the legal context of abortion influenced neither their perception of PAC nor the manner in which they delivered services. They located PAC within the continuum of professional maternal health care duties, no different from practicing prenatal care, delivering babies, and prescribing contraceptives. Dr. Sarr at l'Hôpital de Ville explained that while Senegalese society may frown on abortion, treating complications was somewhat of a "banal," everyday affair for health workers because they were "often confronted with these cases." Nevertheless, health providers were quick to distinguish their role in managing abortion complications from that of law enforcement officials. Police officers actively investigated the possibility that an illegal abortion had occurred. In contrast, health workers understood themselves as technical experts who treated patients regardless of the type of abortion (spontaneous or induced). "Even if the patient had an induced abortion," Mme Kanté, a midwife in a district hospital in the first study region, explained, "it's not my problem. The obligation of a midwife is to care for the patient."

Various professional and legal frameworks require health workers to respect the patient's right to confidential medical care. In 2005, the National Assembly passed a reproductive health law that entitles all patients, regardless of gender, age, or marital status, to confidential reproductive health care. Article 7 of the national professional code of medical ethics requires providers to maintain patient confidentiality. Although the national penal code prohibits the practice of abortion, it does not obligate medical providers who treat complications of induced abortion to notify law enforcement officials.

Many of the health workers I interviewed believed that alerting the police was stressful, wasteful of limited human resources, and beyond the purview of their medical duties. Dr. Sarr at l'Hôpital de Ville complained that "denouncing" women to the police siphoned away time and resources from treating patients. For him, interrogating a patient about her social and sexual life was "on the margins of medicine." During my fieldwork at l'Hôpital Médina, Mme Diop, the head midwife, revealed that she was serving as an expert witness in a case of illegal abortion under prosecution at the regional tribunal. The police had requisitioned her to examine a woman who was suspected of having procured an illegal abortion at a private clinic. Going back and forth between the hospital and the courthouse in the regional capital not only disrupted her work but also incurred transportation costs, which she paid out of pocket. Instead of reporting an illegal abortion to the police, Mme Diop said, it was preferable to "manage" the case at the hospital by treating and subsequently releasing the woman.

Some health workers articulated a public health rationale for treating complications without notifying the police. Dr. Diatta, the head gynecologist at l'Hôpital Senghor, indicated that reporting cases to the police would discourage other women from seeking care for abortion complications at the hospital. For him, reporting women not only violated the professional obligation to respect confidentiality, but in the long run also deterred health workers from exercising their primary responsibility, which was "simply to treat."

In practice, however, health workers confronted a number of challenges in protecting their patients' confidentiality as they treated abortion complications. While national norms and protocols for reproductive health care offered technical guidelines for managing abortion complications, they did not explain how to handle confirmed or suspected cases of illegal abortion. District, regional, and national health officials assured me that MVA training seminars (almost always organized and financed by international NGOs) instructed health workers on how to handle such cases. Not all health workers in government hospitals who practice MVA have participated in these trainings: among the twenty-three midwives I interviewed, over half had received uterine evacuation training in school or on the job. Reporting confirmed or suspected cases of induced abortion to the police was ultimately a matter of discretion for individual health workers. Women bore the brunt of this lack of professional guidance as medical providers determined whether they would leave the hospital of their own free will or in police custody.

The greatest challenge to observing the ethic of the global PAC model and national regulations on confidential medical treatment was the lingering threat of police involvement at the hospital. Although the national penal code does not require health workers to notify the police when they encounter suspected or confirmed cases of induced abortion, law enforcement officials often expected them to do so. Among the four police officials I interviewed in the region of Dakar, all believed that medical providers were legally obligated to report such cases and that failure to do so might be interpreted as a form of complicity that could result in legal proceedings.[1] At the same time, police officials did not rely solely on health workers' formal reports in their investigations of illegal abortion, but also followed up on anonymous tips from individuals working in the hospital, as well as from the neighbors, family members, and acquaintances of suspected women. "We have many sources of information," M. Kane, an official from a police station in the Médina neighborhood of Dakar, assured me. "Our own sources, the police, and other people. We have our ways of getting information. We are very well informed. If I'm investigating a case, I'll get to know all the important people in the neighborhood—the Imam, for example, or the neighborhood delegate."

To illustrate the utility of these multiple "sources," M. Kane described a case where he had "heard" about a divorced woman who became pregnant but had illegally procured an abortion. He approached the neighborhood delegate, told him he was looking "for such and such woman," and asked if he could tell him where she lived. With this information, he went to her house in an unmarked car, "so as not to be conspicuous," and waited for her. When she arrived, he told her who he was and why he was there and asked her if she would come to the police station with him. He said that it was her choice: "She could either come with me discreetly or she could make a scene and then everyone would know why I was there." The woman went to the police station with him, at which point he asked her about the abortion. "She denied it," according to M. Kane, "saying that she had not been pregnant." Determined to resolve the situation, he requisitioned a doctor to examine her. The doctor pronounced that the woman had not been pregnant and therefore could not have aborted. M. Kane, however, remained suspicious because during a subsequent interrogation, the woman "had stains on her shirt in front of her breasts as if she were breastfeeding." My research assistant and I watched uncomfortably as M. Kane animatedly demonstrated how he had asked the woman to "pinch" her breasts to determine if she was lactating. As a final measure, he requisitioned another doctor to examine the woman, and asked him to "push the interrogation." This time, the doctor reported that the woman had been pregnant, allowing M. Kane to move forward with an arrest.

Police officials may take the initiative to investigate a case without waiting for formal notification from health workers or tip-offs from civilians. "Sometimes," explained Mme Diousse, an official from a police station in the Bel Air neighborhood of Dakar, "I pursue the case myself, without being notified by family members or health providers. If I hear rumors, I may just go ahead and send a requisition to the hospital."

Under these circumstances, some health professionals felt pressured to report cases of induced abortion and to comply with police investigations lest they be viewed as accomplices. Over a span of two months, between September and October 2011, the press reported three cases in which medical providers notified the police of women with complications of illegal abortion at the hospital ("Avorte-ment," 2011; Diedhiou, 2011a, 2011b). One of these cases, published on Septem-ber 22, 2011, in *L'Observateur*, involved a nineteen-year-old woman, Penda Seck, who had been "locked up" two days earlier for illegal abortion. The article reported that a gynecologist at l'Hôpital Roi Baudouin in Dakar had alerted the police of a young woman being treated at the facility for severe bleeding after a two-month absence of menstruation. After two days of observation, the hospital ambulance transported Penda to the police station, where she admitted that she had, with the help of her boyfriend, procured an abortion from a nurse at a hospital in the region of Louga ("Avortement," 2011).

On April 26, 2012, *L'Observateur* reported the case of a young woman, N. Kanté, who had been evacuated to a hospital in the region of Tambacounda. Kanté had developed complications after ingesting pills that she had received from a *guéris-seur* (healer), who claimed they would bring on her monthly period. The physi-cian and the midwife who first encountered the patient at the regional hospital contacted the police. After receiving treatment, N. Kanté was taken to the police station, where she admitted to having procured an illegal abortion. She was sub-sequently sentenced to three months in prison (Diallo, 2012).

Police reports from cases of illegal abortion prosecuted by the regional tribu-nal of Dakar offer further insight into what happens when some women receive PAC in public hospitals. At 11:37 P.M. on March 17, 2009, the physician on call at a district hospital called the police to notify them of a young woman who had been evacuated to his facility with complications of abortion. The police imme-diately went to the hospital to interrogate the nineteen-year-old patient, Mlle (abbreviation of Mademoiselle) Diedhiou, who admitted to swallowing several pills of Spasfon[2] to commit suicide after learning she was pregnant. The police came to the hospital, interrogated the patient, and the next day escorted her to another health facility to conduct a sonogram to obtain more conclusive evi-dence of induced abortion. After conducting the sonogram, the second hospital issued a certificate, displayed in figure 3.1, that confirmed the patient was preg-nant and had attempted to induce abortion. The certificate offers no details regard-ing the length of gestation, the state of the woman's uterus, or the viability of the fetus. Although the woman was arrested and prosecuted, this lack of precision may have contributed to the court's subsequent decision to acquit her.

At l'Hôpital Senghor, l'Hôpital Médina, and l'Hôpital de Ville, health workers described a chain of responsibility with respect to contacting the police. Midwives in the delivery ward brought suspicious cases to the attention of the senior gynecologist, who made the final decision regarding whether to notify the police. Providers who worked in primary health care facilities explained that they referred suspect cases to the hospitals. Only l'Hôpital de Ville, however, appeared to actively alert the police in cases where the woman admitted to procuring an abortion. This

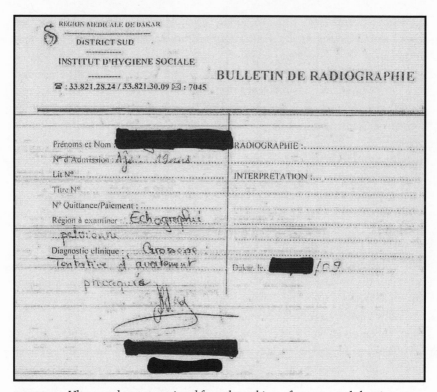

FIGURE 3.1. Ultrasound report, retrieved from the archives of a prosecuted abortion case, confirming the defendant had "attempted abortion."

was the only facility where I observed a file of medical certificates that were transmitted to the police as confirmation that an induced abortion had occurred. "We do the medical certificate when there's absolutely no doubt," Dr. Fall, the head gynecologist at l'Hôpital de Ville, explained as he showed me the file. "I won't take risks. I'm not obligated to send if there's suspicion, but not evidence. But if there's evidence, I will send. I have to protect myself."

During my fieldwork at l'Hôpital de Ville, Mme Diarsso, a member of l'AJS, told me about a young woman currently in police custody after being treated at Dr. Fall's facility. When I followed up on the case with Dr. Fall, he showed me the medical certificate he had prepared and sent to the police on May 11, 2011. The case involved a fourteen-year-old girl who had arrived at the hospital with a catheter in her vagina and admitted to procuring an abortion. "Even in cases with such a young girl," said Dr. Fall, "I must write the report. Even if it's due to rape, and I get a lot of rape cases. On days when I have to write these reports, I don't feel well at all. But I can't risk my reputation because of clandestine abortion. It's a real professional dilemma." On May 25, 2011, a newspaper reported that the girl admitted to procuring an illegal abortion after being raped (Bâ, 2011). According to Mme Diarrso, she would face charges, and possibly imprisonment, given that the law does not permit induced abortion in the case of rape.

One explanation for the vigilance over induced abortion observed at l'Hôpital de Ville may be its status as one of the first facilities in the country to provide PAC at a time when senior health officials were still arguing about the difference between PAC and induced abortion. For a while, this facility also served as the national distribution point for MVA syringes. With heightened national scrutiny over PAC practices at this hospital, medical professionals may have experienced a greater incentive to play by the rules (even though the penal code does not require health providers to report cases of abortion). Almost all of the health professionals interviewed at this hospital believed that failure to notify the police might result in charges of complicity in an illegal abortion. Still, as I will explain later in this chapter, health workers at this facility did not systematically bring suspected cases of illegal abortion to the attention of senior gynecologists. Even in a facility that appeared more likely to notify the police, women suspected of illegal abortion were often quietly treated and eventually discharged.

At all three hospitals, the possibility of anonymous tips pressured even those providers who wished to protect their patients' confidentiality into reporting. Mme Camara, a district health official and a midwife in the second study region, described how tip-offs could implicate providers in the criminal prosecution of illegal abortion:

> As long as it stays at the level of the health center, it's not a problem. We don't call the police. We say nothing to the police. But the police can be called by a third person who knows the victim and who knew that this woman was pregnant and who knows that she had an induced abortion. And then this person informs the police. When the police do an investigation, they can come to the maternity ward. There can be problems when the health provider is implicated, when she wrote that she consulted the patient and that she did not see an induced abortion. In these situations, when there's a legal proceeding, they'll call the provider.

Not only did these tips raise the possibility that the health provider had been complicit in an illegal act, but also that she or he was incompetent. Dr. Ndao, a district health official and gynecologist in the third study region, explained:

> I am not obligated to report, but I will never protect someone else before I protect myself. There have been cases where people in the neighborhood went to the police and said this girl had an induced abortion. The police investigate the case and find out she was treated at my hospital. They ask me, "Doctor, what do you think of this girl?" And I say I didn't know it was an induced abortion? What does

it say about my credibility as an obstetrician-gynecologist? It's all well and good to say you shouldn't report such cases, but there are things that happen to you that make you feel smaller than . . . you just want to crawl under the table.

The looming threat of police involvement meant that health workers remained vigilant in identifying suspected cases of illegal abortion. Providers attempted to protect themselves by knowing, or at least by being able to demonstrate that they attempted to learn, the type of abortion, should the police inquire into a case of suspected induced abortion at the hospital. Mme Tall, a midwife at l'Hôpital Senghor, described a situation in which her colleagues were summoned to the police station in an ongoing investigation of a suspected case of illegal abortion. "They asked them questions," she said, shaking her head. "Finally, they saw it was a case of spontaneous abortion. The patient does not always tell you. You always have to know what you're doing, otherwise you're not covered. You have to do complete exams and in-depth interrogations. It's also better to do the ultrasound."

SEEKING ILLEGAL ABORTION IN THE HOSPITAL

It is within this context of uncertainty—about the kind of abortion being treated and the extent to which the police may become involved—that the subject of the expectant mother emerged. Contrary to health workers' claims that their primary responsibility was to treat patients, they were extremely concerned about the kind of abortion the patient had experienced because of the possibility of police intervention at the hospital. Consequently, health workers deployed the interrogation, the clinical exam, and the ultrasound to search women's bodies and behavior for markers of inappropriate sexuality that would signal illegal abortion. They interpreted these markers according to gendered expectations regarding the relationships among marriage, familial obligations, sexuality, fertility, and health-seeking behavior. For most health providers, the typical PAC patient was a married woman suffering complications of miscarriage of a presumably desired pregnancy. Suspicion of induced abortion emerged as health workers perceived that a patient's body and behavior did not align with what they would anticipate of a married, expectant mother.

Medical providers looked for physiological signs of abortion through the vaginal exam and, if the patient was stable, the ultrasound. The vaginal exam, conducted with a speculum, allowed providers to view the cervix and search for tears or foreign objects. With the ultrasound, they evaluated the size, shape, and contents of the uterus and tried to establish gestational age. If providers discerned any incongruence between ultrasound data and the patient's account of her last menstrual period, they could become suspicious that she illegally procured an abortion. Mme Ndour, a midwife at l'Hôpital Senghor, explained the importance of the ultrasound: "Women will never tell you what they did, or they'll tell you 'I didn't see my period in four months.' Meanwhile, the pregnancy is four months if you see the ultrasound."

Providers paid attention to advanced gestational age because unsafe abortions at later stages of pregnancy frequently result in complications. While an estimated 20 percent of pregnancies end in spontaneous abortion, most miscarriages occur before twelve weeks of gestation and less than 4 percent occur during the second trimester of pregnancy (Curtis, 2007; Farquharson, Jauniaux, and Exalto, 2005; Kalumbi, Farquharson, and Quenby, 2005). In places with restrictive abortion laws, teenagers and low-income women are more likely to pursue later-term abortion because of barriers in accessing safe first-trimester abortion. Nearly 60 percent of unsafe abortions in Africa occur among women under twenty-five years of age (Warriner and Shah, 2006). In Ghana, most life-threatening abortion complications result from unsafe abortions performed after the first trimester of pregnancy (Payne et al., 2013).

At the same time, health workers recognized the challenges of identifying induced abortions during earlier stages of pregnancy. "Especially in the first trimester," explained Mme Dieng, a midwife at l'Hôpital de Ville, "it may be harder to detect an induced abortion if a woman uses a method like drinking a décoction that doesn't leave traces or traumatize the cervix."

Although physiological markers offered strong evidence of illegal abortion, simpler clues often first elicited health workers' suspicions. These markers could be perceived quite soon after the woman arrived at the facility, and did not require the technological assistance of the speculum and the ultrasound. During l'interrogation, health workers sought physiological information such as the date of the last menstrual period and the duration, intensity, and sequence of symptoms such as bleeding and abdominal pain. Additionally, this process established a sociodemographic profile by requiring patients to reveal their age, number of pregnancies, deliveries, and living children, marital status, occupation, and residence. Health workers observed women's behavior and social interactions over the course of their treatment, including time of arrival, cooperation with health workers, and the extent to which they received care from accompanying relatives. Perceptions of the woman's emotional reaction to the interruption of pregnancy were also important. These were the clues, having little to do with the physiological state or biomedical treatment of the woman's body, that initially raised health workers' suspicions that she might have experienced something other than a miscarriage, and prompted them to seek additional information. Commonly known as "pushing the interrogation," these techniques began at the moment of triage and continued throughout the course of treatment.

Mme Mbaye, the head midwife at l'Hôpital Senghor, explained that pushing the interrogation sometimes involved detaining women at the hospital: "We don't let them leave. If they don't tell us when they first come in, we wait until the next day and then we push the interrogation further." Sometimes health workers detained women at the hospital in case the police became involved. "We keep the woman under observation for seventy-two hours," said Mme Mbaye, "because someone could notify the police. Maybe someone knows she had an induced abortion, and could notify the police. We don't want to lose her." Mlle Touré, a midwife at l'Hôpital de Ville, emphasized the importance of keeping an eye on suspected patients: "Until the problem is resolved, we can't let her escape. She needs to be watched." Although providers spoke of "keeping" women at the hospital in such cases, their capacity to detain women was somewhat limited. Providers may have watched suspected women more carefully, but they did not hold them captive. Once a woman recovered from treatment and settled her bill, she could leave the hospital.

Some health workers explained that they threatened to withhold care from women until they explained the circumstances of the abortion. Mme Sidibé, a nurse at l'Hôpital Médina, explained: "The midwives may tell the woman they won't treat her until she admits to what she did. When there's pain, women will talk." While I did not observe any health workers engaging in this form of obstetric violence against women suspected of abortion, these threats directly contradict the treatment ethic of the global PAC model, which calls on providers to treat all patients regardless of abortion type.[3]

Although all Senegalese citizens are entitled to reproductive health care, many people, including health professionals, believed these services were most appropriate for married women who desire or already have children (Foley, 2007). Consequently, single women nearly always caused health workers to think about the possibility of illegal abortion. "If it's a single woman," Mlle Touré at l'Hôpital de Ville explained to me, "rest assured that the interrogation will be more intense, because we think it may be an induced abortion." Women who appeared to be beyond the sexual control of men—through divorce, widowhood, or because their husbands lived and worked in other countries—raised health providers' suspicions of abortion. At l'Hôpital de Ville, Dr. Sarr explained to me that in the district where he previously worked, women with husbands abroad "frequently" requested health workers to terminate pregnancies from extramarital relationships. Such women, according to Mme Mbaye at l'Hôpital Senghor, sought abortion to avoid the possibility of divorce. "Even for married women," she said, "we ask if the husband is there." Although marriage to men who migrate for work is becoming an increasingly attractive option for women within a broader context of economic instability (Hannaford and Foley, 2015), the sexuality of unsupervised women may be perceived as suspicious (Hannaford, 2014). Similar anxieties around married women with absent husbands have been documented in a study of unsafe abortion in Malawi, where men frequently migrate to neighboring countries for work (Levandowski et al., 2012).

Despite the importance of marital status in providing insight into the possibility that a patient had procured an illegal abortion, health workers could not always identify whether a woman was single, cohabiting, married, widowed, or divorced. Providers thus relied on other characteristics to determine marital ties. Women who arrived at the hospital alone, whether or not they self-identified as married, immediately raised suspicion. Family members frequently accompanied women to the hospital for various forms of obstetric care and paid for treatment and medication. In situations where women required hospitalization for obstetric complications, family members cared for them by bringing meals, changes of clothing, and clean bedsheets. The family's investment in the woman's health, and their efforts to prevent such "reproductive mishaps" (Bledsoe, Banja, and Hill, 1998) from reoccurring, signaled the embeddedness of her fertility within a network of conjugal and kinship relationships. Providers perceived women who lacked sufficient food or appeared disheveled to be without familial support, and therefore more likely to have attempted abortion.

For example, one morning, while I was observing Dr. Thiam treat a patient in the MVA room at l'Hôpital de Ville, he mentioned that there was a woman in the recovery room of the maternity ward whom the midwives suspected of induced abortion. Later that afternoon, after obtaining permission from Mme Sène, the head midwife, my assistant and I examined the woman's file. She had arrived four days earlier, was twenty-one years old, and self-identified as married with two children. An ultrasound conducted the same day suggested an incomplete abortion had occurred. Although she was treated shortly thereafter, the physician on call, Dr. Nahm, instructed midwives to "re-orient the interrogation" because there were "no accompanying individuals on the premises."

Health workers scrutinized the patient's time of arrival to the facility. They believed that women who arrived very late at night or early in the morning were more likely to have experienced an illegal abortion. Arrival outside of regular consultation hours was interpreted as an attempt to seek discretion when the hospital was less crowded with staff members and possibly even family members, neighbors, and other acquaintances. Health workers believed women who arrived during such hours without family members were even more likely to have had an illegal abortion. During an early-morning staff meeting at l'Hôpital Senghor, Dr. Diatta instructed midwives to re-interrogate a single, eighteen-year-old woman who had arrived alone earlier that morning with complications of abortion. For each of the remaining abortion cases discussed during the meeting, he inquired about the patient's time of arrival.

Patients who offered "incoherent" details regarding their abortion raised suspicion among providers. The description of symptoms such as the chronology of bleeding or pain, as well as the patient's report of her response to these symptoms, had to make sense to health workers. Midwives explained that in cases of induced abortion, pain frequently preceded bleeding. In contrast, they found that women with spontaneous abortion usually first experienced bleeding and then pain. When patients reported a symptom narrative that did not line up with this symptomology, or who seemed confused, anxious, or uncooperative, health workers began to suspect the patient had procured an illegal abortion. "Women who have had a miscarriage," explained Mme Ndour at l'Hôpital Senghor, "are more cooperative and at ease than the others. They have nothing to hide." In contrast, she said, "those with induced abortions are more difficult to manage. They know what they've done is illegal."

Women sometimes demonstrated multiple markers of suspicion. At l'Hôpital Senghor, Dr. Diatta asked midwives to re-interrogate a woman who had arrived the night before with complications of abortion. The woman was in her early thirties, was unmarried, and had an eleven-year-old child. She had arrived without family members. She reported bleeding after taking a décoction. Mme Ndour, the midwife who conducted the interrogation, laughed skeptically as she told me the woman reported taking the décoction to "clean her stomach because she was feeling ill." Although the woman told the midwives she did not know she was pregnant, they believed the results of the ultrasound procedure—which revealed the presence of an inanimate fetus with an estimated gestational age of seventeen weeks—offered strong evidence that she had procured an illegal abortion.

Pushing the interrogation included making inquiries into women's occupational and socioeconomic status. Providers believed students were particularly likely to procure clandestine abortions to remain in school. Mme Coly, a midwife at l'Hôpital Senghor, explained that "we ask the woman's profession because often these students will do anything to terminate an unwanted pregnancy." Dr. Sarr at l'Hôpital de Ville spoke to me about a case involving a woman who self-identified as a student pursuing a master's degree. He later questioned his decision to release the patient after treatment. "That girl," he mused, "shouldn't I have interrogated her a bit more? She's a master's student, and she's pregnant." Here, the intersection of the patient's youth, singlehood, and student status led Dr. Sarr to suspect she had illegally procured an abortion.

Providers viewed women who had difficulty paying for treatment and medication with suspicion. They were particularly suspicious of low-income, unmarried patients, as such women were thought to be likely to terminate unwanted pregnancies they could not care for without the support of a husband and extended family members. At l'Hôpital de Ville, Mme Sène, the head midwife, described a patient who had been accompanied to the gynecological unit by the facility's social worker. The woman was in a "very difficult social situation" and therefore unable to pay for services. She was divorced and admitted to being pregnant outside of marriage, although it was unclear whether the man who impregnated her was her ex-husband or another individual. She and her five children lived with her parents. She had hidden the pregnancy from her parents because she was reluctant to "burden them further." Immediately suspicious, Mme Sène insisted on interrogating the patient personally.

Health workers closely observed women's emotional affect during PAC, expecting displays of sadness and regret over pregnancy loss. Such emotions were thought to be a natural response to the miscarriage of a presumably desired pregnancy, even for unmarried patients who normally would be suspected of induced abortion. At l'Hôpital de Ville, Mme Mbengue, a midwife, interrogated a young woman with abortion complications who self-identified as single. While she initially believed that the woman may have had an illegal abortion, Mme Mbengue later told me that the patient was so distraught—"Did you not see her crying in the delivery room?"—that it was more likely that she had experienced a miscarriage. The absence of "flagrant" signs of induced abortion further strengthened her belief that the patient had miscarried. Although Dr. Sarr at l'Hôpital de Ville was skeptical of the student's story, the sadness she expressed over pregnancy loss, as well as her willingness to identify the man who impregnated her, convinced him that this was indeed a case of miscarriage.

Through these processes of interrogation and surveillance, health workers sorted women into two possible categories: expectant mothers with complications of miscarriage, and suspect women who had likely procured an illegal abortion. Assignment into either category depended on the extent to which providers' interpretation of women's symptoms, narratives, and family situations aligned with normative expectations that bind women's sexuality to procreation within marriage. Patients with complications of miscarriage were usually married and lived with their husbands. They arrived at the hospital during regular consultation hours and were accompanied by immediate or extended family members, who were responsible for the cost of treatment and medication. Normal PAC patients cooperated with questioning and treatment and articulated coherent descriptions of symptoms and care-seeking practices.

Medical providers' expectations did not always align with the conjugal, reproductive, and health care realities of Senegalese women. An estimated 32 percent of Senegalese women in union are in polygamous marriages (ANSD and ICF, 2018) and may not always live in the same household as their husbands (Duffy-Tumasz, 2009; Hannaford and Foley, 2015). Whether or not they live with their husbands' in-laws, women married to migrant men may not see their husbands for years at a time (Hannaford, 2014; Hannaford and Foley, 2015). Multiple factors influence when and how women reach the hospital, including availability and cost of transportation, influence of family members in care-seeking decisions, and the actual onset and acknowledgment of symptoms such as bleeding, pain, or fever. Women may also seek care from a variety of informal practitioners before coming to health facilities (CEFOREP, 1998b). Differences in age, ethnicity, and socioeconomic status between women and health professionals may limit women's willingness to disclose sensitive information during consultation and treatment (Jaffré and Prual, 1994). Additionally, the desirability of pregnancy for married women may shift over time and in relation to changes in their status throughout the course of marriage (Bledsoe, 2002).

Remarkably, being insufficiently attached to a husband did not immediately assign women to the category of suspected induced abortion. Unmarried women who fulfilled other expectations of typical PAC patienthood, such as complying with instructions, arriving at the hospital during the daytime, or receiving family support, could be assigned to the category of miscarriage. The same was true for unmarried women who displayed an appropriate emotional response to pregnancy loss. While some women may risk clandestine abortion rather than carry a premarital pregnancy to term, unwed motherhood is not entirely unprecedented in Senegalese communities. On average, one in five pregnancies in sub-Saharan Africa occurs before marriage (Garenne and Zwang, 2006). In Senegal, 15 percent of births among women aged fifteen to thirty-five occur before the woman's first marriage (Guilbert and Marazyan, 2013). In the capital city of Dakar, premarital births increased from 8 percent to 23 percent for women born between 1942 and 1956 and those born between 1967 and 1976 (Adjamagbo, Antoine, and Delaunay, 2004). Health workers, thus, were not entirely unaccustomed to encountering unwed mothers, and exercised considerable flexibility in their interpretation of bodily and behavioral markers to determine abortion type. The presumption of expectant motherhood, even for unmarried women, facilitated health providers' capacity to categorize suspected cases of induced abortion as miscarriage. In the next section, I describe how this process of renaming abortion unfolded.

DISGUISING INDUCED ABORTION IN THE HOSPITAL

In 2009 and 2010, health workers documented eleven and seven cases of induced abortion, respectively, in the PAC registers at the three study hospitals. Table 3.1 shows that at each hospital, nearly all PAC cases were identified as cases of spontaneous abortion or miscarriage.

If health workers actively sought out cases of induced abortion, why did so few cases appear in hospital records? During formal interviews and informal conversations, most health workers indicated that miscarriage accounted for the bulk of their PAC caseload. Yet, epidemiological studies from other African countries with restrictive abortion laws suggest that induced abortion may account for over half of the PAC caseload in public hospitals: 60 percent in Nigeria (Bankole et al., 2015), 63 percent in Malawi (Levandowski et al., 2013), and 77 percent in Uganda (S. Singh, Prada, Mirembe, and Kiggundu, 2005). One explanation for lower percentages of induced abortion among PAC cases in Senegal is lower abortion incidence. At 17 abortions per 1,000 women, Senegal's abortion incidence is lower than the regional rate for West Africa (28 per 1,000 women) (Sedgh, Sylla,

TABLE 3.1. Types of abortions treated at three hospitals, 2009–2010

Year	Hospital	Total abortions treated	Spontaneous abortions	Induced abortions
2009	Hôpital Senghor	403	400	3
	Hôpital Médina	443	442	1
	Hôpital de Ville	1467	1460	7
2010	Hôpital Senghor	361	360	1
	Hôpital Médina	389	387	2
	Hôpital de Ville	1091	1087	4

Philbin, Keogh, and Ndiaye, 2015). In contexts with restrictive abortion laws, however, reluctance among women and health workers to disclose abortion may result in underestimated abortion incidence. In what follows, I explore how hospitals' accounts of PAC are produced at the intersection of competing professional jurisdictions in a political arena hostile to abortion.

Hospital records, and the processes of medical inscription, are important tools of professional boundary work. Medical records organize the accomplishment of clinical work (Timmermans and Berg, 2003), including the production of new knowledge about the body (Foucault, 1973; Mol, 2002), the distribution of labor within the clinic, and the transmission of information to other institutions involved in health planning, social and economic welfare, and law enforcement (Berg and Bowker, 1997; Heath, 1982). Hospital records do more than simply represent events that occurred in the clinic. Rather, they offer a selective, standardized account of events—a "preferred account" (Berg and Bowker, 1997, p. 525)—that justifies the course of action taken between diagnosis and treatment, thereby limiting health workers' liability (Berg, 1996; Hughes, 1988). Although records are created through verbal consultations with patients, health workers carefully "edit out" parts of patients' stories to produce records that present only "the important stuff" to audiences within and, if required, outside the hospital (Good, 1994, pp. 78, 79). For example, midwives in West African hospitals often complete the partograph, a labor-monitoring tool, after rather than during delivery, to "rewrite" this event in a way that minimizes responsibility in the case of poor maternal and newborn outcomes (Jaffré, 2012).

My review of the 2009 and 2010 PAC registers at l'Hôpital Senghor, l'Hôpital Médina, and l'Hôpital de Ville, conducted in tandem with interviews and observation of PAC services, suggests that while medical providers may search for induced abortion, they simultaneously disguise suspected cases in the record as miscarriage. At each of the study hospitals, health workers—usually midwives—recorded cases in a register dedicated solely to PAC.[4] The PAC register collected sociode-mographic information retrieved during l'interrogation, including age, occupation, marital status,[5] parity, and gestational age. Health workers documented multiple aspects of clinical treatment, including the type of uterine evacuation, the name of the provider who administered treatment, and whether the woman received family planning counseling or methods. Additionally, the register required the provider to clearly state the type of abortion treated (spontaneous or induced). Although I did not directly observe or learn retrospectively of any situations in which the police seized or reviewed the PAC register, providers involved in investigations of illegal abortion would presumably draw on the data included in this document. In other words, the PAC register would be an important starting point for determining not only what kind of therapy the patient had received and by whom, but also the kind of abortion that occurred.

The reclassification of suspected induced abortion occurred in a number of ways. First, health workers explained that they designated cases as induced abortion in the register only if the woman "confessed," during l'interrogation or treatment, to having attempted to terminate pregnancy. They deemed the confession as the ultimate "proof" that an induced abortion had been attempted or completed. Without the woman's admission, they managed and recorded the case as a spontaneous abortion. "The first proof is an admission of the induced abortion, without coercion. This is not Guantanamo," quipped Dr. Fall, the head gynecologist at l'Hôpital de Ville. "'Madame, what happened?' 'I was pregnant and my boyfriend didn't want it, so I went to a man who gave me something to swallow, or who used an instrument on me.' It's formal . . . we don't try to discuss further, she admitted."

This method of determining the type of abortion echoes abortion classification schemes deployed in an epidemiological study of abortion in four Senegalese hospitals during the mid-1990s. Investigators classified as "definite" induced abortions women who admitted having procured the procedure. Cases of "probable" induced abortion referred to women who presented with clinical signs of pregnancy termination but did not admit to having an abortion. "Possible" cases of induced abortion referred to situations in which only one of the two preceding conditions was met. Women who did not show signs of definite, probable, or possible induced abortion or who affirmed that the pregnancy was desired or expected were classified as spontaneous abortion (F. Diadhiou, Faye, Sangaré, and Diouf, 1995). Among the health workers I interviewed, "probable" and "possible" cases of induced abortion were by default classified as cases of spontaneous abortion.

Providers considered physiological conditions observed during the vaginal exam or the ultrasound procedure as evidence of induced abortion. Even in the presence of such clinical observations, however, health professionals expressed reluctance to categorize a case as induced abortion without the woman's admission. Dr. Fall at l'Hôpital de Ville explained: "You do the exam, and you find a foreign object in the vagina. That's happened plenty of times. Sometimes it's compresses, cannulas, stalks, pills. She won't admit what it is, but you, you're sure that something . . . it's caustic soda, bleach, or permanganate pills. So you have a bunch of elements that tell you that it's strongly suspicious, but if she hasn't admitted, she hasn't admitted. You stick to that." Drawing on this logic, the eighteen cases of abortion documented in table 3.1 likely represent women who, at some point during their hospital stay, and in response to interrogation procedures, admitted to having an illegal abortion.

Other reclassification techniques included the use of clinically ambiguous terminology and selective omission of data (examples from the PAC registers are displayed in table B.1 in appendix B). Despite the presence of a column in the PAC register requiring providers to explicitly categorize cases as induced or spontaneous, they often used clinical terms that did not differentiate between the two. Examples of such terminology include "late abortion," "hemorrhagic abortion," "fetal abortion," "incomplete abortion," and "stopped pregnancy." At l'Hôpital Senghor in 2009, providers identified a case as simply an "abortion," which refers to *any* pregnancy loss before the twenty-fourth week of gestation (Farquharson et al., 2005; WHO, 2008). At l'Hôpital de Ville in 2009, health workers noted a patient who was eighteen years old, single, and a primigravida. Although gestational age was omitted, the case was classified as a "late abortion." At l'Hôpital de Ville in 2010, a midwife documented a single, eighteen-year-old woman who "expulsed two stillborn fetuses" at four months of gestation as a "fetal abortion." The woman at l'Hôpital Senghor who ingested a décoction to "clean her stomach" was classified as a "late abortion." At l'Hôpital de Ville, Maimouna Diallo, the woman who lingered in the recovery room for four days with no accompanying family members, was categorized as an "incomplete abortion." Such cases would be considered spontaneous abortions in any retrospective reviews of the register, because they were not classified as definite induced abortions.

Omissions usually appeared in the form of a blank entry or a question mark. Providers omitted the type of abortion as well as sociodemographic and clinical data. To be sure, my retrospective review of the registers limited my ability to determine the circumstances contributing to such omissions. For example, did the patient refuse to provide information to the medical worker during the interrogation? Did the health provider make a deliberate decision to withhold information that might foster suspicion about the case, such as marital status? Or did the omission merely reflect the administrative oversight of an overstretched health worker with a heavy patient caseload? While we can only speculate about why health providers omitted certain indicators from the register, such cases were generally less likely to be classified as induced abortions. In a case at l'Hôpital Senghor in 2009, the only information the provider included was the patient's age (thirteen). The attending provider was not identified and abortion type was omitted. At l'Hôpital de Ville in 2009, the attending midwife inserted "?" for marital status for a fourteen-year-old patient who "expulsed" a fetus with a gestational age of two months. The midwife did not identify abortion type. At l'Hôpital Médina in 2010, providers omitted gestational age and abortion type for a case involving a sixteen-year-old who self-identified as married. Because these cases were not marked as induced abortions, by default they would be classified as spontaneous abortion in any retrospective inspections of the register. Cases formally documented as induced abortion, however, appeared to have fewer omissions. Among four cases of induced abortion documented at l'Hôpital Médina and l'Hôpital de Ville, only one case at l'Hôpital de Ville in 2010 was missing information (gestational age).

To what extent did health workers *deliberately* apply these techniques of reclassification when they suspected a patient had illegally procured an abortion, and why? After all, without clinical signs of unsafe induced abortion such as uterine perforation, or objects in the cervix or uterus, health workers might have genuinely experienced difficulty in differentiating between induced and spontaneous abortion, especially during the first trimester of pregnancy. In places with restrictive abortion laws, women may be reluctant to reveal a pregnancy termination out of fear of arrest (Gerdts, Tunçalp, Johnston, and Ganatra, 2015; WHO, 2011). Clinical studies of PAC in Burkina Faso and Ghana have documented differences in the ways that health workers and patients report abortion type, with women being more likely to classify an abortion as spontaneous (Dao et al., 2007; Taylor, Diop, Blum, Dolo, and Winikoff, 2011). Even in places with more liberal abortion laws, like the United States, women may limit the disclosure of induced abortion to health professionals because of the stigma of abortion (E. Jones and Forrest, 1992; Udry, Gaughan, Schwingl, and van den Berg, 1996).

Conversations with health workers suggested that their desire to circumvent the involvement of law enforcement officials motivated them to deliberately classify suspected cases of induced abortion as miscarriage. "Sometimes we're not sure if it's a case of induced or spontaneous abortion," Mme Bâ at l'Hôpital Médina explained. "But the midwife may write spontaneous if she's not sure, or even if she knows it's an induced abortion because of the possibility of being called to testify. It happens often." Another midwife at l'Hôpital Médina, Mlle Kebe, pointed out that it was "rare" for the provider to classify a case as an induced abortion, because this would require the production of a formal medical certificate proving that an illegal abortion had taken place. "You have to do an investigation to say why you recorded an induced abortion. It's just easier to write spontaneous abortion," she said. "You won't have to be bothered with all that. It's better to let some cases go."

Even if some providers understood such actions as complicity in an illegal act, this was preferable to stepping beyond the boundaries of their duties as medical professionals. "We know that most of them lie," explained Dr. Ly at l'Hôpital Senghor. "But if she says it's spontaneous, you can't write induced, you have to write spontaneous. We record what the patient tells us. We write the words of the patient. We are not the police. We don't do investigations."

M. Sall, the head nurse at a primary health care facility in the same region as l'Hôpital Médina, described how the legal context of abortion encouraged providers to preemptively record PAC cases as spontaneous abortions. "We record them all as spontaneous abortions," he said, "knowing induced abortion is illegal. Therefore, there can't be any induced abortions. So we consider them as spontaneous abortions, and we record them as such."

I asked: "But is it possible that there are induced abortions among these cases?"

"Yes," M. Sall impatiently replied, "but as long as there are no complications, we can manage the situation." For M. Sall, the term "complications" did not simply refer to obstetric complications but also signaled a variety of situations that may constrain health workers' ability to manage a suspicious case without police involvement. For example, a health worker might uncover "flagrant" signs of abortion during treatment that prompt her to notify her supervisors, who in turn alert the police. Mme Seck, the midwife at M. Sall's facility, described a situation at her previous job—a district hospital—that illustrates a cascade of administrative disclosures that shift professional authority over PAC cases away from medical providers:

> When I worked at the health center, I got a case once. I was with a nurse at the time. It was 7 A.M. in the morning when she came. I knew immediately that it was an induced abortion because there was a catheter in the uterus. I called the head nurse. He called the doctor, who did the interrogation until she confessed. She said she'd done it in Dakar, and the person told her to go to the nearest health facility if she started to feel pain. We took out the catheter and treated the woman. But the doctor said we couldn't just treat it like any case, otherwise people might think that we did the abortion at the hospital! The doctor prepared a report and sent it to the police. The woman was in prison, and they were still looking for the guy who did the abortion.

In this situation, the presence of the nurse during the initial exam may have pressured Mme Seck into alerting the head nurse, who in turn notified the doctor. Concerned about the hospital's reputation, the physician referred the matter to the police.

The involvement of other institutions may limit providers' capacity to categorize suspicious cases as spontaneous abortions. Two cases of induced abortion—one at l'Hôpital Médina in 2009 and another at l'Hôpital de Ville in 2010—were referred by health workers from neighboring health facilities. In 2010 at l'Hôpital Médina, health workers classified as induced abortion a patient who was escorted to the facility by police officers from a neighboring town. At l'Hôpital Senghor, I identified a case of induced abortion recorded in December 2010, just one month before I began my fieldwork at this hospital. When I asked Mme Traoré, a midwife at l'Hôpital Senghor, to explain the circumstances of the case, she recalled that a nurse at the primary health care facility where the woman first sought treatment for complications had reported her to the police. The police escorted the woman to the hospital for treatment and demanded a medical report that confirmed the induced abortion. Mme. Traoré deplored the nurse's decision to involve the police, explaining that a basic referral would have allowed the hospital to treat and release the woman.

The desire to circumvent police involvement at the hospital was not the only reason health workers classified suspected cases of induced abortion as miscarriage. Although most health workers were not in favor of induced abortion, many empathized with women desperate enough to seek clandestine abortions. When asked if midwives at her facility alerted the police to suspected cases, Mlle Touré at l'Hôpital de Ville replied: "Normally we're supposed to, but it's a question of humanity. We try to understand the woman. It depends on the situation. What happened to her?" Others expressed reluctance to contribute in any way to the arrest and imprisonment of women. "Have you ever seen the inside of a women's prison in Senegal?" Dr. Fall, the head gynecologist at l'Hôpital de Ville, asked me. "When you see the conditions there you'll understand why it's hard to write and send these reports, because you know what the woman will experience, and it's very difficult." Mme Diop, the head midwife at l'Hôpital Médina, echoed Dr. Fall's discomfort when she explained that "the interrogation should help us decide if it's an induced abortion. So when we're not really sure, and we know that these women, if they are denounced [to the police], that they'll be in prison for two years or more, then we try to manage the emergency and the rest is not our problem." By reclassifying suspected induced abortions as miscarriage, health workers attempted to protect not only themselves but also their patients from the threat of police investigation.

CONCLUSION

Although treating abortion complications was an important part of obstetric practice in Senegalese hospitals, these services were not entirely the "banal" affair Dr. Sarr at l'Hôpital de Ville claimed them to be. To the contrary, PAC required health workers to negotiate a complex set of expectations regarding obstetric care on the part of global health organizations, donor agencies, national health authorities, and the criminal justice system. The production of the typical PAC patient, an expectant mother suffering complications of miscarriage of a desired pregnancy, emerged from these daily negotiations and was instantiated in hospital records that identified most cases as spontaneous abortion.

The contradictory practices of seeking out and obscuring suspected induced abortion illustrated what institutional ethnographers have called "the organizing power of texts" (DeVault, 2006; D. Smith, 1993). The medical record sought out induced abortion by requiring health professionals to identify the type of abortion and, unlike other registers in the maternity ward for delivery and family planning, the patient's marital status. Motherhood, ideally within marriage, was the primary reproductive identity that provided the basis for assessing women's sexual and reproductive propriety. Women who did not conform to providers' expectations regarding good motherhood were singled out for further questioning and, in some situations, detention at the hospital. The punitive nature of these attempts suggests that even if providers do not always report women to the police, they may still humiliate them during treatment for the possible moral failure of abortion.

At the same time, the medical record and its processes of inscription produced a "preferred account" of PAC that suggested that most cases were a result of miscarriage, thereby protecting health workers and many of their patients and families from police scrutiny. This account rendered invisible the highly subjective—and at times violent—practices involved in seeing, speaking, and writing (Atkinson, 1995; Good, 1994) women's bodies and behavior as providers attempted to differentiate between induced and spontaneous abortion. The act of record keeping obscured the very practices of interrogation—not unlike the techniques employed by the police—that contradicted the treatment ethic of the global PAC model but remained crucial to the protection of medical authority over abortion.

The "preferred account" of PAC represents a "public secret" (Taussig, 1999)—knowledge about what happens in hospitals and the kinds of women treated there—that must be strategically articulated, if it is articulated at all. The typical PAC patient *has* to be an expectant mother, otherwise the entire premise of the intervention, and the involvement of health workers in public hospitals, can be called into question in a country where induced abortion is prohibited under any circumstance; where there remain lingering questions about the difference between PAC and induced abortion; and where one of the primary donors of reproductive health aid, USAID, does not support abortion-related activities. By portraying PAC as the medical management of miscarriage, health workers maintained the legitimacy of their clinical work within this political context and remained "accountable" (Sullivan, 2017) to national health officials, religious leaders, and international NGOs and donors that invest in maternal and reproductive health care.

In the long run, however, providers' record-keeping practices, and the public secret of PAC, contribute to what has been termed the "prevalence paradox of abortion" (Kumar et al., 2009), in which underreporting of induced abortion engenders epidemiological "truths" (V. Adams, 2005), within and beyond the hospital, about the low incidence of abortion. The prevalence paradox generates a vicious cycle of obstetric violence in which women with unwanted pregnancies resort to clandestine and frequently unsafe abortion services and are then subjected to discrimination and harassment if and when they seek medical care for obstetric complications. These instances of obstetric violence are further obscured as most PAC patients end up being classified in hospital records as cases of miscarriage.

PAC performs multiple forms of reproductive governance through daily obstetric practice, including protecting health workers' jurisdictional authority over abortion and facilitating medical surveillance of sexually active women. It offers a clinical platform for the intersection and mutual reinforcement of national and global discourses that valorize motherhood as women's primary reproductive identity. In the next chapter, I explore how hospital data have been pragmatically assembled in ways that simultaneously align the intervention with national and global safe motherhood discourses, thereby suppressing political will to relax the national abortion law. These data play a critical role in conveying not only that most PAC patients are expectant mothers but also that such women are most deserving of affordable obstetric care, and that PAC is the only kind of abortion care to which women should be entitled.

4 · WHEN ABORTION DOES NOT COUNT
Interpreting PAC Data

There is no evidence that PAC works in Senegal. In public health terms, this means that no nationally representative data exist showing a statistical relationship between PAC services and a decline in maternal mortality. The absence of such data is by no means a secret among reproductive health experts. Even high-level officials within the DSR acknowledged that, nearly twenty years after the introduction of PAC to the health system, few data were available to suggest that the intervention had reduced maternal mortality. Yet, PAC was widely considered an effective maternal mortality reduction strategy among health workers, health officials, and national and international NGO stakeholders. Additionally, most Senegalese reproductive health experts asserted that the majority of cases treated in hospitals were related to miscarriage. In this chapter, I explore how Senegalese health experts established claims about the impact of PAC and the kinds of women treated by the intervention in government hospitals. I illustrate how, in a global health landscape that has increasingly mandated statistical data on impact and cost-effectiveness, and has prioritized the RCT in particular as the "gold standard" of such evidence (V. Adams, 2013, 2016), these actors have negotiated the meaning of evidence, of what "works" in reducing maternal mortality, and even of what happens during PAC in government hospitals.

Critical scholars of global health have demonstrated that "evidence-based" policy making—the translation of scientific method into practice—is far from a linear, objective process. The acceptance of global health interventions by national governments does not immediately translate into widespread coverage and acceptance at the local level (Feierman, Kleinman, Stewart, Farmer, and Das, 2010; Ogden, 2003). National policy makers, academic researchers, and district and regional health officials negotiate the salience of evidence-based health interventions for local health systems. With increasing pressure from donors and global health organizations to adopt interventions that are based on "global" evidence (V. Adams, 2013) derived from RCTs, national governments may deprioritize locally produced evidence and national professional expertise (Feierman et al., 2010). Despite pressures to enact rationalistic, evidence-based policy, health decision-making often unfolds within highly context-specific and competing political goals and financial considerations among multiple stakeholders. Spending money on an intervention may in fact be more critical to establishing political credibility within a short period of time than rigorously determining the intervention's cost-effectiveness over longer time intervals. (Hunsmann, 2012). Additionally, gaps, inconsistencies, and other problems related to data are deliberately "unknown" (Geissler, 2013) or managed in ways that maintain accountability to national and global priorities (Sullivan, 2017). Even imperfect data can be overstated as or "fetishized" (Oni-Orisan, 2016; Wendland, 2016) into markers of progress and impact that are recognized and rewarded through lucrative development contracts, grants, and political opportunities. While the strategic interpretation and deployment of data facilitate health and development work across multiple uncertainties and inequalities, these practices do not necessarily reflect or meet the health needs of those targeted by "evidence-based" policies and interventions (Lambert, 2013; Pfeiffer and Nichter, 2008).

The global PAC model is "accountable" (Sullivan, 2017) to various political, programmatic, and clinical paradigms within the fields of global maternal and reproductive health. Given that abortion complications are among the five leading direct causes of global maternal mortality (Say et al., 2014), PAC has been recognized as part of a constellation of lifesaving obstetric services promoted by the global SMI since its inception in 1987. In 1994, the ICPD acknowledged access to quality PAC as a "reproductive right" for women in countries with restrictive abortion laws. Although the fifth MDG calls on governments to improve maternal health, it was only in 2005 that universal access to "reproductive health"—a concept that is often negatively associated with abortion—was adopted as a subtarget (Glasier, Gülmezoglu, Schmid, Moreno, and Van Look, 2006). PAC is compatible with the funding policies of USAID and the Bill & Melinda Gates Foundation, two of the most prominent donors of global reproductive health aid, both of which categorically refuse to support abortion.

In this chapter, I explore how PAC champions in Senegal demonstrated accountability to and compliance with various global regimes of reproductive governance through the strategic production and deployment of abortion and PAC data between the mid-1980s and the late 2000s. I illustrate how the arrival of the global PAC model introduced new categories of evidence that rendered the public health problem of abortion complications legible as a safe motherhood issue to Senegalese health authorities and other stakeholders. I argue that this transnational legibility hinged on pragmatic interpretations of available data by health professionals in which the definition of PAC as the medical management of miscarriage assumed greater importance than the statistical reliability or precision of the data themselves. A focus on hospital metrics—specifically, the number of women receiving PAC and the percentage treated with MVA—has transformed a politically controversial procedure into a set of clinical conditions that can be managed by professionals at the hospital with support from USAID and celebrated as part of the government's commitment to protecting women's reproductive rights by lowering maternal mortality. By demonstrating how various stakeholders negotiate clinical, demographic, and epidemiological data in the formulation of population problems and solutions, I illustrate how PAC data enact reproductive governance.

PAC AND THE GLOBAL POLITICS OF MATERNAL HEALTH

Competing claims about the meaning of PAC data and the intervention's impact on maternal mortality in Senegal must be situated in the broader field of global maternal health, which suffers from what has been called "the measurement trap" (Graham and Campbell, 1992). This term refers to the vicious cycle between a lack of sufficient statistical data on maternal death and weak political will to improve maternal health. The gold standard of scientific research, the RCT, requires large samples to produce reliable and precise measures of association between health interventions and outcomes. Large samples generate higher levels of statistical significance, which increase the investigator's confidence that the results observed are not due to chance. Maternal deaths[1] tend to be smaller in number than infant deaths or deaths from infectious diseases such as malaria, and are especially difficult to capture in contexts where a significant percentage of births take place outside the hospital. Even when maternal deaths occur in hospitals, misclassification of cause of death may result in underreporting of these events in national vital registration systems (Béhague and Storeng, 2013; Shiffman and Smith, 2007; WHO, 2004). These factors have complicated maternal health scientists' ability to obtain rigorous statistical data showing that certain interventions lead to reduced maternal death, which in turn has suppressed political prioritization of maternal health in comparison with global health initiatives for infectious diseases such as HIV, tuberculosis (TB), and malaria. For some maternal health advocates, the persistent neglect of maternal health mirrors broader gender inequalities that minimize the importance of women's health. In particular, the proximity of maternal health to abortion and reproductive health, which have long been contentious topics in the fields of health, population, and development, has fostered reluctance among policy makers and donors to invest in this area of global health (AbouZahr, 2003; Storeng and Béhague, 2014).

Part of this measurement trap stems from disagreement over what works in reducing maternal mortality and morbidity. Measuring impact is particularly difficult in this subfield as declines in maternal mortality often cannot be associated with a single intervention. In high-income countries such as Sweden and Britain, maternal deaths declined drastically in the late nineteenth and early twentieth centuries because of a confluence of social, professional, and institutional factors: advocacy by doctors, professionalization of midwives, improved clinical techniques for cesarean section, more effective medication for infection prevention, and better blood banking systems (Högberg, Wall, and Broström, 1986; Loudon, 1992). Unlike infant mortality and adult deaths from infectious disease, maternal mortality does not decline with improved living standards and socioeconomic status (Maine and Rosenfield, 1999). In fact, medical professionals in nineteenth-century western Europe observed that wealthy women were somewhat more likely to experience poor pregnancy and birth outcomes because they had greater access to the interventionist techniques of physicians (Loudon, 2000). Starting in the mid-twentieth century, countries such as Malaysia and Sri Lanka dramatically reduced maternal mortality by investing in professional training for rural midwives and by improving the quality of care in public hospitals (Liljestrand and Pathmanathan, 2004).

The SMI, an association of UN agencies and NGOs,[2] was founded in Nairobi, Kenya, in 1987, nearly ten years after the Alma-Ata Declaration of 1978, which called on governments to invest significantly in primary health care to reduce disparities in health outcomes between high- and low-income populations (Basilico, Weigel, Motgi, and Bor, 2013). From its inception, the SMI has expressed commitment to reversing the gendered social injustice of maternal mortality and morbidity, which primarily affected women in developing countries with limited access to quality reproductive health care (AbouZahr, 2003; S. Smith and Shiffman, 2016). Maternal health experts drew on historical evidence from developed countries such as Sweden and Britain as well as more recent data from countries such as Malaysia and Sri Lanka to advocate for multisector approaches to reducing maternal mortality, including strengthening health systems and investing in midwifery training and professionalization (Béhague and Storeng, 2013). At a time when population control, in the form of family planning, was widely understood by development experts as the key to reducing poverty in the global South, the SMI argued that a disproportionate focus on fertility reduction overlooked deplorable global disparities in the safety and quality of services for pregnancy and delivery. In some contexts, investment in maternal health services by donor agencies like USAID was critiqued as a highly medicalized form of family planning that did not adequately respond to women's broader reproductive needs (Morsy, 1995). The SMI advocated for the inclusion of maternal health in the ICPD's declaration of reproductive health as a human right. In 1994, the ICPD's Platform of Action established demographic targets for reducing global maternal mortality: by 2015, countries were supposed to reduce 1990 estimates of maternal mortality by 75 percent (CRR and UNFPA, 2013).

Despite the incorporation of maternal health into the global reproductive rights agenda, debates about what works in reducing maternal mortality continued to unfold alongside broader shifts in what counts as evidence in the field of global health toward selective, disease-specific approaches (V. Adams, 2013, 2016). The global economic crisis of the late 1970s and early 1980s had called into question the financial feasibility of the 1978 Alma-Ata Declaration. The vision of primary health care for all seemed incompatible with the growing embrace of neoliberal economic thought—which argued for the privatization of social services like health and education—by influential donor countries and global financial institutions like the IMF and the World Bank. In addition to promoting user fees for health services in developing countries, this approach called for narrowing primary health care to a selected cluster of interventions such as breast feeding, oral rehydration therapy, and immunization that were cost-effective (low in cost but high in impact, or saved lives) (Basilico et al., 2013).

Against this increasingly neoliberal backdrop of global health governance, and at a time of economic scarcity, NGOs and national health authorities were increasingly held accountable to donors who desired statistical measures of cost-effectiveness of the interventions and programs they funded. Many donors considered the breadth of the SMI, which arguably included family planning, antenatal care, primary health care, obstetric care, and gender equity, to be nearly impossible to implement and measure reliably (Maine and Rosenfield, 1999). In response, some maternal health experts advocated for targeted interventions such as training traditional birth attendants and investing in antenatal care to screen pregnant women for risk of obstetric complications (Béhague and Storeng, 2008). By the late 1980s and into the 1990s, however, the effectiveness of these interventions was increasingly called into question (Langwick, 2012; Pigg, 1997). Trained traditional birth attendants could not manage or avert obstetric emergencies in the same manner as skilled professionals such as nurses, doctors, and midwives working within a health system (Béhague and Storeng, 2013; Béhague, Tawiah, Rosato, Some, and Morrison, 2009). Additionally, maternal health scientists found that while most obstetric complications can be effectively treated in the hospital, very few can be successfully predicted during antenatal care (Maine and Rosenfield, 1999; Rosenfield and Maine, 1985).

By the early 1990s, some maternal health advocates were expressing discomfort with the SMI's use of social justice and feminist arguments to promote investment in maternal health. In addition to appearing insufficiently "scientific," such approaches polarized the movement from conservative donors and governments that were concerned that safe motherhood was a backdoor approach to promoting or, even worse, legalizing "the 'a' word" (AbouZahr, 2003)—abortion. Like other global health initiatives, the SMI needed "neutral" statistical data that could clearly demonstrate the relationship between specific interventions and reductions in maternal mortality (Storeng and Béhague, 2014).

Consequently, maternal health experts began to push for hospital-based interventions such as EmOC (AbouZahr, 2003; Maine and Rosenfield, 1999).[3] Even with this new approach, challenges arose in producing reliable evidence of effectiveness because EmOC involves various components of the health system[4] and cannot be collapsed into a single intervention. EmOC advocates drew on results from observational and quasi-experimental studies (Paxton, Maine, Freedman, Fry, and Lobis, 2005) that are considered less rigorous than RCTs in determining causality because they lack the element of random assignment. For example, anthropologist Vincanne Adams describes a safe motherhood project in Tibet that sought donor funding for a longitudinal, quasi-experimental study of the impact of midwifery training on maternal mortality. Over a period of five years, investigators aimed to compare maternal mortality between two counties that received the midwifery training program and two counties that did not. The proposal was rejected because "not enough women die in Tibet to get a good power calculation" (V. Adams, 2005, p. 76). In other words, the sample size was too small to produce statistical significance. Additionally, the donor expressed concern that the study design itself did not adequately separate the treatment and control counties. The possibility of "cross-contamination," in which individuals from the control county receive the same intervention as individuals in the treatment county, threatened to invalidate statistical results. To secure donor support in a global health landscape that prioritizes statistical evidence, some maternal health experts are indeed conducting RCTs for highly targeted interventions, such as the use of magnesium sulfate to treat pre-eclampsia and eclampsia, or the use of misoprostol to prevent or treat PPH (Béhague and Storeng, 2008; Storeng and Béhague, 2014).

The PAC model presented a timely opportunity for government health authorities and NGO stakeholders to collect "objective," hospital-based indicators of abortion and treat complications of incomplete abortion while observing the Mexico City Policy and the Helms Amendment. During a Skype interview in 2011 with Dr. Perez, a senior member of a reproductive health NGO, she explained how PAC introduced novel categories of obstetric care that resonated with global abortion policy frameworks: "We created a category. We made it something that people can count. And so all of a sudden you have data . . . that says, the number of PAC cases is going down or up, or not changing, what does that mean? Why are there so many PAC cases in this hospital? It just raises all these questions, and that's only because we're actually capturing this data. So yeah, I think it . . . has allowed organizations that get USAID funding to remain active in abortion, otherwise abortion would have been completely dismissed and taken out of the reproductive health continuum. It's not complete, obviously, but it's there."

PAC offered new ways of measuring the clinical management of incomplete abortion at the hospital. Process indicators such as the number of women treated and the percentage treated with MVA technology provided statistical insight into the availability and quality of obstetric services. Health professionals could evaluate cost-effectiveness by calculating the extent to which MVA treatment reduced expenses for patients and facilities in comparison with dilation and curettage. Given that PAC was compatible with U.S. restrictions on abortion, health professionals and NGOs funded by USAID could engage in abortion-related research and programming while remaining eligible for U.S. funding for other global health activities, including child health, malaria, TB, and HIV/ AIDS. For example, USAID contracted MSH to implement the Prevention of Maternal Mortality and Morbidity Project (PREMOMA) in Senegal between 2003 and 2006. This project supported not only family planning and PAC but also EmOC, malaria prevention in pregnant women, and prevention of mother-to-child HIV transmission (MSH, 2006).

The SMI's focus on hospital-based interventions, including PAC, has been remarkably successful. Maternal health was recognized as a global health and development concern in the fifth MDG, which reiterated the ICPD's call for a 75 percent reduction in the maternal mortality ratio by 2015. In 2015, the third SDG, to "ensure healthy lives and promote well-being for all at all ages," called for further reductions in global maternal mortality ratios to fewer than 70 deaths per 100,000 live births by 2030.

Global funding for maternal, newborn, and child health increased significantly from $2.6 billion in 2003 to $8.3 billion in 2012. Assistance to maternal, newborn, and child health accounts for more than 60 percent of all global funding for reproductive, maternal, newborn, and child health, estimated in 2012 at $12.8 billion (Arregoces et al., 2015). Some have attributed this prioritization of global maternal health to the forging of alliances between maternal and child health experts. In 2005, the Safe Motherhood Interagency Group joined the Healthy Newborn Partnership[5] and the Partnership for Child Survival[6] to form the Partnership for Maternal, Child, and Newborn Health. Although some maternal health experts and feminist advocates were wary of linking women's health to children's and newborns' health, they recognized the benefits of affiliating with global health initiatives that were less politically controversial than maternal and reproductive health (AbouZahr, 2003; S. Smith and Shiffman, 2016).

In 2007, nearly 2,000 maternal health advocates and scientists from 115 countries convened in London for a meeting called "Women Deliver." Held on the twentieth anniversary of the SMI in Nairobi, Kenya, the conference aimed to review lessons learned in improving maternal health and to renew political commitments to global maternal mortality reduction based on "evidence-based advocacy" (Storeng and Béhague, 2014). In contrast to the 1987 meeting in Nairobi, which revolved around a comprehensive health system–strengthening approach to women's health, Women Deliver emphasized hospital-based, technological maternal mortality reduction interventions that could produce statistical data on impact and cost-effectiveness for donors. Remarkably absent from the meeting was the feminist, social justice orientation that highlighted maternal mortality as one of the greatest disparities between the developed and developing worlds. The rationale for investing in maternal health was articulated not as a matter of reproductive justice for women but rather its potential to measurably contribute to and improve other areas of social and economic development, such as child health and environmental sustainability.

Feminist historian Michelle Murphy (2017) has referred to this harnessing together of "life, reproduction, and capital" as an "economization of life" that emerged in the post–World War II period as demographers, economists, and "First World" policy makers conceptualized contraception as a technology of economic development in decolonizing nations in the "Third World." Later in the twentieth century, this neoliberal logic of investing in girls and women for future economic gain has broadened beyond contraception to include education, health care, and microcredit programs for female entrepreneurs. Anthropologists Dominique Béhague and Katerini Storeng argue that the Women Deliver initiative has similarly economized the value of preventing maternal death. The official slogan of the 2007 Women Deliver conference, which now occurs every three years, aptly captured this neoliberal dimension of maternal mortality reduction as a gendered development project: "Invest in Women: It Pays" (Storeng and Béhague, 2014). The new "reproductive subject" (Morgan and Roberts, 2012) of the contemporary global campaign to reduce maternal mortality is the modern woman who not only responsibly uses contraception to avert unplanned pregnancies but also carefully seeks out obstetric care to reduce the risk of maternal death (Bhatia et al., 2019; MacDonald, 2019). Donors and governments will be motivated to "invest" in her rational and self-actualizing behaviors because of their potential contributions to improved health and environmental outcomes.

Some progress has been achieved in global efforts to reduce maternal mortality. The WHO recently estimated a 35 percent decline in the total number of maternal deaths between 2000 and 2017 (WHO, 2019). Trends in the distribution and causes of maternal mortality, however, suggest that some of the same problems identified by the SMI in 1987 continue to plague this global health issue. In 2014, only sixteen countries (seven of which are developing countries) were estimated to meet the fifth MDG by 2015 (Kassebaum, Bertozzi-Villa, and Coggeshall, 2014). Almost all maternal deaths (66%) occur in sub-Saharan Africa, followed by South Asia (20%) (WHO, 2019). Nearly three-fourths (73%) of maternal deaths are related to direct causes such as hemorrhage, pre-eclampsia and eclampsia, sepsis, and unsafe abortion. A growing percentage of maternal deaths (27%) are related to indirect causes such as chronic disease (Say et al., 2014). Although the percentage of maternal deaths related to HIV has declined from 2.1 percent in 2005 to 1 percent in 2017, almost all (89%) HIV-related maternal deaths occur in sub-Saharan Africa (WHO, 2019).

In 1985, public health scholars Alan Rosenfield and Deborah Maine published an article in *The Lancet* titled "Maternal Mortality, a Neglected Tragedy: Where Is the M in MCH?" to highlight the role of functioning health systems in treating and preventing obstetric complications. More than thirty years later, trends in global funding for reproductive, maternal, newborn, and child health raise troubling questions about the extent to which donors' goals and priorities align with pregnant women's needs. Although HIV accounts for the least amount of maternal deaths worldwide (Kassebaum et al., 2014), in 2011 and 2012 over 80 percent of global funding for reproductive health was earmarked for HIV (Arregoces et al., 2015). A thirty-two-fold increase was observed in the percentage of funding earmarked for projects explicitly involving newborns, suggesting a shift in focus from women to infants and children (Arregoces et al., 2015). The increase in family planning funding, from $63 million to $462 million between 2009 and 2012, is likely related to advocacy leading up to FP 2020 (Arregoces et al., 2015). USAID's influence as the most significant donor of global reproductive health aid (Hsu, Berman, and Mills, 2013), however, ensures that little of this funding can support abortion-related activities despite the fact that complications of unsafe abortion are among the top five causes of maternal death. And while the SMI initially argued for comprehensive, health-systems-strengthening approaches to reducing maternal mortality, funding for reproductive, maternal, newborn, and child health has been increasingly funneled into stand-alone projects rather than the general budget and sector support preferred by recipient governments (Arregoces et al., 2015). While I do not contest the importance of HIV, newborn and child health, and family planning within the spectrum of reproductive health care, the increase in funding to these areas relative to obstetric care suggests how women's health continues to be narrowly operationalized according to donors' priorities.[7]

Paradoxically, the primary indicator used to measure progress on the MDGs and SDGs, the maternal mortality ratio, offers very limited insight into the technical environment in which health professionals administer obstetric services and the quality of care subsequently experienced by women. The indicator itself is composed of "wobbly" estimates of maternal death generated in countries with weak vital registration systems that are designed to "fill in data that don't exist, smooth out data that do, and throw out data that are such a poor fit that they are deemed unlikely to be true" (Wendland, 2016, p. 69). Yet, perceived reductions in the maternal mortality ratio can facilitate or leverage numerous political and professional opportunities among those who claim responsibility for this accomplishment, such as securing grants for hospitals or health programs or strengthening political careers. In Malawi, for example, a reduction in maternal mortality from 675 to 460 per 100,000 live births was widely attributed in 2013 to

President Joyce Banda's investments in safe motherhood programs. Absent from these laudatory reports, however, was any recognition that the data were based on surveys that had been administered before her presidential tenure or that nearly three-quarters of deaths in Malawi are never recorded anywhere (Wendland, 2016). In 2010, IHME released global estimates of maternal mortality that were lower than those of WHO (Graham and Adjei, 2010; Hogan et al., 2010). Such variations have not only challenged WHO's technical expertise in measuring maternal mortality but also generated concern among maternal health scientists and NGOs that global health donors will deprioritize maternal health (Storeng and Béhague, 2017). In what anthropologists Adeola Oni-Orisan (2016) and Claire Wendland (2016) call the "fetishization" of data, the production and deployment of maternal mortality data acquire greater significance within a neoliberal global health landscape that prioritizes statistical data over the quality of the interventions themselves, and the extent to which they make a meaningful difference in women's lives and health.

Anthropologists have illustrated how global health actors pragmatically manage various kinds of "unknowns" (Geissler, 2013)—including absences of or inconsistencies in data and fragmented priorities among donors, NGOs, and health authorities—to maintain not only the daily operation but also the political legitimacy of clinical research or program implementation (Hunsmann, 2012; Sullivan, 2017). Safe motherhood data co-constitute global forms of reproductive governance through strategic interpretations of maternal mortality ratios that lend themselves to the production of particular kinds of women patients. While maternal mortality ratios reveal little about how or why women end up in hospitals (or not), the quality of care they receive, or what happens to those who survive "near-miss" obstetric events (Storeng et al., 2008; Storeng and Béhague 2017), they generate a portrayal of maternal suffering that resonates with a neoliberal ethic of "investing in women" that in turn has recently led to renewed commitments to maternal health. In 2010, for example, at the second Women Deliver conference in Washington, DC, the Bill & Melinda Gates Foundation (BMGF, 2017) committed $1.5 billion between 2010 and 2014 to expanding access to existing, cost-effective interventions and developing new tools, technologies, and treatments that can be "rigorously evaluated" (BMGF, 2010).[8]

High maternal mortality ratios galvanize policy makers and donors to invest in vertical, hospital-based obstetric care interventions that can statistically illustrate how they protect selfless mothers as they bring new life into the world (Kumar, Hessini, and Mitchell, 2009; Rance, 1997). It is precisely these women's willingness to risk their own well-being for their children that makes them deserving of quality obstetric care. In this model of safe motherhood, miscarriage is the most appropriate reason why a woman would require EmOC for treatment of incomplete abortion. In contrast, the woman who seeks induced abortion, owing to her selfish rejection of motherhood, appears less deserving of care than the self-less expectant mother.

In the remainder of this chapter, I explore how Senegalese health professionals made PAC services and patients legible as part of the national safe motherhood program through strategically negotiating information about the effectiveness of PAC and the kinds of women treated for complications of abortion in government hospitals. I argue that while health professionals were actively producing data about women with abortion complications well before the introduction of PAC, the intervention offered a new clinical lexicon for managing abortion that maintained the legitimacy of these services in a transnational policy landscape highly hostile to abortion.

ABORTION SCIENCE IN SENEGAL, 1973 TO 2003

Senegalese health scientists, primarily epidemiologists, demographers, and public health physicians in large urban hospitals, collected data on induced and frequently unsafe abortion from the mid-1980s until the mid-2000s. Abortion research took a variety of forms, including retrospective reviews of hospital data and national health and fertility surveys, doctoral theses by medical students, maternal death audits, and reviews of existing literature. In this section, I review the results of nine abortion-related studies covering a thirty-year period between 1973 and 2003.[9] These studies varied widely in their methodologies and estimates of induced abortion, and none yielded national estimates of abortion incidence. Still, they illustrate that well before the arrival of PAC in the late 1990s, Senegalese health professionals were accountable to the global SMI, which in 1987 had counted unsafe abortion among the top five causes of maternal death. Given that the Senegalese government had ratified the 1994 ICPD Platform of Action, these health professionals were also committed to reducing the maternal mortality ratio. By investigating unsafe abortion and its contribution to maternal mortality, they located themselves in regional and global networks of research and advocacy related to improving maternal health.

At a time when the national penal code prohibited induced abortion, decisions to conduct scientific research on a criminalized procedure reveal considerable interest in defining the parameters of medical authority over abortion. Epidemiological research represented an opportunity to medicalize abortion, or gain professional control over this procedure. By constructing abortion as a medical rather than legal problem, health professionals aimed to "depoliticize" (Conrad, 1992) a highly controversial, yet not uncommon reproductive experience. Using the scientific tools of epidemiology, these professionals began to piece together the social, political, and economic landscape of induced abortion in Senegal. Patients suffering complications of unsafe abortion tended to be young, unmarried women from precarious socioeconomic backgrounds in rural, urban, and peri-urban zones. Despite their efforts to medicalize abortion, Senegalese health scientists were among the first to construct abortion as a multifaceted, gendered problem related to women's constrained bodily autonomy, limited access to education and professional opportunities, and subsequent economic dependence on men. Indeed, at the end of a 1995 study of abortion complications conducted in collaboration with WHO at CHU Le Dantec in Dakar, investigators called for increased "geographic, financial, and cultural" access to contraception. They suggested that abortion complications weighed heavily on a health system already constrained by "structural adjustment policies and currency devaluation," and called for a "multidisciplinary, multidimensional, and multisectoral" debate on legalizing abortion (F. Diadhiou, Faye, Sangaré, and Diouf, 1995, p. 49).

In 1985, medical student Pierre-Claver Nimbona's doctoral thesis entailed a retrospective review of hospitalized abortion patients between 1973 and 1983 at CHU Le Dantec (CEFOREP, 1998b). He found that among 12,254 abortions treated over a period of ten years, only 136 (1%) were recorded as induced abortions. Nearly 70 percent of patients classified as having procured an abortion were between fourteen and twenty-three years old, and for the majority of them (58%), it was their first pregnancy. Nimbona questioned the low number of induced abortions identified over a ten-year period, suggesting that the omission of marital status from individual patient records complicated his ability to differentiate between induced and spontaneous abortion. Although my own review of hospital records found women who self-identified as married among those who were classified as cases of induced abortion, his observation underscores the significance of marital status in determining abortion type well before the introduction of PAC.

Four years later, in 1989, Papa Demba Diouf conducted a retrospective review of abortion data in Pikine, a district in the region of Dakar. Using data from the Senegalese Fertility Survey and the Survey on Infant Mortality in Pikine, Diouf estimated that the percentage of women reporting abortions increased from 10 percent in 1978 to 30 percent in 1986 (CEFOREP, 1998b). Remarkably, neither of Diouf's sources differentiated between induced and spontaneous abortion. Additionally, the increase in reported abortions between 1978 and 1986 possibly reflects different data collection strategies used by the two surveys. Nevertheless, it is important to note that Diouf's study received support from USAID and the Ford Foundation. The involvement of these institutions in an abortion-related study should not be surprising given their roles in researching and developing contraceptive technologies for the global South during the 1960s and 1970s (Murphy, 2012; Takeshita, 2012). While USAID actively disseminated contraceptives during this period, its ability to engage in abortion-related research was severely constrained by the 1973 Helms Amendment, and again by the 1984 Mexico City Policy. Despite this legislation, population and health experts within

USAID maintained interest in reducing fertility to catalyze economic development (Dixon-Mueller, 1993). A major component of USAID's health strategy for Senegal, before the establishment of safe motherhood interventions such as EmOC and PAC, involved "decreasing fertility" (Acedo, 1995; Robinson, 2017). A study on abortion in a high-fertility context, therefore, would not entirely fall beyond the agency's scope of interest.

In 1991, medical student Filbert Koly reviewed twelve months of obstetric records at CHU Le Dantec between 1988 and 1989 (CEFOREP, 1998b). Among 2,020 hospitalized abortions, he found 133 explicitly identified as clandestine induced abortions. Koly's study, thus, estimated a greater percentage of induced abortions among hospitalized cases than Nimbona's 1985 study at the same hospital (6.5% versus 1%, respectively). Additionally, Koly estimated that induced abortion accounted for 1.3 percent of maternal death during the study period. Half of hospitalized abortion cases involved young women and girls between the ages of fourteen and twenty-two, and nearly 40 percent of these patients already had a living child. Almost 60 percent of patients treated at CHU Le Dantec resided in working-class neighborhoods of Dakar. Nearly three-quarters of procedures had been initiated by the introduction of a catheter to the uterus. While nearly all women (69%) had procured the abortion from a paramedical professional, 15 percent performed the procedure themselves, and only 6 percent had received services from a skilled practitioner. Women reported a variety of reasons for terminating pregnancy, including fear of parents, financial insecurity, and the desire to finish schooling.

In 1995, Senegalese physicians F. Diadhiou, Faye, Sangaré, and Diouf (all members of the Clinique Gynécologique et Obstétricale of CHU Le Dantec), in collaboration with WHO, published a report based on data collected between 1993 and 1994 from CHU Le Dantec and three additional referral hospitals in Dakar. They identified five kinds of abortions: (1) definite induced abortion, in which the patient admits to having procured an abortion; (2) probable induced abortion, in which the patient does not admit to having procured an abortion but there are clinical signs of induced abortion; (3) possible induced abortion, in which only one of the first two conditions is present; (4) spontaneous abortion, in which none of the first three conditions are present or the patient affirms that the pregnancy was desired or expected; and (5) therapeutic abortion, in which, in line with the code of medical ethics, termination of pregnancy is necessary to preserve the pregnant woman's life (CEFOREP, 1998b). Health professionals like Dr. Fall, the head gynecologist at Hôpital de Ville, continued to draw on this classification scheme as they attempted to determine abortion type during the daily provision of PAC.

The study yielded the greatest estimate to date of the percentage of induced abortion among hospitalized abortion cases at government health facilities: between 19 and 24 percent. Up to 60 percent of induced abortion patients were less than twenty-five years old, and three-quarters indicated they were not married. The majority of these patients (68%) came from urban areas, a quarter were from the working-class neighborhoods of Dakar, and only 6 percent were from rural zones (F. Diadhiou et al., 1995). Sepsis was the most common cause of death among women hospitalized for complications of induced abortion (Goyaux, Alihonou, Diadhiou, Leke, and Thonneau, 2001). The contribution of abortion to maternal death ranged from 3 to 13 percent (F. Diadhiou et al., 1995).

In 1997, medical student Tidiane Touré published a review of therapeutic abortion in Senegal. Although the penal code forbids abortion under any circumstance, Touré reminded his readers that the code of medical ethics permits abortion if a pregnancy threatens the pregnant woman's life. He identified eight patients who were presented as candidates for therapeutic abortion at CHU Le Dantec between 1989 and 1996. Among these patients, two women had cancer; one patient had been involved in a traffic accident that left her paralyzed from the waist down; two women were diagnosed with severe mental illness; one had an autoimmune disease; one had a neurological disease; and one was co-infected with HIV and TB. Six of these patients were identified as married, and of the two women diagnosed with mental illness, one was single and the other was divorced.

All but two of the patients, one of whom was diagnosed with cancer and the woman involved in the traffic accident, received therapeutic abortions. Physicians recommended a therapeutic abortion for the woman with advanced cancer of the hypopharynx when she was approximately twenty-nine weeks pregnant. Touré suggested that the woman refused the intervention, and delivered via cesarean section a few weeks later. Although her child survived, the woman died a few months later. It is not clear from Touré's report why the second woman, the victim of the traffic accident, did not receive a therapeutic abortion. Although medical professionals submitted a request to the "medico-legal" specialist at CHU Le Dantec, her file shows that she eventually expulsed a dead fetus. She died a year later (Touré, 1997).

Touré's study illustrates how physicians determined, on a case-by-case basis, and in consultation with several other medical experts, the candidate's eligibility for therapeutic abortion. They authorized therapeutic abortions for infectious diseases like HIV and TB and chronic conditions like mental illness. At the same time, physicians demonstrated considerable concern over the sexual behavior of the two unmarried patients, suggesting a certain symmetry between therapeutic abortion and PAC in the surveillance of women's bodies during reproductive health care.

A year later, in 1998, researchers at CEFOREP and CHU Le Dantec collaborated with two USAID-funded NGOs—the Population Council and JHPIEGO—to publish a literature review of unsafe abortion (CEFOREP, 1998b). The authors drew on previous scientific studies and contemporary accounts of abortion in the national press to frame unsafe abortion as a public health and socio-legal problem. Acknowledging that their review of hospital-based studies represented only "the tip of the iceberg" (CEFOREP, 1998b) with respect to the epidemiological scope of abortion, the authors called for national studies of abortion incidence and qualitative research on the social and economic causes and consequences of unsafe abortion. While they did not call for a revision of the abortion law, they indicated that the best way to reduce unsafe abortion, given the importance of fertility within Senegalese society and widespread perceptions that induced abortion violates Islamic and Catholic principles, they urged policy makers to increase women's access to contraception. Finally, they stressed the need for operations research in hospitals to improve the clinical management of abortion complications.

Maternal death audits, which involve retrospective reviews of hospital records to determine cause of death, offer insight into the challenges of capturing abortion data in Senegalese hospitals. In 2002, scientists published a study that reviewed data collected between 1984 and 1988 from eighty-three villages in three rural zones of the country. Two-thirds of maternal deaths were due to direct obstetric causes, with hemorrhage as the leading cause of death. The cause of death in about 22 to 30 percent of cases was unknown (Kodio et al., 2002). In a study of maternal death conducted at a large referral hospital in the region of Dakar, 50 percent of deaths were related to hemorrhage, 26 percent were related to pre-eclampsia, and up to 20 percent of cases were "unknown" (Dumont et al., 2006). It is precisely the retrospective methodology used in these studies that limits their capacity to accurately identify all direct causes of death. Consequently, a significant percentage of mortality remains unaccounted for. Although these audits suggest that abortion accounted for very little mortality, global reproductive health experts suggest that abortion is often misclassified as hemorrhage or sepsis (Khan, Wojdyla, Say, Gülmezoglu, and Van Look, 2006).

In 2007, Senegalese physicians Cissé, Faye, and Moreau published an article in the journal *Médecine Tropicale* that reviewed abortion data from CHU Le Dantec between 2002 and 2003. Although the main purpose of the article was to assess the effectiveness of MVA technology in treating complications of first-trimester abortion, it differed from earlier and subsequent reports of PAC operations research by offering an estimate of the percentage of abortion cases related to induced abortion: 5.6 percent. Similar to Nimbona, the authors acknowledged that they likely underestimated the scope of induced abortion given their retrospective review of hospital records.

Although Senegalese health professionals assembled evidence in ways that primarily framed unsafe abortion as a public health problem, they also highlighted broader sociocultural, economic, and legal dimensions of reproduction that led women to seek clandestine and frequently unsafe abortion services. They recognized how methodological challenges related to collecting data limited their evidence base on abortion. While these demographers, clinicians, and epidemiologists offered many important recommendations for future research to better understand and address the problem of unsafe abortion, the Senegalese MSAS prioritized one recommendation in particular: operations research on the clinical management of first-trimester abortion complications. This series of research projects, conducted in collaboration with NGOs contracted by USAID, would become the scaffolding for the national PAC program.

A NEW CLINICAL LEXICON FOR ABORTION

The introduction of PAC, through a series of operations research projects starting in 1997, signaled a new ethic of obstetric care in which the health worker was no longer concerned with the kind of abortion the patient had experienced. Instead, what mattered was that the woman had been treated, that she had been treated with MVA rather than dilation and curettage or digital evacuation, and that she had received family planning counseling and methods during or after treatment.

Consequently, Senegalese health providers and health officials began to collect new kinds of abortion data in operations research on PAC. In contrast to previous studies that focused specifically on abortion type, they collected PAC *process indicators*—data that allowed them to monitor various dimensions of obstetric care without specifying what kinds of abortions were being treated. Health officials and their NGO partners deployed these indicators to demonstrate not only the feasibility of integrating this model of reproductive health care into the health system, but also that it would be limited to treating complications of abortion. In a country where abortion is altogether prohibited and one of the main donors of health aid, USAID, does not support abortion, reproductive health experts were compelled to define PAC as a safe motherhood intervention by establishing conceptual, clinical, and technological boundaries between PAC and induced abortion.

In chapter 2, I described how health officials and NGO personnel involved in early PAC research negotiated widespread concerns about introducing the MVA syringe to Senegalese hospitals. The dual capacity of the device to treat complications of abortion and to terminate first-trimester pregnancy raised anxieties that PAC would devolve into a de facto form of abortion in public hospitals. With hospital-based process indicators, PAC champions hoped to dispel policy makers' fears by distinguishing between PAC and induced abortion.[10] PAC process indicators dramatically conveyed a public health success story of a new set of lifesaving obstetric services and technologies. Increases in the number of patients treated at district hospitals indicated that midwives could offer these services at lower levels of the health system. Every patient treated represented the aversion of a potential case of maternal death. Concomitant increases in the percentage of cases treated with MVA suggested faster, more affordable, and safer treatment for women in rural zones. In other words, these hospital metrics suggested that decentralizing PAC to lower levels of the health system could lead to reduced rates of abortion-related mortality and morbidity. The careful measurement of process indicators generated a new lexicon to describe the clinical object of PAC—"complications of abortion"—which did not distinguish between induced abortion and miscarriage. Although the term "post-abortion care" does not appear in the title of the final report of the first pilot project, the term "abortion complications" does: *Introduction of Emergency Obstetric Care and Family Planning for Patients Presenting with Complications of Incomplete Abortion* (CEFOREP 1998a). "When presented with all this information," Dr. Dème (a DSR official) told me, "the decision-makers could not make any objections" to PAC.

PAC experts carefully included de-identified "abortion complications" with other kinds of obstetric complications that led to maternal mortality and morbidity. Mme Mbow, a midwife who worked with a maternal health and family planning NGO contracted by USAID, illustrated the clinical coherence between abortion complications and other obstetric complications: "The Ministry's post-abortion care strategy is favorable to the population. It solves the problem. . . . It's part of the larger strategy to reduce maternal mortality and morbidity by 2015, which is part of the MDGs. By stopping hemorrhage, which accounts for 25 percent of pregnancy-related mortality in Senegal—if we can stop hemorrhage we can reduce maternal mortality." By offering an estimate of the contribution of hemorrhage to maternal death,[11] Mme Mbow highlighted the urgency of PAC as a maternal mortality reduction strategy. She selectively drew on global maternal health knowledge to align PAC clinically with safe motherhood and the MDGs. Global health experts have identified hemorrhage and complications of unsafe abortion as two of the top five causes of global maternal death (Khan et al., 2006). While maternal health scientists recognize that abortion complications may be classified as hemorrhage, Mme Mbow did not make such distinctions in her claims about the clinical object of PAC.

In her research on maternal health politics in Tibet, anthropologist Vincanne Adams is reluctant to label such claims about numbers as "lying." Instead, she argues that health professionals, health authorities, and NGO stakeholders negotiate multiple ways of "locating truth" within a particular political and scientific context (V. Adams, 2005). Similarly, Mme Mbow's selective deployment of statistics regarding abortion complications illustrates strategic forms of "unknowing" (Geissler, 2013), of managing uncertainties or silencing truths that maintain the political and professional legitimacy of PAC (Sullivan, 2017). In a context where national policy makers and prominent donors do not support abortion, de-identified abortion complications merge with other obstetric complications to form a quantifiable risk of maternal death that can be addressed through PAC.

The new lexicon of "abortion complications" facilitated the integration of PAC into existing policy and program frameworks for maternal mortality reduction. Dr. Wade, a regional MSAS official, asserted that treatment of abortion complications was one of various safe motherhood strategies to reduce maternal mortality, including birth spacing, prenatal care, skilled birth attendance, cesarean sections, and postnatal care. Dr. Diallo, a physician who worked for a multilateral agency, described how PAC falls under the technical umbrella of EmOC: "Post-abortion care is part of the program that we integrated into everyday practice. To single out post-abortion care, I think we've moved beyond that. You will never see in Senegal a document that talks about EmOC without talking about post-abortion care. If you read the documents before, they said EmOC including post-abortion care. That 'including,' it should be removed. Post-abortion care is included in the package of services for EmOC." Indeed, after the end of the first operations research project in 1998, the MSAS integrated PAC into national protocols for maternal and reproductive health (M. Diadhiou et al., 2008). The new object of clinical action, de-identified abortion complications, permitted the location of an abortion-related intervention alongside other politically acceptable biomedical interventions for reducing maternal mortality.

The introduction of PAC signaled an important shift in the kinds of evidence collected in health professionals' efforts to define and act on abortion as a public health problem. Unlike the abortion science conducted by health professionals until the mid-2000s, very few operations research projects—almost all of them funded by USAID—sought to determine what kinds of abortions were being treated in hospitals. Instead, these projects aimed to depoliticize a new model of reproductive health care by generating statistical metrics of the health system's capacity to offer emergency treatment for abortion complications. They produced a new vocabulary for the object of clinical action that aligned the intervention with existing programs and policy frameworks related to safe motherhood. As long as the health system had the capacity to treat complications of abortion, it did not matter what kind of abortion a woman had experienced. By equipping hospitals and training health professionals to provide these services, the MSAS demonstrated its commitment to national and global frameworks for maternal mortality reduction.

INTERPRETING PAC DATA

After the introduction of PAC and its new indicators, health professionals and officials were tasked with interpreting hospital data across multiple levels of the health system in ways that established the intervention's legitimacy in a political context hostile to abortion. Elsewhere, I have described how statistics on digital evacuation, collected carefully by medical workers in government health facilities, are rendered invisible in national and global accounts of PAC technologies that focus on MVA (Suh, 2020). Here, I offer two examples in which Senegalese health professionals have drawn on local, pragmatic, "common-sense" (Béhague et al., 2009) knowledge and expertise to make evidentiary claims about the national PAC program. First, these actors have interpreted hospital data in ways that suggest that spontaneous abortions account for the majority of hospitalized abortions. Second, they have relied on empirical, context-specific data to make claims about the effectiveness of PAC in reducing maternal mortality. In each case, these actors have carefully assembled data to align PAC with national and global frameworks and discourses related to safe motherhood. These data formulations have been "imbued" (Oni-Orisan, 2016; Wendland, 2016) with various kinds of power that have facilitated the national scaling up of PAC and established Senegal as a PAC leader in West Africa. Additionally, these data have come to represent not only the kinds of women being treated in hospitals but also the kinds of care to which women should be entitled. In this sense, processes related to producing and handling data are not simply mundane forms of applied public health work, but also represent local forms of reproductive governance as health professionals, health officials, and other stakeholders attempt to regulate the kinds of services available in health systems and the kinds of women deserving of this care. Numerical representations of appropriate care and deserving women, however, are not always aligned with the reproductive realities and experiences of women who seek care (or not) in hospitals.

Types of Abortions Treated in Hospitals

In chapter 3, I illustrated how data collection practices in hospitals produce an account of PAC that suggests that most hospitalized cases of abortion are related to miscarriage. Here, I describe three examples that illustrate how these practices are reproduced institutionally through selective interpretations of hospital data across multiple levels of the national health information system.

First, the MSAS plays a critical role in producing narratives about what happens in hospitals by requiring health professionals to report the total number of cases treated—but not the type of abortion—in periodic statistical reports. At each study hospital, the head midwife assembled quarterly reports with data from the registers in the gynecological ward. She sent these reports to hospital administration, which in turn compiled annual reports and transmitted them to district, regional, and national MSAS authorities. I examined annual reports of PAC at each hospital between 2004 and 2010. Disaggregated data on abortion type were available for only two years, 2005 and 2006, at l'Hôpital Senghor.[12] Outside of this exception, all three hospitals reported only the total number of abortions treated between 2004 and 2010. Additionally, annual reports provided information on the percentage of patients treated with MVA, dilation and curettage, digital evacuation, and EVA. At l'Hôpital Médina, the annual report included the number of PAC patients who had received a family planning method. L'Hôpital Senghor and l'Hôpital de Ville did not offer information on family planning in their annual reports.

Central and regional MSAS officials offered pragmatic explanations for not collecting data on abortion type. Mme Niang, a DSR official, explained: "We are not interested in the type of abortion, because we are not here to crack down on women. We do not differentiate in the collection of data. We look at abortions that took place within the first three months that benefited from MVA. And even if we tried to differentiate between the two, there wouldn't be any data. Why? Because people won't admit they've had an abortion because it's forbidden by the law. So we restrict the data to the number of MVA aspirations to see how often MVA was used . . . and also the total number of abortions." Table 4.1 displays data from l'Hôpital Senghor, l'Hôpital Médina, and l'Hôpital de Ville on the total number of PAC patients treated and the percentage treated with MVA. The data show, for the most part, relative stability in the total number of cases treated after an initial increase, and an increase in the percentage of cases treated with MVA. Hospital accounts of PAC yield data that MSAS officials like Mme Niang can use to track and convey to donors and other stakeholders the progress of the national program without specifying what kinds of abortions are being treated. Especially when accountable to donors like USAID that not only "want numbers" but "want to see the numbers go up" (Sullivan, 2017, p. 200), MSAS officials can use these data to add evidentiary (and emotional) heft to the notion that PAC "works" in saving mothers. At the same time, they recognize a legal context of abortion that undermines the collection of reliable abortion statistics.

Dr. Wade, a regional health official, suggested that a focus on process indicators rather than abortion type diverted attention from PAC's connection to illegal abortion. When I asked him why the MSAS did not differentiate between induced and spontaneous abortion, he replied, "No, we can't do it, because abortion is illegal. We can't do it, we can't say that we did induced abortion, it's illegal. If we did something that's illegal, normally people have to do investigations. So we don't differentiate, and the Ministry doesn't either."

I asked: "What about for the purposes of research, to understand the scope of abortion?"

"In that case, you could do a survey, I think," said Dr. Wade. "But we can't make inquiries about this information at the level of the official system."

"Because it's illegal?" I pressed.

"That's the problem with induced abortion," Dr. Wade sighed. "We know it exists but since it's reprehensible, we can't even document it. We can't even say, I saw in such and such facility, that there were so many abortions. Because you're giving information that merits investigation. Giving information about induced

TABLE 4.1. Total abortions and percentage treated with MVA in three hospitals, 2004–2010

	2004		2005		2006		2007		2008		2009		2010	
	N	% MVA	N	% MVA	N	% MVA	N	% MVA	N	% MVA	N	% MVA	N	% MVA
Hôpital Senghor	NA*	NA	377	57.5	531	52.3	582	69.6	451	66.1	456	64.2	405	48.6
Hôpital Médina	121	34.7	160	29.3	211	40.7	248	43.9	339	52.8	415	61.9	384	77.3
Hôpital de Ville	NA	NA	NA	NA	1769	52.1	1743	58.6	1438	65.2	1197	71	678	64.3**

*Data unavailable from annual hospital records.

**This number represents data from January to June 2010. Data for July to December 2010 were unavailable because of the national *rétention des données*, or data strike.

abortion is very problematic, unless it's legalized. If it were legalized, we could do it. If it's not legalized we can't do it."

Like M. Sall, the nurse at a primary health care facility in chapter 3 who asserted that "there can't be any induced abortions" at his facility because of the legal status of the procedure, Dr. Wade preempts the possibility of collecting data on abortion type from government hospitals. His observations about the kinds of data that can be collected illustrate continuities across various levels of the health system in the measures undertaken to strategically manage abortion data. MSAS officials, like health providers in public hospitals, must also fend off inquiries into obstetric care by criminal justice authorities through the manipulation of data. Finally, Dr. Wade suggests how, even among health officials, there remain lingering ambiguities about the conceptual, clinical, and technological boundaries between PAC and induced abortion. Like the health experts who carefully selected process indicators to demonstrate the legitimacy of PAC during the phase of operations research, health officials must carefully collect and interpret hospital data in the routine surveillance of an established reproductive health intervention that remains uncomfortably close to induced abortion.

Second, MSAS officials and NGO personnel readily acknowledged the limitations of national surveys or earlier hospital-based studies in determining the incidence and fatality of induced abortion, and filled in gaps in the data with a "vague gut feeling" (Hunsmann, 2012, p. 1482), based on professional experience, of the scope of abortion. Consider how Dr. Keïta, an official involved in the research sector of the DSR, reflected on the 2005 DHS estimates of the contribution of abortion to maternal mortality:

> In Senegal, abortion complications account for 4 percent of maternal death. So maybe we could say that the number is small, but I think it's as they say, it's the tip of the iceberg, because we know that a lot of abortions happen in the community.... Don't forget also that there are lots of factors that cause these abortions, like malnutrition in adolescents. It's obvious that malaria causes a lot of abortion. But even if people say that there is a lot of unsafe abortion in Senegal, I think that spontaneous abortion takes the cake. There are many factors that can cause it, such as anemia and malaria, and we see that in our country.

While the 2005 DHS estimates the maternal mortality ratio, it does not calculate the contribution of abortion complications to maternal death. At this time, apart from the DHS, there had been no national studies on the causes of maternal mortality in Senegal; thus it is unclear where Dr. Keïta obtained this statistic.[13] Nevertheless, he offered context-specific, "common-sense" (Béhague et al., 2009) information to support his claim that most maternal mortality caused by abortion complications is related to spontaneous abortion.

When I asked M. Gueye, a demographer at a reproductive health research NGO, whether induced abortion was an important factor in maternal mortality and morbidity in Senegal, he expressed reservations: "Quite frankly, I can't say because the research I've done and the research that I've read and consulted doesn't really show that there's a high rate of clandestine abortion. There are no studies that show that there's a high rate and there are no studies that show the burden of abortion. Even if we say it's because of the methodology, I haven't seen any studies that show the contribution of clandestine abortion to maternal mortality and morbidity." Although M. Gueye draws on previous abortion science to bolster his claims about the preponderance of spontaneous abortion, he elides the observations of investigators like Nimbona, F. Diadhiou and colleagues, and Cissé and colleagues regarding the difficulty of differentiating between induced and spontaneous abortion in retrospective reviews of hospital records. Through this claim, he asserts that what appears in hospital records can be understood as a form of truth about the kinds of women treated. Dr. Mane, a physician who worked with a multilateral health organization, expressed a similar understanding of the kinds of abortions treated in hospitals. "It's mostly spontaneous abortion," she told me. "There are induced abortions, but at the level of the public system, it's spontaneous abortions that account for most cases." In this sense, the preferred account of PAC, generated through health workers' clinical and record-keeping practices that obscure suspected cases of induced abortion, accomplishes its goal within and beyond the hospital. By portraying PAC as the medical management of miscarriage, health workers minimize police scrutiny of what happens in the gynecological ward. At the same time, health workers' accounts of PAC are deployed beyond the hospital by MSAS officials and NGO personnel in the establishment of facts regarding what the national PAC program does and whom it treats.

These circular, interpretive logics about the kinds of abortions treated in hospitals reinforce the erasure of induced abortion from PAC. Health officials and NGO stakeholders strategically articulate and obfuscate data (Sullivan, 2017) related to abortion in their efforts to render PAC legible as a safe motherhood intervention. Precisely because of the restrictive abortion law, the MSAS does not require hospitals to differentiate between spontaneous and induced abortion in reports of PAC. Yet, accounts of PAC generated by health workers are widely accepted by PAC experts as accurate representations of the types of complications treated in hospitals. If induced abortion is not legible in the record, it does not exist in the hospital. Record-keeping practices across multiple levels of the national health information system, in tandem with flexible logics of interpretation about what happens in hospitals, engender the portrayal of PAC as an intervention concerned primarily with treating complications of miscarriage. These interpretations of data are not simply mundane forms of public health work.

FIGURE 4.1. Abortions treated in three hospitals over twenty-four months between 2009 and 2010.

Instead, by producing selective narratives about the kinds of women treated in hospitals (expectant mothers), these practices reinforce gendered and classed expectations of sexuality, fertility, and the circumstances under which women may legitimately seek obstetric care.

Finally, practicing health workers, like health officials and NGO stakeholders, also exercise local, commonsense scientific knowledge about their patient population in their interpretation of the kinds of abortions treated in hospitals. Diseases such as anemia and malaria are known to increase the risk of miscarriage (Curtis, 2007). In 2017, an estimated 54 percent of Senegalese women were anemic (compared with 28% of men), and over half (68%) of pregnant women were anemic (ANSD and ICF, 2018). Only 62 percent of pregnant women sleep under mosquito nets (ANSD and ICF, 2018). Health professionals' perceptions of the frequency of miscarriage among pregnant women owing to such diseases reinforced the notion that most PAC cases are due to miscarriage. Many believed the risk of miscarriage was elevated during the rainy season, when women were more likely to be exposed to mosquitoes infected with malaria. When I shared figure 4.1, which displays abortion cases over a period of twenty-four months at the three study hospitals, with health providers at l'Hôpital de Ville, several pointed out that at all three facilities, the number of cases increased during the months of the rainy season (roughly between June and October) and declined precipitously during the dry season (roughly between November and April).

Such commonsense explanations for abortion draw simultaneously on scientific evidence regarding the causes of miscarriage and gendered notions of motherhood as vulnerable and in need of protection, thereby aligning the treatment of incomplete abortion with national and global discourse regarding the need to keep mothers safe.

Despite common understandings of the frequency of miscarriage within their patient population, the professional threat of induced abortion loomed large in health workers' professional imaginations. When Dr. Fall, the senior gynecologist at l'Hôpital de Ville, saw this graph, he explained that his hospital treated nearly three times as many cases as the others because his facility was located in a more densely populated area.[14] Still, he expressed considerable unease with the graph, urging me to explain the broader demographic context when sharing it with others. Otherwise, I risked portraying the hospital to MSAS officials and NGO stakeholders as a place "where all they do is treat abortions." His concerns revealed that nearly twenty years after the introduction of PAC to Senegal, health workers continued to negotiate public and professional anxieties about the slippage between the treatment of incomplete abortion and induced abortion in government hospitals.[15]

The Impact of PAC

Although PAC indicators can reveal progress in meeting hospital-based targets, they are less helpful in estimating whether and to what degree PAC services lead to a reduction in abortion-related mortality. The omission of data on abortion type further complicates the possibility of calculating the contribution of induced abortion to maternal mortality. Consequently, health professionals have used a combination of population data, program indicators, and anecdotal information to estimate the impact of PAC on maternal mortality.

National estimates of maternal mortality have been generated by DHS conducted in 2005 and in 2010–2011, which yielded maternal mortality ratios of 434 and 392 deaths per 100,000 live births, respectively (N'Diaye and Ayad, 2006; ANSD and ICF International, 2012). The 2017 DHS estimates the maternal mortality ratio at 273 deaths per 100,000 live births (ANSD and ICF, 2018). Although these estimates suggest that maternal mortality has declined, they do not indicate the percentage of maternal deaths that can be attributed to abortion. The maternal mortality ratio was calculated using an indirect survey technique known as the "sisterhood" method of verbal autopsy, in which people provide information about sisters who have died during pregnancy or childbirth.[16] This technique does not specifically inquire about abortion. In fact, by requiring respondents to establish that the woman was pregnant at or around the time of death, this method may systematically underreport abortion deaths. It may also lead to underestimation of deaths related to ectopic or early pregnancy. In places with strict abortion laws and high levels of abortion stigma, people may be reluctant to report abortion-related deaths in sisterhood verbal autopsy surveys of maternal mortality (Aa, Grove, Haugsjå, and Hinderaker, 2011; Doctor, Findley, and Afenyadu, 2012; Olsen et al., 2000).

Still, health authorities and NGO personnel used commonsense knowledge about program data to attribute part of this decline in maternal mortality to PAC. They explained that greater access to and availability of PAC, through sensitizing communities, training health providers, and decentralizing services to lower levels of the health system, had reduced mortality related to abortion. Mme Camara, a district health official in the second study region, spoke enthusiastically about training health workers to sensitize communities on early referral of women to health centers. "This has reduced the complications of abortion," she said, "because now everyone who has bleeding or after a lateness comes to the health facilities. So we can prevent complications." Mme Camara offers a grassroots or "bottom-up" (Jaffré and Suh, 2016) public health success story. By increasing awareness of obstetric danger signs at the community level, measures can be implemented, such as transportation systems, that ensure rapid referral of women to health facilities equipped to handle complications. Consequently, the risk of mortality or morbidity from abortion complications is lowered. Omitted from this narrative, however, is any baseline measure that would facilitate calculation of the extent to which complications have been reduced over time. Additionally, it is unclear where Mme Camara has observed this decline in complications: in the hospital (which would account only for women who seek treatment) or in the larger population.[17]

Dr. Sané, a physician who worked with a health NGO funded by USAID at the time of my fieldwork but had previously been a care provider at a regional hospital, echoed Mme Camara's description of the public health impact of PAC when she explained: "There are many more places now where complications can be treated. In 2005, when I was working in Region X,[18] it was only done at the hospital. Now, there are nine health centers in the region that can do it. The technology has been decentralized. And by 2009, we were receiving fewer complications at the hospital. Even the mortality rate related to abortion complications has gone down. It's not so high anymore." In contrast to Mme Camara, Dr. Sané identified the regional hospital as the site of an observed decline in abortion-related complications and mortality. Although she convincingly illustrated how this decline could be generated by the distribution of patients to other facilities equipped with MVA, she cannot estimate the extent to which abortion complications or mortality has declined within the larger population.

For some health professionals, community-based work played an important role in reducing abortion-related mortality. According to Mme Diakhaté, a member of a USAID-contracted NGO that focused on child welfare, the organization's community-based work was accomplished in the form of "conferences, sensitization campaigns, songs, slogans, poems, and skits." When I asked her to describe the results of these activities, she explained that their community agents had reported important "progress" in reducing cases of abortion complications: "They say that when you do an evaluation in certain zones, there's been a reduction [of cases], or there aren't any more. It's a bit premature to say this, but we go by these statements." Similar to Mme Camara and Mme Sané, Mme Diakhaté notes an impact without specifying a denominator for abortion complications: Were reductions observed in villages, hospitals, or health districts? Additionally, she does not specify who is observing these reductions (community agents, health workers, or health officials), or the period of time over which this decline occurred.

High-level officials in the DSR acknowledged a lack of data that showed a statistical association between reduced mortality and PAC. They drew on empirical information from hospitals and districts to bolster claims that PAC "worked." Dr. Keïta, who worked in the research sector of the DSR, explained: "I suppose that when there's a greater offering of services, there is improvement, but currently there aren't health statistics to prove this." One reason for a lack of PAC data was the rétention des données that took place from July 2010 to March 2013, in which health workers, demanding better working conditions, withheld patient data from the MSAS while performing their routine duties (Tichenor, 2016). Nevertheless, Dr. Keïta believed that a situational analysis of unsafe abortion conducted between April and May 2010, in collaboration with Ipas and WHO (DSR, 2010), illustrated the impact of PAC: "Providers told us that there's an improvement in PAC services, and the MVA syringes are available. Even the health committees[19] are purchasing them. This leads to an improvement of services."

Dr. Ndiaye, another high-level official of the DSR, concurred with Dr. Keïta's assessment and offered additional anecdotal evidence to support claims that PAC effectively reduced abortion-related mortality: "It's been a long time since we've had these statistics, but in a general fashion, people really appreciate these services in the health facilities. I think it relieves them. I rarely hear nowadays of cases of mortality or morbidity related to abortion. We are in the process of going in the right direction. I don't have the data to say things have changed between 2009 and 2010, but I can say in an empirical sense that things are evolving in the right direction." In the absence of statistics, word-of-mouth reports of lowered rates of abortion-related mortality and morbidity—or no reports at all—signaled the impact of PAC. Similar to other health workers, health officials, and NGO stakeholders, Dr. Ndiaye relied on a hunch, drawn from his experience as a health professional, that maternal mortality due to abortion must be on the decline.

In a global health landscape where donors increasingly prioritize health initiatives that can demonstrate a statistical association between an intervention and improved health outcomes, these observations reveal a striking degree of ambiguity in the "facts" (V. Adams, 2005) that are deployed to convey PAC's effectiveness. The operations research conducted between the late 1990s and the mid-2000s entailed quasi-experimental projects[20] rather than RCTs. Although these projects yielded data that permitted the MSAS to measure the impact of PAC by "counting" (V. Adams, 2013) how many women had been treated, they could not demonstrate that the intervention reduced abortion-related mortality. In other words, because there was no randomization of study hospitals or study subjects, there was no way to prove that any reduction observed was due to the intervention or other unmeasured variables. Health professionals extrapolated reductions in maternal mortality and morbidity loosely in terms of increased coverage of services and both an increase and decrease in the number of abortion complications treated in hospitals.

Remarkably, PAC advocates have translated these quasi-experimental data, and even anecdotal accounts—the "worst" kind of evidence in the world of science (V. Adams, 2013)—into a narrative of PAC's impact on maternal mortality that has secured programming contracts with at least nine international NGOs that have provided critical technical and financial support for technologies and services throughout the country since the late 1990s. Among these NGOs, six received funding from USAID to support the MSAS in scaling up PAC. In 2002, Senegal joined the Francophone Regional Post-Abortion Care Initiative, a global consortium of organizations involved in safe motherhood, including thirteen international health NGOs, USAID, the Swedish International Development Cooperation, and the Rockefeller, Ford, and Packard Foundations. Senegal hosted a regional meeting the same year to disseminate lessons learned from PAC programming in four countries that was attended by over 200 representatives from fourteen African countries and international organizations (Thiam, Suh, and Moreira, 2006). A year later, in 2003, Senegal was one of seven countries selected by USAID to receive funding to support the expansion and institutionalization of PAC over a period of five years (Curtis, 2007). In October 2013, Senegal hosted a second regional meeting for disseminating lessons learned from PAC, with seventy-six representatives from eight African countries in attendance. Throughout the West African region, Senegal is known as a "pioneer" of PAC because of the Ministry's pragmatic approach to introducing, scaling up, and institutionalizing these services (M. Diadhiou et al., 2008; Dieng, Diadhiou, Diop, and Faye, 2008).

In addition to securing donor funding for PAC and highlighting Senegal's role as a PAC leader in the region, PAC data enact reproductive governance by suppressing political will to engage in reform of the abortion law. Dr. Ndiaye, a high-ranking DSR official, told me that "in Senegal, I'm not sure that we're ready to adopt a law that will authorize abortion generally." Although he did not rule out the possibility of legal reform, he believed that "there was fundamental work that has to be done," and "that it will take time." M. Malick Ibnou Anass Camara, a Senegalese judge who has presided over cases of infanticide, expressed support for abortion law reform in a 2017 interview with *The New Yorker*. At the same time, he echoed Dr. Ndiaye's cautious approach to legal change, calling for "strict conditions" because "we must not leave the door open for abortion anarchy" (Gaestel and Shryock, 2017). Similarly, health workers and health officials in Burkina Faso believed that their society was "not ready" for abortion law reform, not only because of religious opposition but also because of the health system's limited capacity to provide safe services (Storeng and Ouattara, 2014).

Expatriate PAC stakeholders explained that people supported PAC because it was less controversial than legal reform. "People are steeped in PAC," Dr. Jones, a regional official of an international reproductive health NGO, explained to me, "especially in Francophone Africa." Dr. Ayo, also a regional official of a reproductive health NGO, believed that PAC data could show that "people have been trained," that "equipment has been procured here and there," and that "maybe severe morbidity has been reduced to some extent." These data, he argued, had "blinded countries, because people think that now that they are providing PAC they don't need to do anything more."

A conversation with M. Mbacké, the director of a national demographic research NGO, revealed how PAC data exercise reproductive governance by shaping perceptions of the kinds of interventions that effectively reduce maternal mortality. For M. Mbacké, the decline in the maternal mortality ratio from 435 to 320 maternal deaths per 100,000 live births between 2005 and 2010 indicated that PAC could reduce maternal mortality *without* reforming the abortion law. "I'm not sure that in Senegal, even if we have a good PAC program, that it means that we will eventually legalize abortion," he explained. "I think it's not related. You can have a good PAC program that has been implemented and accepted, with quality services and with results on the impact on maternal mortality without a revision."[21]

Despite a lack of statistical precision, PAC data have been carefully negotiated by health workers, health officials, and NGO stakeholders in ways that demonstrate their accountability to national and global safe motherhood discourses and policies. Data from hospitals convey that the imperative to reduce the maternal mortality ratio is being carefully addressed: health workers have been trained, health facilities have been equipped, and complications of abortion are being treated. Numbers related to these indicators may go up or down, but they offer political credibility to PAC by showing that things are being "done" (Hunsmann, 2012; Sullivan, 2017). At the same time, interpretations of PAC's effectiveness suppress political will to move beyond harm reduction, thereby foreclosing opportunities to engage in processes of abortion law reform observed in other African countries such as the Democratic Republic of Congo, Ethiopia, Mozambique, and Rwanda (PRB, 2020; Rwirahira, 2018; Durr, 2015; Guttmacher Institute, 2012; Holcombe, Berhe, and Cherie, 2015).

CONCLUSION

This chapter has explored the practical and political complexities of interpreting PAC data in Senegal. Similar to other contexts in sub-Saharan Africa (Biruk, 2012; Geissler, 2013; Hunsmann, 2012; Jaffré, 2012; McKay, 2012; Rossier, Guiella, Oué-draogo, and Thiéba, 2006; Sullivan, 2017), Senegalese hospital and health system data are often imperfect, and part of the process of producing evidence for policy making involves filling in gaps with estimates and less "scientific" information such as hunches and anecdotes. At times, the production of evidence unfolds through deliberately obscuring what happens in hospitals and the kinds of patients who seek care. The production and interpretation of data co-constitute health gover-nance through generating evidence of the kinds of interventions that work and should therefore be scaled up, and the kinds of women who will benefit from (and are deserving of) these services.

The strategies undertaken by PAC experts in Senegal to deploy data are part of a longer global health project of maternal mortality reduction, in which evidence of what "works" has significantly narrowed to hospital-based, vertical interventions that can approximate RCTs in their production of rigorous statisti-cal metrics. Hospital statistics—and national indicators like maternal mortality ratios that are often derived from unwieldy estimates—take on a social life of their own as they are deployed to demonstrate commitment to national and global frameworks for reducing maternal death. Since the late 1970s, a neoliberal rationale for "investing" in health, in tandem with increasingly anti-abortion reproductive health funding policies from the United States, has narrowed the scope of women worth saving to those who are already or expect to become mothers.

Although the PAC model legitimated abortion as a cause of maternal death within the global SMI, in Senegal it led to a shift in the kinds of evidence that mattered in addressing abortion-related mortality and morbidity. Starting in the mid-1980s, reproductive health experts in Senegal attempted to increase the vis-ibility of induced abortion as a clinical, legal, and social problem. They were interested not only in finding more effective ways to manage abortion complica-tions but also in identifying the reasons why women ended up in hospitals with complications of unsafe abortion in the first place. With the introduction of the global PAC model, the MSAS narrowed the focus of data collection to hospitals' capacity to treat de-identified abortion complications. Selective interpreta-tions of these data have fetishized the extent to which the intervention works. In turn, the MSAS has been rewarded by donor agencies and NGOs with financial and technical support for more PAC services and technologies throughout the country.

Despite the impressive national scale-up of PAC, significant gaps remain between what PAC indicators purportedly measure and the social realities of abortion and obstetric care for women patients. These gaps raise troubling questions about whether and how PAC works, and for whom. If we think about *what* counts from the perspective of an increasingly "technocratic" (Storeng and Béhague, 2014), hospital-based SMI, an increase in PAC indicators such as the total number of patients (read: expectant mothers) treated and the percentage of patients treated with MVA conveys impact. While these indicators represent simple counts rather than statistical measures of effectiveness, they suggest that PAC is reaching the community. And without a doubt, PAC is "better than bad" (Roe, 2005): no emergency treatment for abortion complications at all.

But if we are interested in *who* counts in reproductive health, a different kind of "truth" (V. Adams, 2005) about PAC, and about what it does and does *not* do in hospitals and health systems, comes into view. Although Dr. Perez recognized how PAC offered new opportunities for measuring and acting on abortion-related complications within the global field of reproductive health, she also highlighted its limitations as a form of harm reduction:

> But you know that post-abortion care is actually an indicator of failure, right? Something has failed the woman if she is seeking post-abortion care.... It is completely inadequate. Post-abortion care is an indicator that a woman did not get the information that she needed. She didn't find the contraception she needed. She did not find the safe abortion care she needed. And because of those factors and many others, she has actually . . . resorted to an unsafe means of terminating a pregnancy. And that's why she's a post-abortion care case. Post-abortion care is a colossal, systemic failure. It's an emergency, and you shouldn't be having this number of thousands of emergencies like this.

For Dr. Perez and other stakeholders from international NGOs, PAC was a "failure" because it represented a curative response to a preventable health problem. Each PAC patient represented gaps in the health system that failed to provide women with affordable contraception and safe abortion that would prevent the need for EmOC following an unsafe clandestine abortion.

In Senegal, PAC has proliferated significant amounts of data that have linked health professionals to a global field of maternal and reproductive health dominated by influential donors who do not support abortion as a reproductive right. These data have simultaneously obfuscated the material reality of reproduction in which many women, regardless of marital status or obstetric parity, seek to terminate unwanted or ill-timed pregnancies, but few can afford safe, discreet abortions. Instead, selective interpretations of hospital data suggest that most PAC patients are expectant mothers who have experienced miscarriage. As a model of reproductive health care, PAC has reduced women's embodied experiences with pregnancy and abortion to hospital metrics that can be used to measure the capacity of the health system to keep them alive. PAC metrics offer little insight into how obstetric violence unfolds in maternity wards through the interrogation of patients, delays in care, and the persistence of digital evacuation. PAC represents a profoundly unjust form of reproductive governance in which women's reproductive bodies, experiences, and choices do not count until after the emergence of life-threatening obstetric complications that can be mundanely recorded and managed as miscarriage, and ultimately fetishized as markers of commitment to national and global road maps for reducing maternal mortality.

CONCLUSION
Evidence, Harm Reduction, and Reproductive Justice

In July 2019, nearly ten years after the completion of my fieldwork, I returned to Senegal to conduct exploratory research on misoprostol and reproductive health care. Through my conversations with representatives of NGOs and the DSR, I learned of recent changes in PAC norms and protocols to improve women's access to quality obstetric care. First, although MVA remains outside of the PNA, the MSAS has authorized MVA use by both midwives and nurses in primary health care facilities. Second, health facilities may purchase new MVA kits directly from DKT International, an NGO that specializes in social marketing of reproductive health commodities. Between 2018 and 2019, DKT sold over 1,300 MVA kits in Senegal (DKT International, 2018). A 2016 national survey of health services suggests that these revisions in PAC protocols have led to greater availability of MVA throughout the health system: an estimated 73 percent of facilities (including national hospitals, district hospitals, and primary health care facilities) reported the provision of MVA services in the past three months (ANSD and ICF, 2016). When I asked Mme Niang, a midwife and MSAS official, about digital evacuation, she told me with confidence that this technique had been effectively "banished" from Senegalese health facilities.

These changes in PAC policy suggest that Senegalese health authorities remain accountable to the continuing significance of PAC in global efforts to reduce maternal mortality and morbidity. In 2016, the journal *Global Health: Science and Practice* published a review of over 500 studies on PAC, published between 1994 and 2013, that concluded there was "strong evidence" that the intervention improved organization and quality of obstetric care, increased uptake of post-abortion family planning, and raised awareness of obstetric emergencies within the community (Huber, Curtis, Irani, Pappa, and Arrington, 2016). In 2018, an article published in the *Lancet Global Health* identified PAC as a "missed opportunity" for improving women's reproductive health and urged governments to increase provision of quality PAC

(Temmerman, 2018). Senegal was among ten developing countries included in a survey of PAC between 2007 and 2017 that revealed persistent gaps in the quality and availability of PAC worldwide (Owolabi, Biddlecom, and Whitehead, 2018).

As long as access to safe abortion is restricted, PAC is needed to reduce the burden of abortion-related mortality and morbidity. And in a global health landscape where the most influential donor of reproductive health aid, the U.S. government, has demonstrated unprecedented hostility to abortion outside the United States, PAC has never mattered more as a politically acceptable intervention for the reduction of abortion-related mortality. On his third day in office in January 2017, President Donald Trump not only reinstated the Mexico City Policy (despite a lack of evidence that it achieves its goal of reducing abortion incidence in countries that receive family planning aid from USAID) but also extended it to NGOs that receive USAID funding for treatment and prevention of infectious diseases like HIV, Zika, malaria, and TB (J. Singh and Karim, 2017). In his remarks to the UN General Assembly Press in September 2019, Alex M. Azar II, the secretary of health and human services and U.S. representative to the UN High Level Meeting on Universal Health Coverage, reminded the global community that "there is no international right to an abortion and these terms should not be used to promote pro-abortion policies and measures" (Health and Human Services, 2019). These remarks were later developed into a Joint Statement on Universal Health Coverage that was signed by twenty-one countries[1] in advance of the twenty-fifth anniversary of the ICPD in Nairobi, Kenya, in November 2019.

Several months into the global COVID-19 crisis of 2020, the Trump administration threatened to defund the UN's Global Humanitarian Response to the global pandemic because of its alleged "promotion" of abortion. On May 18, 2020, President Trump wrote to Dr. Tedros Adhanom Ghebreyesus, director general of WHO, and threatened to withdraw U.S. funding from the organization because of its "failed response" to the COVID-19 crisis (Borger and Rourke, 2020). The same day, John Marsa, acting administrator of USAID, sent a letter to António Guterres, UN secretary-general, reminding him of the role of the United States as the "largest donor of global health and humanitarian assistance" and noting USAID's contribution of $650.7 million to combat the pandemic. Marsa argued that the UN was using the global pandemic to "promote abortion" as an "essential service" by "cynically placing the provision of 'sexual and reproductive health services' on the same level of importance as food-insecurity, essential health care, malnutrition, shelter, and sanitation" and by supporting "the widespread distribution of abortion-inducing drugs and abortion supplies." The letter demanded that the UN "remove references to 'sexual and reproductive health' and its derivatives from the Global Humanitarian Response, and drop the provision of abortion as an essential component of the UN's priorities to respond to the COVID-19 pandemic" (USAID, 2020). Despite the U.S. government's mounting hostility to abortion outside the United States, PAC remains exempt from the Mexico City Policy because it entails obstetric care after women have experienced abortion. Even in places where abortion is permitted under certain circumstances, PAC may represent the only form of abortion care that can be legitimately connected to maternal and reproductive health initiatives eligible for USAID funding.

In this book, I have shown that while PAC demonstrates public health impact, or "works," by keeping women alive, it does not achieve reproductive justice. PAC exposes women, and young, unmarried, and low-income women in particular, to discriminatory treatment by health workers and the threat of criminalization. While some health workers may protect their patients from the police by misclassifying suspected cases of illegal abortion as miscarriage, in the long run these recording practices generate an epidemiological account of PAC that suppresses political will to revise a colonial-era abortion law that abandons the most vulnerable women to clandestine, unsafe procedures. Efforts to keep MVA syringes secure, both at the national level and in health facilities, have compromised the quality of PAC, exposing women to digital evacuation, overused syringes, and delays in care, and have transferred the cost of referral from primary health care facilities to hospitals to women and their families. Despite widespread acceptance of PAC as a harm reduction intervention, PAC harms socially and economically vulnerable women in contexts with restrictive abortion laws.

PAC is not only harmful but also extremely expensive for hospitals, health systems, women, and their families. An estimated $232 million is spent on PAC every year in developing countries (S. Singh and Maddow-Zimet, 2016). In sub-Saharan Africa alone, the cost of PAC is estimated at $117 million a year (Vlassoff, Shearer, Walker, and Lucas, 2008). In Ethiopia, PAC costs amounted to $47 million in 2008 (Vlassoff, Fetters, Kumbi, and Singh, 2012). A study in Zambia found that women paid 2.5 times more for PAC than for safe abortion (Parmar et al., 2017). A study in Nigeria estimated that women paid nearly four times more for PAC than for safe abortion (Henshaw et al., 2008). In Uganda, PAC patients reported experiencing a loss of economic productivity and a deterioration in their economic circumstances, and observed negative consequences for their children (Sundaram et al., 2013).

In 2016, the average cost of PAC for Senegalese patients was $24.72, and they shouldered 20 percent of all health system costs for PAC in the form of fees. The average cost of PAC does not account for other, nonmedical costs such as transportation, child care, and lost wages due to missed work. Considering that the legal minimum hourly wage in Senegal is under a dollar, PAC poses an enormous financial burden on economically vulnerable women and their families. The cost of providing PAC in Senegal in 2016 was nearly $500,000. This underestimates the cost of PAC if the health system were providing care to all those who need it.

An estimated 42 percent of women with complications of abortion do not receive medical treatment. If these women's PAC needs were met, the annual cost of PAC would be more than $800,000 (Lince-Deroche, Sène, Pliskin, Owolabi, and Bankole, 2020).

While PAC's contribution to maternal mortality reduction may be difficult to quantify, global health experts have long been aware of the public health impact of safe, legal abortion. Very little abortion mortality occurs in countries where abortion is broadly legal. Data from developed countries (United States, England, Sweden, and Romania) suggest that access to safe abortion leads to declines in abortion mortality. More recently, declines in abortion mortality have followed abortion law reform in countries such as Nepal, Guyana, and South Africa (Faúndes and Shah, 2015). In South Africa, where abortion was legalized upon request in 1996, abortion-related mortality declined by 91 percent between 1994 and 2001 (Guttmacher Institute, 2012). Three years after Ethiopia relaxed its abortion law in 2005, a study estimated that a little over 25 percent of all pregnancy terminations were safely and legally performed in health facilities (Guttmacher Institute, 2012). Several studies have found reductions in abortion-related deaths in Ethiopia since the early 1990s (Berhan and Berhan, 2014; Tessema et al., 2017).

It should come as no surprise that existing evidence on abortion and maternal mortality has not been translated widely into relaxed abortion laws to improve women's access to safe procedures and reduce the cost of PAC. Even in wealthy countries like the United States, where abortion mortality plummeted after the legalization of abortion in 1973, individual states continue to propose and enact laws that restrict women's access to services (R. Jones and Jerman, 2017). The pathway between evidence and policy making is hardly linear, but rather a highly political process in which various actors negotiate what counts as evidence (V. Adams, 2013; Lambert, 2013; Parkhurst, Ettelt, and Hawkins, 2018), and data are manipulated— "cooked" (Biruk, 2018) or deliberately "unknown" (Geissler, 2013)—to attract donor support in a highly competitive global health landscape and to meet the objectives of national and global stakeholders. Biruk's (2018) study of HIV/AIDS data in Malawi demonstrates how "good, clean" data, normally the gold standard for evidence-based policy making, may at times lose favor over less reliable data that resonate more closely with local forms of knowledge about risk groups and practices. In Zambia, despite a relatively permissive abortion law, provincial and district data on abortion and PAC are scarce, while indicators directly associated with the SDGs, such as the maternal mortality ratio, facility deliveries, and contraceptive use, are widely deployed by health professionals and officials (Haaland, Haukanes, Zulu, Moland, and Blystad, 2020).

PAC data in Senegal cannot definitively establish that the intervention contributes to maternal mortality reduction; additionally, they offer limited insight into the quality of care. Although the 2016 report showing that 73 percent of health facilities have MVA (ANSD and ICF, 2016) is encouraging, these data say little about how many (functional) devices are available at each facility or the percentage of PAC patients that are treated with digital evacuation. When I asked Mme Sankharé, a midwife who used to work with the MSAS and now worked with an international NGO, whether digital evacuation had indeed been banished from health facilities, she said she suspected it still happened in facilities that lacked MVA syringes or staff trained in MVA.

My conversation with a representative of DKT International, which now sells MVA syringes directly to health facilities, raised further questions about the extent to which this new supply system has contributed to improved quality of care in health facilities. Although DKT International has sold an impressive number of syringes, the individual acknowledged that sales occur primarily in urban areas in a select group of administrative regions. In rural areas, or even in urban zones far away from DKT International's headquarters in Dakar, health facilities may still struggle to renew MVA syringes in a timely fashion, meaning that women may still be exposed to overused syringes, delays in care, and digital evacuation. Additionally, lingering concerns about keeping MVA secure may discourage timely renewal of the device. The individual revealed that the organization was required to send the DSR a list of health facilities that had purchased the device.

Despite these shortcomings, PAC data serve an important political purpose by establishing facts about what PAC technologies do in hospitals and the kinds of abortions that are treated by PAC services. These facts demonstrate PAC stakeholders' accountability to various regimes of reproductive governance, including the national prohibition on abortion, the government's commitment to global accords on maternal and reproductive health, and the Mexico City Policy. Data showing that something is being "done" about life-threatening abortion complications, deployed alongside data suggesting that most PAC patients have experienced miscarriage rather than induced abortion, exercise power by foreclosing opportunities to revise the national abortion law. In other words, these data enact reproductive governance by establishing claims not only about what works in reducing maternal death but also about the kind of care that Senegalese women are entitled to. PAC data and counting techniques allow people to "see exactly what they intend to see" (Biruk, 2012, p. 348) about the kinds of obstetric services that should be in place. Yet another striking example of these pragmatic PAC counting techniques is the absence of digital evacuation in national and global accounts of PAC (Suh, 2020), despite the persistence of this technique in daily practice described in chapter 2.

Calls for more PAC (Temmerman, 2018), despite a lack of "gold standard" evidence that it works in reducing maternal death, reveal how PAC data open up considerable professional, financial, and technological opportunities to a variety of national and global stakeholders. Here, I am reminded of anthropologist Susan Erikson's (2015) advice to "follow the money" in the financing of global health programs and commodities to determine who benefits, and how, and the extent to which global health interventions strengthen or erode public health systems and improve or threaten access to quality health care services. Since the introduction of PAC to Senegal in the late 1990s, at least nine international NGOs have collaborated with Senegalese health authorities on PAC training, services, provision, or equipment distribution. In 2003, Senegal was one of seven countries that received special funding from USAID to implement its global PAC strategy.

Although contraception has been a fundamental component of PAC since the inception of the global model in the early 1990s, more recently there has been interest in harnessing the intervention toward the achievement of global and national family planning targets related to FP 2020. In response to advocacy by USAID showing increased contraceptive uptake following PAC in fifteen countries, the Gates Foundation incorporated post-abortion family planning into its approach (Curtis et al., 2019). Senegal was one of several testing sites in sub-Saharan Africa for Sayana Press, a self-injectable LARC that has been promoted by FP 2020. As a member of the Ouagadougou Partnership, Senegal benefited from a special low price ($0.85/dose) for FP 2020 countries, negotiated with Pfizer by the Gates Foundation (Bendix, Foley, Hendrixson, and Schultz, 2019).

Senegal's extension of Sayana Press to lower levels of the health system, like its extension of PAC from tertiary to district hospitals and primary health care facilities, is heralded as a "success story" in the region (Intrahealth, 2018). In 2017, injectables accounted for an estimated 37.8 percent of Senegal's contraceptive method mix. Since the launching of FP 2020 in 2012, Senegal's modern contraceptive prevalence rate has doubled not only among married women but among all women (Track20, 2019).[2] Undoubtedly, this contraceptive success story has benefited organizations involved in the sale and social marketing of contraceptive technologies. PATH[3] and Marie Stopes International (MSI)[4] were involved in the administration of 120,861 doses of Sayana Press between 2014 and 2016 (nearly 500,000 doses were administered in Senegal, Uganda, Burkina Faso, and Niger during this time) (PATH, 2018). Between 2017 and 2018, DKT International (2018) sold 4,524 IUDs in Senegal.

At the same time that PAC offers lucrative links to recently reinvigorated interest in global family planning, it also offers a critical entry point to self-managed or medication abortion as the latest frontier of abortion-related harm reduction. Misoprostol, manufactured under the brand name Cytotec by Pfizer, has been available on the global market for treating gastric ulcers since the 1980s. Misoprostol may also be used for obstetric purposes, including PAC, labor induction, treatment and prevention of PPH, and termination of first-trimester pregnancy. The drug has been on WHO's LEM, along with mifepristone, for abortion since 2005. WHO placed misoprostol on its LEM for treatment of incomplete abortion in 2009 and prevention and treatment of PPH in 2011 and 2015, respectively. In 2018, WHO's manual for the medical management of abortion recognized misoprostol alone as an alternative to the recommended combination treatment (mifepristone and misoprostol) for both treatment of incomplete abortion and termination of pregnancy. Increasingly available at lower cost under generic brands, misoprostol does not require refrigeration (when stored in its original blister packaging), can be administered by nonphysicians, and requires no anesthesia, sterilization, or equipment. In response to data from various countries showing that misoprostol reduced the rate and severity of complications related to unsafe abortion, global reproductive health advocates have framed the medication as a harm reduction response to improve women's health, especially in low-resource settings (Erdman, Jelinska, and Yanow, 2018; Hyman, Blanchard, Coeytaux, Grossman, and Teixeira, 2013; Kulczycki, 2016).

Senegalese health authorities have collaborated with international NGOs since the late 2000s to test the effectiveness of misoprostol for PAC and PPH (M. Diadhiou et al., 2011; Diop et al., 2016; Gaye, Diop, Shochet, and Winikoff, 2014; Schochet et al., 2012). In 2011, MSI registered a form of misoprostol under the name Misoclear with the Senegalese government. DKT International is also in the process of registering its version of misoprostol in Senegal (and various other West African countries). In 2013, the government placed misoprostol on its national LEM for labor induction, management of PPH, and PAC. Given the national prohibition on abortion, termination of pregnancy is not among the authorized obstetric indications for which misoprostol may be used. Nevertheless, several health professionals expressed to me during my fieldwork, and during my most recent visit to Senegal in July 2019, that women were using misoprostol, obtained from health workers, private pharmacies, or informal pharmaceutical vendors, to induce abortions. Some health workers believed that misoprostol was responsible, in part, for reductions in the number of "flagrant" complications of unsafe abortion, such as uterine perforation, treated in government hospitals.

Like MVA, misoprostol can be used by midlevel providers at primary health care facilities for PAC. Unlike MVA, misoprostol has been integrated into the PNA, meaning that it can be procured directly from regional and district depots rather than purchased from distributors like DKT International. The incorporation of misoprostol into public and private supply systems has contributed to sales of reproductive commodities. According to a report commissioned by the Reproductive Health Supplies Coalition, MSI sold at least 514,800 tablets of misoprostol in Senegal between 2017 and 2018 (Mann Global Health, 2019). Although I could not find sales data specific to Senegal, DKT International (2018) sold over 15 million units of misoprostol worldwide in 2018.

Despite these important developments in misoprostol as a form of harm reduction, a restrictive national abortion law means that women and health workers still face significant barriers in accessing misoprostol for abortion and PAC. Although misoprostol can be procured through the PNA, a 2015–2016 survey of obstetric care revealed that only 3.4 percent of referral facilities carried the drug (MSAS, CEFOREP, and UNFPA, 2017). A 2013 study conducted among pharmacists in Dakar found that despite high levels of knowledge about misoprostol (72% had heard of the drug), only 35 percent of pharmacists stocked the drug. Furthermore, most misoprostol sales were related to gastric ulcers (70%), with only 8 percent of sales related to PAC or abortion (Reiss et al., 2017). Concerns about legal restrictions on abortion contribute significantly to pharmacists' reluctance to stock misoprostol, let alone sell it for the purposes of abortion. At least one pharmacist has reportedly been imprisoned for selling misoprostol to a nurse with a fake prescription, who gave the medication to a woman who later died of complications (Mann Global Health, 2019).

Even if women are able to obtain misoprostol, with or without a prescription, they may not receive accurate information about dosage and gestational limits. Data from low- and middle-income countries suggest that women often receive inaccurate information about misoprostol (Footman et al., 2018). Recent studies from Tanzania (Solheim, Moland, Kahabuka, Pembe, and Blystad, 2020), Burkina Faso (Drabo, 2019), Brazil (De Zordo, 2016), and Kenya (Izugbara, Egesa, and Okelo, 2015) illustrate that low-income women are at greater risk of receiving incorrect information or fake medication that lead to complications, thereby increasing the likelihood that they will end up in government hospitals in need of PAC. It seems reasonable to assume that in Senegal, rural and low-income women face similar barriers to accessing quality services and information related to misoprostol (Suh, 2019).

Here, I return to Mbembe's concept of necropower (Mbembe and Meintjes, 2003) to highlight the imbrications of violence and care in PAC as a model of maternal health harm reduction. The global PAC model promised to reduce harm related to clandestine, unsafe abortion. FP 2020 frames family planning, including post-abortion family planning, as a way of averting pregnancies that might result in unsafe abortions or maternal deaths. For example, in 2019, FP 2020 estimated that contraceptive use in Senegal would avert 112,000 unsafe abortions and 690 maternal deaths. Self-managed abortion has been framed by global reproductive health NGOs such as Ipas as a form of harm reduction against unsafe abortion, with PAC as a backup if complications arise.

Women's health is only one—and not always the first—consideration in the achievement of national and global targets related to maternal and reproductive health, recognition of good health governance in the global community, and the expansion of pharmaceutical markets. Regardless of the national abortion law—or perhaps because of it—pharmaceutical companies, NGOs, government health authorities, and other national and global stakeholders benefit from harm reduction research and programming for Senegalese women who represent new populations for clinical experimentation on contraceptive and abortive technology and are actual or potential consumers of commodities and services related to family planning, PAC, and delivery care. Although maternal health harm reduction in the form of technological magic bullets (misoprostol, MVA, and LARCs) keeps women alive, it does not necessarily translate into quality health care. In fact, Leigh Senderowicz's (2019) study of family planning in an unidentified country in sub-Saharan Africa illustrates how health workers, under pressure to meet local and national FP 2020 targets, may resort to coercive service provision practices, such as pressuring women to adopt or refusing to remove LARCs.

I wish to be clear: I am not calling for a termination of PAC or other harm reduction strategies related to maternal health. As long as abortion laws remain strict and abortion stigma remains high, there will be a need for PAC. The need for PAC under these conditions applies to wealthy countries in the global North as well as low- and middle-income countries in the global South (Suh, 2019). In 2012, Savita Halavanappar died of septicemia in an Irish hospital because health workers refused to terminate her pregnancy while the fetus was still alive (Specia, 2018). In 2015, Anna Yocca was taken to an emergency room in Murfreesboro, Tennessee, after she used a coat hanger in an attempt to terminate her pregnancy of twenty-four weeks (Eckholm, 2015).

I advocate for a commitment to reproductive justice that critically situates PAC within multiple and contradictory regimes of national and global reproductive governance in which various actors, including government health authorities, multilateral, bilateral, and philanthropic donors, NGOs, and pharmaceutical companies, are motivated to achieve goals that are not always aligned with women's needs and interests. PAC's capacity to keep women alive does not mean we should *not* be critical of how interventions that are "better than bad" (Roe, 2005) may foreclose opportunities for reproductive justice that put women first. An approach that understands survival of abortion complications as "good enough" for women, and women in the global South in particular, suggests that such women do not matter enough to be entitled to high-quality services and information that prevent unsafe abortions from happening in the first place. Put differently, PAC entrenches race, gender, geographic, age, and class inequalities in the achievement of reproductive well-being.[5]

Reproductive justice is not limited to abortion law reform, which does not automatically result in improved access to safe abortion. In South Africa, where abortion upon request has been legal since 1996, a study conducted in forty-seven public hospitals in 2004 found that while the number of abortion-related deaths had declined, there was little change in abortion morbidity, suggesting that women, and young women in particular, continued to resort to clandestine and potentially unsafe procedures (Jewkes, Rees, Dickson, Brown, and Levin,

2005). In Ethiopia, the government revised the criminal code in 2005 to permit abortion in the case of rape, incest, or fetal malformation or if the pregnant woman is under the age of eighteen. The law further specifies that a woman's "word" is sufficient to establish her age or that she was a victim of rape or incest (Blystad et al., 2019). Despite these important developments, at least a third of abortions among adolescent girls are estimated to be clandestine and possibly unsafe (Sully, Dibaba, Fetters, Blades, and Bankole, 2018). Although abortion-related mortality has declined since 1990, in 2013 unsafe abortion accounted for nearly 20 percent of maternal mortality (Tessema et al., 2017).

Studies in Ethiopia and Rwanda (where the law was relaxed in 2012) suggest that clandestine and unsafe abortions persist because even if women are aware of legal reform, their desire to avoid abortion stigma may discourage them from openly seeking abortion services, including misoprostol, from health workers. Other factors that limit women's access to safe services include conscientious objection among trained professionals and a lack of trained health workers who are willing to provide abortions. Access is further restricted by health workers' lack of knowledge about legal reform, their concerns about criminalization due to lingering ambiguities in eligibility criteria for legal abortion, and their reluctance to be known among their colleagues and within the community as an abortion provider (Påfs et al., 2020; McLean, Desalegn, Blystad, and Miljeteig, 2019).

In Senegal, l'AJS bravely works toward achieving reproductive justice at multiple levels of society. The organization lobbies the government to harmonize the abortion law with international and regional human rights treaties such as CEDAW and the Maputo Protocol that call for legal abortion if pregnancy threatens the woman's mental or physical health and in cases of incest or rape. In several regions of the country, l'AJS provides free legal advice in *boutiques de droits* (legal drop-in centers) on matters related to property rights, access to land, paternity, forced marriage, and abandonment. The organization works directly with youth groups, religious leaders, health professionals, police officers, and journalists to raise awareness about the causes and consequences of unsafe abortion and to advocate for medicalized abortion (Archer, Finden, and Pearson, 2018). Since 2008, l'AJS has trained over 1,000 *parajuristes* (legal laypeople) to identify and advocate for girls and young women who have attempted to induce abortion. On several occasions, the organization has pressured the government to cover the medical expenses of young survivors of rape or incest who were denied a legal abortion and forced to carry their pregnancies to term. In 2011, l'AJS paid for the cesarean section of a nine-year-old who had been raped, impregnated, and denied a legal abortion. She died several months after the procedure (A. Smith, 2014). Unfortunately (but unsurprisingly), members of l'AJS have become targets of anti-abortion sentiment. In July 2019, a member of l'AJS who is part of the national task force on medicalized abortion revealed to me that she has experienced harassment and insults, such as being called *une avorteuse* (a female abortionist) both at work (for example, on the air during a radio spot) and in her private life by people in her neighborhood.

Mme Fatou Kiné Camara, professor of law at l'UCAD and president of l'AJS between 2013 and 2015, highlighted interlocking systems of inequality that place low-income women at greatest risk of death or injury related to unsafe abortion: "The greatest unfairness is that the poor are the victims of our archaic legislation. Anyone with enough money can easily have an abortion at a private clinic. But if you are poor you are expected to go through the legal motions or risk your life in a backstreet clinic" (A. Smith, 2014). Although the code of medical ethics permits therapeutic abortion with the certification of three doctors, Professor Camara notes that "poor people in Senegal are lucky if they see one doctor in their lifetime, let alone three" (A. Smith 2014).

PAC completes a vicious cycle of gender and class inequality, abortion stigma, and inadequate or thoroughly absent obstetric care for the most socially and economically vulnerable Senegalese women. A colonial-era law limits safe abortion care to those who can afford it in the private sector. The exclusion of abortion from the spectrum of legitimate reproductive health care is amplified by anti-abortion policies such as the Mexico City Policy that force NGOs to abandon abortion-related activities in order to maintain eligibility for USAID's family planning and global health funding. At the intersection of these transnational regimes of reproductive governance, PAC has been cemented as a harm reduction approach to reducing maternal death. Although PAC data generate support for more PAC, they obscure the incidence of abortion, thereby dampening political will to liberalize the abortion law. Until the reproductive lives and bodies of all women truly matter, last-resort approaches to obstetric care like PAC will not only remain necessary but also celebrated and quantified as good care.

APPENDIX A
Methodology

HOSPITAL FIELDWORK: OBSERVATION OF SERVICES AND REVIEW OF RECORDS

Fieldwork observations at l'Hôpital Senghor, l'Hôpital Médina, and l'Hôpital de Ville entailed shadowing health workers and engaging them in informal conversation as they moved between the delivery room, private consultation offices, and, at l'Hôpital Senghor and l'Hôpital de Ville, the MVA room. While observing clinical care or recordkeeping, I asked them to explain what they were doing or to comment on my observations of other health workers' actions. About every thirty minutes, I stepped out of the maternity ward to jot down my observations in a notebook. At the end of each day, I typed up my field notes into Word documents.

After shadowing health workers for several weeks, I began to divide my time between observing PAC services and reviewing PAC records. At each hospital I reviewed several years of PAC registers from the maternity ward and PAC and delivery statistics in annual hospital reports and transferred selected data into an Excel spreadsheet, where I generated descriptive statistics of PAC that appear throughout the book. At l'Hôpital Senghor and l'Hôpital de Ville, I obtained district and regional data on the number of PAC patients and the number treated with MVA.

Most of the clinical PAC data that appear in this book are from the 2009 and 2010 registers at l'Hôpital Senghor, l'Hôpital Médina, and l'Hôpital de Ville. Older PAC registers were often missing pages or missing entirely. At l'Hôpital Médina, for example, I was unable to locate the 2008 PAC register. At l'Hôpital Senghor, before 2009, providers recorded cases treated by digital evacuation and MVA in different registers. At l'Hôpital de Ville, physicians recorded MVA cases in a separate register that were then transferred to the main PAC register by the head midwife.

To ensure comparability in PAC register data across the three study hospitals, I focused on PAC cases recorded over twenty-four months between 2009 and 2010. For each PAC case that appeared during these months, I recorded the method of uterine evacuation, the professional identity of the health worker who treated the patient, and the type of abortion recorded as well as other terminology used to describe the case. During formal interviews and informal conversations, I asked health workers to explain terminology used to classify and describe abortion as well as omissions in the register. Drawing on these conversations and my observations of PAC services, I highlighted cases with indicators (or omissions) in the register that would likely have been considered suspicious. Examples of such indicators include marital status, age, type of abortion, time of arrival, profession, related complications, and length of gestation.

Some of my observations occurred outside the study hospitals. First, during fieldwork at l'Hôpital Médina, I accompanied several community health workers from an international NGO on a field trip to a primary health care facility and a *case de santé* or health hut in a neighboring district. During this trip, I spoke with the community health workers about the NGO's PAC strategies and interviewed the head nurse at the primary health care clinic. Second, in June 2011, I attended a meeting organized by Ipas to disseminate the results of a situational analysis on unwanted pregnancy and unsafe abortion that was coordinated by the DSR. Many of my study participants from local and international NGOs and the MSAS were in attendance, and I listened with great interest to these stakeholders discussing "next steps" with respect to advocacy for abortion law reform. Third, after an interview with a key informant who was the head of the national professional nursing association, I had the opportunity to speak informally with several nurses who happened to be at the association's headquarters for a meeting. What started as an interview with one nurse turned unexpectedly into an informal group discussion with about ten nurses.

INTERVIEWS

I conducted in-depth interviews with eighty-nine individuals: sixty-seven of these individuals were directly involved in PAC clinical practice, program implementation, or policy development, and twenty-two were key informants. I used theoretical or purposive sampling (Bernard and Ryan, 2009) to identify the sixty-seven PAC practitioners according to specific categories of interest, such as gender, profession, region of practice, type of health facility, and type of uterine evacuation training. Unlike studies that rely on statistical sampling, in which data collection occurs before analysis begins, theoretical sampling occurs alongside data collection and analysis (Becker, 1998; Corbin and Strauss, 2008; Lofland and Lofland, 2006). I began to analyze data immediately after the first few interviews conducted with NGO personnel and MSAS officials. These data, along with my

TABLE A.1.   Number, profession, and institutional affiliation of health
professionals interviewed in three regions

Region	Type of health facility		Number and type of health provider	Total number of interviewees by region
Region 1	Interviewing and observation site	Hôpital Senghor	2 doctors 8 midwives	12
	Interviewing site only	District hospital	1 midwife	
		Primary health care facility	1 midwife	
Region 2	Interviewing and observation site	Hôpital Médina	1 doctor 2 nurses 4 midwives	11
	Interviewing site only	Tertiary level regional hospital	1 doctor	
		Primary health care facility	1 nurse 1 midwife	
		Primary health care facility	1 midwife	
Region 3	Interviewing and observation site	Hôpital de Ville	6 doctors 7 midwives 1 nursing assistant	14
Total number of interviewees				37

review of the literature, informed the selection of study sites and shaped the questions I asked health workers who were directly involved in PAC service delivery. In turn, my interviews with health workers and observation of services shaped the questions I asked of other PAC stakeholders.

Among the thirty-seven health workers interviewed, five worked at health facilities where I did not conduct direct observation, including a district hospital and a primary health care facility in the first study region and a regional hospital and two primary health care facilities in the second study region. Table A.1 displays the number and type of health professionals interviewed in each region according to health facility.

Included in the subsample of PAC practitioners were thirteen officials from district, regional, and central levels of the MSAS and seventeen individuals from national and international NGOs and donor agencies. The average age of PAC participants was approximately forty-six, and most (70%) were women. Midwives accounted for 62 percent of the subsample of health workers.

I used purposive sampling to recruit twenty-two key informants according to their professional knowledge and experience related to the social, legal, and political aspects of abortion. This subsample includes professors from l'UCAD, members of l'AJS and the Ministry of Gender and Culture, police officials from the region of Dakar, and members of professional nursing and physician associations.

With the exception of five interviews (one in Wolof, four in English), all interviews with PAC practitioners and key informants were conducted in French. Most interviews (56%) were recorded with a digital recorder. At l'Hôpital Senghor, l'Hôpital Médina, and l'Hôpital de Ville, I conducted interviews with health workers in private offices, consultation rooms, or the delivery room. All other interviews were conducted at the participant's place of work, and in a few cases, via Skype.

ARCHIVAL REVIEW OF ILLEGAL ABORTIONS

Between August and September 2011, after obtaining authorization from the regional tribunal of Dakar, I identified and reviewed forty-two cases of illegal abortion prosecuted by this unit between 1987 and 2010. These cases were stored in boxes in the archival unit in the basement of the regional tribunal, alongside other infractions of the penal code, including theft, embezzlement, driving while inebriated, sale of narcotics, pedophilia, and homosexuality (described as "acts against nature"). They included cases in which women were solely prosecuted for procuring an illegal abortion and cases involving practitioners and accomplices. I made photocopies of each abortion case and logged case details in an Excel file.

Each abortion case entailed a summary of the court proceedings. Only three cases included more extensive documentation such as transcripts of police interviews with the suspect and copies of medical documents. Most cases in the archival room were much more circumscribed, detailing the case in just a few paragraphs. All cases stated the defendant's name, age, and in some instances, profession. They also outlined the court's decision (acquittal or jail sentence and/or fines). Information from these court cases appears throughout the book. Additionally, I share accounts of illegal abortion reported by the Senegalese press.

PAC AND ABORTION LITERATURE REVIEW

During the fieldwork period, I reviewed copies of operations and clinical research on PAC at CEFOREP's library. I read epidemiological studies of abortion complications, theses on abortion by medical students at CHU Le Dantec, reports of national and regional PAC conferences, and NGO reports on reproductive health. Many sources of demographic and clinical information were available online, such as Demographic and Health Surveys (DHS), studies published by members of the faculty of medicine at l'UCAD in academic journals, and reports published by international NGOs. Additionally, study participants who worked for the MSAS, NGOs, and professional associations generously furnished me with a great deal of literature. For example, MSAS officials gave me a copy of reproductive health norms and protocols, a draft of a study on unwanted pregnancy and unsafe abortion funded by Ipas, and PowerPoint presentations from MVA training seminars. Key informants from l'AJS sent me electronic copies of the 2005 reproductive health law, the penal code, and the code of medical ethics. Throughout the book, I compare my ethnographic data with global data on PAC and abortion published before, during, and after the fieldwork period.

RESEARCH ASSISTANCE AND DISSEMINATION OF RESULTS

At each study hospital, I worked with a research assistant to observe PAC services and review PAC records. I identified the research assistants, all of whom were young women pursuing graduate degrees at Senegalese universities, through local networks of friends and colleagues. These women accompanied me to interviews and field visits outside the hospitals. They approached women patients and requested, in Wolof, their consent to be observed during treatment. During fieldwork, they frequently translated exchanges in Wolof between health workers and patients into French. Over time, the research assistants felt confident enough to directly participate in interviews with health workers and key informants by asking questions, and one conducted an interview with a key informant on her own in Wolof. One of the women helped me with the archival review of court documents at the regional tribunal of Dakar. Additionally, she transcribed interviews that had been conducted in French.

At the end of the fieldwork period at each hospital, I shared preliminary findings with supervisory staff in the gynecological ward. Few of these individuals expressed surprise when I suggested that cases of induced abortion may be underreported. They were more interested in discussing my findings related to family planning counseling and the organization of services. At the end of the research period, I submitted a report of preliminary findings to the Comité National d'Ethique pour la Recherche en Santé [National Ethics Committee for Health Research], the DSR, and other stakeholders.

APPENDIX B

Cases of Admitted and Suspected Induced Abortions

Table B.1 displays twenty-six cases that appeared in PAC registers at three hospitals between 2009 and 2010. These cases include confirmed induced abortions as well as cases with indicators that providers likely considered suspicious. For each year, I present selected indicators of cases that providers at each hospital recorded over the course of one month, including marital status (column A), age (column B), gestation/parity (number of pregnancies / number of live births) (column C), gestational age (column D), mode of uterine evacuation (column E), practitioner (column F), and the type of abortion recorded in the PAC register (column G). To protect confidentiality, I do not reveal the month. Months are in no particular order and may not correspond across all three hospitals.

TABLE B.1. Cases of admitted and suspected induced abortions in six months of PAC register data in three hospitals, 2009–2010

Month of observation in each hospital	Case number	Marital status (A)	Age (B)	Gestation/ Parity (C)	Gestational age (D)	Mode of uterine evacuation (E)	Practitioner (F)	Type of abortion recorded in PAC register (G)
2009 Hôpital Senghor	1	Single	18	2/1	20 weeks	Expulsion, digital evacuation	Midwife	Abortion
	2	None listed	13	0/0	None listed	None listed	None listed	None listed
Hôpital Médina	1	Married	26	2/0	1 month	MVA	Midwife; "patient referred from Clinic X"	Induced abortion
	2	None listed	30	1/1	2 months	Digital evacuation	Midwife	Spontaneous
	3	"?"	18	1/0	2 months	Digital evacuation	Midwife; "patient referred from Clinic X"	Spontaneous
Hôpital de Ville	1	Single	18	1/0	None listed	Expulsion	Midwife; "patient referred from Clinic X"	Late abortion
	2	Single	19	1/0	2 months	MVA	Physician	Incomplete abortion
	3	Single	18	1/0	None listed	MVA	Physician	Molar abortion
	4	Single	19	1/0	None listed	Electric aspiration	Physician	Molar abortion
	5	None listed	26	1/"?"	2 months	Dilation and curettage	Physician	Hemorrhagic abortion
	6	"?"	14	1/0	2 months	Expulsion at home	Midwife	None listed
	7	Single	31	2/1	6 weeks	MVA	Physician	Ovulatory retention
	8	Single	30	4/3	3 months	Expulsion	Physician; "patient referred from Maternity X"	Induced abortion

2010								
Hôpital Senghor	1	None listed	22	3/3	None listed	MVA	Midwife	Incomplete abortion
	2	Single	38	6/4	1 month	Digital evacuation	Midwife	Spontaneous abortion
	3	Single	18	1/0	2 months	Digital evacuation	Midwife	None listed
	4	Single	"?"	2/1	4 months	Digital evacuation; "expulsion of fetus at home, not brought to hospital, according to patient"	Midwife	Spontaneous abortion
Hôpital Médina	1	Married	17	1/0	7 months	Expulsion; hemorrhage	Midwife	Spontaneous
	2	Married	19	1/0	5 months	MVA; complications of infection	Midwife; "patient brought by police of Town X"	Induced abortion
	3	Married	16	1/0	"?"	Manual removal of placenta	Midwife	"?"
Hôpital de Ville	1	Single	22	2/1	None listed	MVA	Physician	Empty sac
	2	Single	23	2/1	None listed	Dilation and curettage	Physician	Induced abortion
	3	Single	19	1/0	None listed	Dilation and curettage	Physician	Hemorrhagic abortion
	4	Married	30	1/0	None listed	MVA	Physician	None listed
	5	Single	18	1/0	4 months	Expulsion of 2 stillborn fetuses	Midwife	Fetal abortion
	6	None listed	23	5/3	None listed	Digital evacuation	Physician	Late abortion

ACKNOWLEDGMENTS

This book about post-abortion care (PAC) would not have been written without the support and generosity of colleagues, mentors, and friends in Senegal. I am grateful to Dr. Philippe Moreira, Dr. Fatim Tall Thiam, and the rest of the Management Sciences for Health (MSH) team in Dakar for welcoming me and giving me a hands-on opportunity to learn about PAC. I wish to thank Dr. Ousmane Sène and the West African Research Association in Dakar for hosting me. I spent countless hours on my laptop in their wonderful reading room and printed all my interview questionnaires in their computer lab. I wish to thank the Centre Régionale de Formation, de Recherche, et de Plaidoyer en Santé de la Reproduction (CEFOREP) for granting me access to its excellent library. I am very grateful to members of the Division de la Santé de la Reproduction (DSR) who discussed PAC with me and shared important documents and reports related to maternal and reproductive health.

I draw inspiration from the fearless advocacy and brilliant scholarship on sexual and reproductive health by Professors Cheikh Ibrahima Niang and Fatou Kiné Camara at l'Université Cheikh Anta Diop (UCAD) and Mme Codou Bop of le Groupe de Recherche sur les Femmes et les Lois au Sénégal. I am enormously grateful to Professor Niang for serving as faculty sponsor during the process of applying for research clearance from the Comité National d'Ethique pour la Recherche en Santé. Thank you for sharing meals with me in your homes, introducing me to your colleagues, and offering important theoretical, methodological, and empirical insights throughout my fieldwork.

I am grateful for the support I received from representatives of national and international organizations involved in maternal and reproductive health in Senegal, including l'Association des Juristes Sénégalaises (AJS), Child Fund, Marie Stopes International (MSI), the Population Council, Ipas, Intrahealth, the Guttmacher Institute, Gynuity Health Projects, United Nations Population Fund (UNFPA), World Health Organization (WHO), and United States Agency for International Development (USAID). Much gratitude is owed to them for sharing documents and reports, aiding with recruitment, and offering excellent advice.

My hospital fieldwork could not have been completed without the assistance of three incredible young women, all of whom were pursuing advanced degrees in sociology and public health at the time of my fieldwork: Rama N., Marie C., and Ngoma F. At each of the study hospitals, these intrepid investigators co-conducted interviews with health workers and helped collect obstetric care data from hospital records. They accompanied me to health facilities and offices of NGOs and health officials to conduct interviews. With Rama's help, I combed through the archives of the regional tribunal of Dakar, searching for cases of illegal abortion. She also co-conducted several interviews with law enforcement officials in Dakar. I am very grateful to Rama for transcribing interviews conducted in French.

In the United States, I wish to thank my mentors at Columbia University, who pushed me to embrace the interdisciplinarity of my work: Constance A. Nathanson, Peter Messeri, and Kim Hopper in the Department of Sociomedical Sciences; Mamadou Diouf in the Institute of African Studies; Gil Eyal in the Department of Sociology; and Wendy Chavkin in the Department of Population and Family Health. Thanks to Elizabeth Bernstein in the Department of Sociology at Barnard College, who encouraged me to start thinking about PAC as a form of governance.

My research was generously supported by an F31 Pre-doctoral Fellowship to Promote Diversity in Health-Related Research from the National Institute of Child Health and Human Development. Additionally, I received support from the Dissertation Proposal Development Fellowship and the International Dissertation Research Fellowship of the Social Science Research Council and the Dissertation Completion Fellowship of the American Council of Learned Societies.

Several chapters of the book were written with funding from the American Association of University Women and the Advancing New Standards in Reproductive Health program of the Bixby Center for Global Reproductive Health (University of California, San Francisco) while I was on the faculty at the University of Minnesota. Thank you to my colleagues and friends in Minneapolis for your kindness and support throughout this project: Aren Aizura, Sugi Ganeshananthan, Maggie Hennefeld, Annie Hill, Zenzele Isoke, Rachmi Diyah Larasati, and Kari Smolkoski. I am enormously grateful for the intellectual community and warm and enduring friendship of Vivian Choi, Susan Craddock, Sonali Pahwa, Elliott Powell, and Terrion Williamson.

At Brandeis University, the African Diaspora Cluster and the Norman Fund for Faculty Research generously supported this work through writing retreats and a book manuscript workshop in 2019. I am immensely grateful to Lynn Morgan, Ellen Foley, and Rachel Sullivan Robinson for their close readings of and critical commentary on the manuscript, and for inspiring me with their scholarship on reproduction. Many thanks to the members of my writing group, Julia McReynolds-Pérez, Elyse Singer, and Jess Newman, for their thoughtful engagement throughout this project. I am eternally indebted to Justin Jiménez, who provided invaluable research, copyediting, and indexing support during the final stages. Thanks to my editor at Rutgers University Press, Kimberly Guinta, for her excellent stewardship of this project, and two anonymous reviewers for their insightful feedback. I am deeply grateful to Lenore Manderson for her vision of this project within the series on health, inequality, and social justice.

To Rebecca Desvaux, Maaike van Min, Patricia Matthew, Althea Anderson, Kirk Grisham, and Tara Bedeau—thank you. I am very grateful to my family—Joseph, Nicoline, Suzie, Leo, Amy, Stella, and Esme—for cheering me on until the last page of this book was written. Most of all, I am indebted to the Senegalese medical workers and women patients who made this book possible through their gracious participation in the study.

NOTES

NOTES TO INTRODUCTION

1. An image of digital evacuation appears on page 175 of *Essential Obstetric and Newborn Care: Practical Guide for Midwives, Doctors with Obstetrics Training and Health Care Personnel Who Deal with Obstetric Emergencies*, a clinical manual of obstetric care published by MSF (2019).

2. Also known as acetaminophen, a pain relief medication.

3. These estimates are from a national study of abortion conducted by the Research Center for Human Development, a national demographic research agency, and the Guttmacher Institute, a U.S.-based reproductive health research agency. Investigators used an indirect technique known as the Abortion Incidence Complications Methodology (AICM), which estimates abortion incidence from the number of women who receive facility-based treatment for complications of induced abortion. These numbers are obtained through nationally representative surveys of facilities that provide PAC and by surveying health experts with context-specific knowledge about abortion provision. The AICM has been used to estimate abortion incidence since the early 1990s in seventeen countries (Argentina, Bangladesh, Brazil, Burkina Faso, Chile, Colombia, Costa Rica, the Dominican Republic, Ethiopia, Guatemala, Malawi, Mexico, Nigeria, Pakistan, Peru, the Philippines, and Uganda) with restrictive abortion laws or where abortion is permitted under certain circumstances but rates of unsafe abortion remain high (S. Singh, Remez, and Targtaglione, 2010).

4. In El Salvador, for example, women have received prison sentences of up to thirty years for "aggravated homicide" following miscarriage. A review of 129 abortion-related investigations conducted in El Salvador between 2000 and 2011 found that not one originated from a private doctor or hospital (Oberman, 2018).

5. Since the 2000s, global reproductive health advocates have also championed misoprostol as a safe and effective PAC technology (Sherris et al., 2005).

6. An image of dilation and curettage appears on page 180 of *Essential Obstetric and Newborn Care: Practical Guide for Midwives, Doctors with Obstetrics Training and Health Care Personnel Who Deal with Obstetric Emergencies*, a clinical manual for obstetric care published by MSF (2019).

7. Another influential funding policy is the Kemp-Kasten Amendment, which withdrew U.S. funding from UNFPA in 1985 because of (unfounded) claims that the organization was supporting China's "coercive" abortion practices under the One Child Policy (Barot and Cohen, 2015). Like the Mexico City Policy, this policy is activated or rescinded along Republican and Democratic party lines.

8. An RCT is an experimental study design that requires random assignment of study subjects to either the test group or the control group. The test group receives the treatment or intervention, while the control group receives a placebo or no treatment. Random assignment ensures that all study subjects have an equal chance of being assigned to either the test or control group, and that there are no systematic differences between the test and control groups at the start of the study. At the end of the study, the investigator measures the effectiveness of the intervention by statistically comparing outcomes between the test and control groups.

9. In addition to wresting control over pregnancy and delivery from African midwives, hospital delivery granted European doctors unfettered access to women's bodies for racialized knowledge production and experimentation. In the Belgian Congo, embryotomies (in which

the fetus is dismembered to facilitate removal from the uterus) were understood as a necessity of "tropical" obstetric care until blood supply systems and antibiotics became more widely available. In Uganda, racial explanations for obstructed labor motivated colonial doctors to unearth the corpses of women who had died during childbirth to measure pelvic shape, long understood as an indicator of the primitive nature of the African race (Bridges, 2011; Briggs, 2000; Hunt, 1999). See Briggs (2000) and Owens (2017) for excellent histories of medical experimentation on enslaved Black women in the United States that illustrate how racialized knowledge was key to the professional consolidation of Euro-American gynecology/obstetrics.

10. Although the 1954 gathering in Rome is officially labeled as the First World Population Conference, an earlier version took place in Geneva, organized by birth control advocate and cofounder of the International Planned Parenthood Federation (IPPF) Margaret Sanger. The Geneva conference aimed to focus international attention on population as an object of political and economic planning that was distinct from the racialized population projects promoted by eugenic science (Murphy, 2017).

11. The 1965 World Population Conference was co-organized by the International Union for the Scientific Study of Population.

12. USAID spending on family planning, including contraceptive research, family planning services, and population training in developing countries, increased from $2.1 million in 1965 to $125.6 million in 1973. The global community was understandably stunned when U.S. delegates to the 1984 conference revealed President Reagan's Mexico City Policy. In a sharp reversal from its earlier stance, in which high fertility was a significant impediment to development, the United States now claimed that free markets, unfettered by government intervention, were necessary to achieve economic growth. Although the United States reaffirmed its commitment to funding family planning programs, USAID's language shifted from emphasizing "informed choice" and "voluntarism" (Dixon-Mueller, 1993, p. 71) to a more conservative discourse of "meeting the interests of families," which included "desire of couples to determine size and spacing of family," "mother and child survival," and "reduction of abortion" (p. 74). During this meeting, the U.S. delegation unveiled the part of the policy that quickly became known as the Global Gag Rule (Dixon-Mueller, 1993).

13. Some donors, like the World Bank, the Global Fund, and USAID, prefer to distribute aid through NGOs (in order to encourage innovation through competition) rather than through government agencies, which are widely viewed as paralyzed by bureaucracy or corruption. Critics argue that this approach leads to highly verticalized landscapes of care and to "parallel health systems" that are inadequately connected to government health systems (Packard, 2016; Pfeiffer, 2013).

14. Founded in 1969 as the Inner City Fund, ICF is a global consulting firm that has contracted with USAID since 1984 to conduct Demographic and Health Surveys (DHS) around the world.

15. In 2007, IHME received grants in the amounts of $105 million and $20 million from the Bill & Melinda Gates Foundation and the University of Washington, respectively, to conduct global health evaluation research. In 2017, IHME announced that it would receive an additional grant of $279 million from the Bill & Melinda Gates Foundation (Butler, 2017).

16. Writing in the late seventeenth century, British cleric Thomas Malthus argued that unchecked population growth (especially among the poor) would deplete the earth's finite resources, leading to political unrest, famine, and disease. The term "neo-Malthusian" describes twentieth-century iterations of his theory of the relationship between population and environment, in which "overpopulation" (primarily in developing countries in the global South) will destroy the planet (Sasser, 2018).

17. Demographic transition theory posits that modernization and urbanization lead to fertility decline. Yet, fertility first began to decline in some of the poorer, less industrialized parts of Europe. Economic factors alone could not account for the diversity of experiences in the amount or speed of fertility decline in Europe or postcolonial countries. The theory did not account for nontechnological forms of fertility control used by "traditional" societies such as abortion, fostering, infanticide, and lactation. It narrowly defined fertility as an entity bounded within the conjugal couple (and the bedroom) rather than a set of relations operating throughout women's reproductive life cycles and situated in broader social, economic, and political relations. At the height of Cold War anxieties about newly sovereign nations in the global South turning to Communism, American demographers argued that high fertility itself impeded economic development, and that birth control was necessary to encourage economic growth and political stability. Social scientists have disputed the theory's conceptualization of the relationship between fertility and poverty, arguing that high fertility is a consequence rather than a cause of poverty. Until large families ceased to represent a viable economic strategy (especially in the face of high childhood mortality), people would continue to value high fertility.

18. Sayana Press is a self-administered form of Depo-Provera, an injectable LARC. For an excellent review of Depo-Provera's troubled history of coercive testing practices on men and women in the United States, read William Green's (2017) book *Contraceptive Risk: The FDA, Depo-Provera, and the Politics of Experimental Medicine*.

19. Joanna Crane's (2013) ethnography of global HIV science in Uganda illustrates how local scientists and medical professionals are keenly aware of structural inequalities in the conduct of research. Although collaborations with Western institutions increased resources related to infrastructure, equipment, and staff, local professionals complained of being relegated to the role of "blood senders" (p. 105), which entailed processing the "raw materials" (p. 105) used in experimental trials without the professional recognition accorded to Western scientists in global scientific arenas.

20. A detailed description of research methods appears in appendix A.

NOTES TO CHAPTER 1: A "TRANSFORMATIVE" INTERVENTION

1. Between 1984 and 2006, the University of Michigan Population Fellows Program, funded by USAID and the William and Flora Hewlett Foundation, provided field placement opportunities for early population professionals to support various family planning and reproductive health organizations in developing countries.

2. The SDM, also known as the Fertility Awareness Method, is a form of natural contraception. Women track their menstrual cycles on a necklace of multicolored beads and abstain from sex or use barrier methods on days when they are ovulating. Developed by the Institute of Reproductive Health (IRH) at Georgetown University in 2001, this method has been implemented worldwide in over twenty-two countries. In Senegal, some reproductive health experts believed that the SDM's multicolored beads would resonate well with other culturally familiar beads, including Islamic prayer beads and women's colorful waist beads (bin-bin).

3. Two of the nurses in my sample of health worker interviewees worked at a district hospital. The other worked at a primary health care facility. A fourth nurse was informally interviewed during an impromptu field trip to a primary health care facility and is classified as a key informant.

4. Hospital administrators at each study facility loaned my research assistant and me white coats. Only individuals wearing special coats, including clinical and janitorial staff, were permitted into the maternity ward.

5. In her ethnography of global HIV science in Uganda, anthropologist Joanna Crane illustrates how structural inequalities between low- and high-income countries extend to the conduct of research. Western researchers are frequently granted access to the bodies of African patients, health facilities, and biomedical data. In contrast, access to Western patient populations, facilities, and data is rarely, if ever, extended to African scientists, health professionals, or students (J. Crane, 2010, 2013).

6. In 1999, AMDD received a $50 million grant from the Bill & Melinda Gates Foundation to support the introduction of EmOC in eighteen low- and middle-income countries (Averting Maternal Death and Disability [AMDD], 2020).

7. Headquartered in New York.

8. Headquartered at Johns Hopkins University in Baltimore, Maryland.

9. Headquartered in Washington, DC.

10. Headquartered in Chapel Hill, North Carolina.

11. Headquartered in Richmond, Virginia.

12. Although the report does not explain how investigators verified women's accounts of the kind of abortion they experienced, this project was one of only two PAC operations research projects that documented abortion type. During the first phase of the project, in a sample of 320 patients, 79.7 percent of cases were identified as spontaneous and 10.3 percent as induced. During the second phase, within a sample of 543 patients, spontaneous abortions accounted for 80.5 percent of cases while 8.3 percent of cases were related to induced abortion. Given that information regarding abortion type was obtained from face-to-face interviews with patients, investigators likely underreported induced abortion.

13. The study estimated that the vast majority of cases (94%) were related to spontaneous abortion. However, 33 percent of patients in the first phase and 28 percent of patients in the second phase reported that their pregnancies were unwanted. In addition to highlighting the problem of unmet contraceptive need among this population, the investigators suggested that the percentage of patients who had procured an induced abortion was likely greater than 6 percent. This would be the final mention of abortion type in reports of operations research on PAC.

14. Headquartered in Chapel Hill, North Carolina.

15. In contrast to previous operations and clinical research that focused on assessing the feasibility of PAC for treating abortion complications in hospitals, this was the first qualitative study of unsafe abortion conducted by health authorities. The study consisted of in-depth interviews and focus groups with health workers, health officials, community representatives, teachers, politicians, religious leaders, and women. Using convenience and snowball sampling, study investigators interviewed a total of 732 people around the country. Many participants believed that clandestine abortion occurred frequently and that lack of access to contraception, especially among young people, was largely to blame. They also recognized the stigma of abortion that drove women to seek services in secret. Although many approved of PAC services, they critiqued the restriction of MVA to regional and district hospitals, urging an extension of the technology to primary health care facilities to increase access to PAC. Responses regarding the national abortion law were mixed. While some informants favored relaxing the law for cases of rape or incest, religious leaders were firmly against induced abortion under any circumstance. The study called on the government to harmonize the abortion law with ratified international human rights treaties, to release norms and protocols for treating abortion complications at the hospital that were in accordance with the law, and to consider revising the law to permit abortion in cases of rape or incest (DSR, 2010).

16. In chapter 2, I describe how PAC stakeholders in Bolivia used similar language to address concerns that the provision of PAC in government hospitals would "promote abortion."

17. Headquartered in New York.

18. Out of the 481 cases included in the study, only one was believed to have resulted from an induced abortion. The authors do not explain how they differentiated between induced and spontaneous abortion.

19. Compressed, sterilized seaweed the size of a matchstick, used to dilate the cervix prior to surgical abortion.

NOTES TO CHAPTER 2: A TROUBLESOME TECHNOLOGY

1. During this time, USAID began to promote natural family planning methods. For example, USAID has supported the development and testing of "fertility awareness methods" (also known as the calendar or rhythm method) at IRH at Georgetown University, a Catholic institution in Washington, DC, since the mid-1980s. One such method is the SDM, which was piloted in several African countries, including Senegal, during the mid-2000s. In 2013, USAID awarded IRH $19.8 million for a five-year fertility awareness and family planning project in sub-Saharan Africa and South Asia (Georgetown University, 2013).

2. In 2016, the PAC Consortium renamed itself the Abortion and Post-Abortion Care Consortium to reflect its commitment to addressing "the full continuum of abortion care," including safe abortion and high quality PAC (PAI, 2018).

3. DKT International is a nonprofit organization headquartered in Washington, DC, that relies on social marketing to distribute condoms and contraceptive and abortion technologies around the world.

4. Concerns about the "ease" with which technologies facilitate the capacity of skilled and unskilled practitioners to perform abortions are not limited to developing countries with restrictive abortion laws. In the United States, anti-abortion groups succeeded in pressuring the Federal Drug Administration (FDA) to ban the importation of mifepristone (RU-486) for personal use between 1989 and 1993. The FDA did not approve the drug for abortion until 2000. Unlike surgical abortion procedures, mifepristone was not limited to clinical settings and could therefore be prescribed by nonphysicians. It was precisely the drug's potential to facilitate women's access to abortion, by placing it in the hands of nonphysicians, that galvanized anti-abortion activists into demanding restrictions over the drug from the federal government. Although the 2000 FDA ruling authorized nonsurgical providers to offer mifepristone (as long as they had the "backup" of a surgical provider in case of emergency [Joffe and Weitz, 2003]), by 2020 up to thirty-two states had restricted the provision of medical abortion to physicians (Guttmacher Institute, 2020).

5. To protect this individual's confidentiality, I am not sharing their pseudonym.

6. The Kemp-Kasten Amendment was passed in 1985, a year after the Mexico City Policy or "Global Gag Rule." It blocked U.S. funding to UNFPA because of the organization's alleged support of coercive abortion practices under China's One Child Policy. Like the Mexico City Policy, the Kemp-Kasten Amendment is reactivated or rescinded along party lines when a new president takes office.

7. In Senegal, although midwives receive theoretical training in MVA in school, hands-on MVA training has taken place primarily during seminars supported by NGOs like MSH and Ipas and through on-the-job training. At the three study hospitals, some of the midwives I interviewed had attended training seminars, and others had been trained on-site by senior midwives and gynecologists.

NOTES TO CHAPTER 3: "WE WEAR WHITE COATS, NOT UNIFORMS"

1. I did not find evidence in the legal archives or in the press that providers were arrested or prosecuted for improper recording of abortion or failure to report abortion to the police. These sources suggest health workers are primarily prosecuted for involvement in procuring illegal abortion. Midlevel and paramedical professionals like midwives, nurses, and nursing assistants appear to be more vulnerable to prosecution. Between 1987 and 2010, not a single physician was among the twenty-three practitioners directly implicated in forty-two cases of illegal abortion prosecuted by the region of Dakar.

2. An antispasmodic drug available in pharmacies.

3. Threats to withhold PAC are reminiscent of the highly coercive "dying confessions" elicited by medical professionals from women with complications of abortion in U.S. hospitals before the legalization of abortion in 1973. The purpose of the dying confession was to uncover the identity of illegal "abortionists." One technique involved withholding care until the woman revealed the abortion provider to health care workers and police officers. Alternatively, physicians would lead women to believe they were near death, and encourage them to "confess" before they succumbed to their injuries (Reagan, 1998).

4. Other registers in the maternity ward included those for deliveries and family planning.

5. Unlike the registers for family planning and delivery, the PAC register required health workers to record patients' marital status.

NOTES TO CHAPTER 4: WHEN ABORTION DOES NOT COUNT

1. The WHO (2019) defines maternal death as "the death of a woman while pregnant or within 42 days of termination of pregnancy, irrespective of the duration and site of the pregnancy, from any cause related to or aggravated by the pregnancy or its management but not from accidental or incidental causes" (p. 8).

2. Founding members included the World Bank, WHO, UNFPA, UNICEF (UN Children's Fund), UNDP (UN Development Program), the Population Council, and IPPF.

3. Basic EmOC entails the administration of parenteral antibiotics, uterotonic medications (to manage PPH), and anticonvulsants (to manage seizures); manual removal of placenta; removal of retained products (this would include uterine evacuation for PAC); and assisted delivery. Comprehensive EmOC includes the basic functions plus cesarean section and blood transfusion.

4. Examples include trained, competent personnel; functioning and available infrastructure, equipment, and technology; information systems; and referral and transportation mechanisms.

5. An initiative of Save the Children.

6. An initiative of UNICEF.

7. For an excellent critique of the racialized neglect of chronic disease relative to HIV/AIDS in sub-Saharan Africa by global health actors, see Julie Livingston's (2012) ethnography of cancer care in Botswana.

8. This was not the first time that the Gates Foundation had invested in highly targeted approaches to maternal health that are compatible with statistical evaluation. In 2007, for example, the Gates Foundation awarded $1.4 million to fund clinical trials conducted by the University of California, San Francisco, in Zambia and Zimbabwe on an "anti-shock" garment meant to decrease PPH (Bole, 2007).

9. I identified the first six studies through an archival review of documents available at CEFOREP's library in Dakar. Additionally, these studies were described in a review of literature on unsafe abortion published in 1998 by CEFOREP. The last three studies were found using an internet search.

10. The introduction of PAC did not entirely cease the collection of data on induced abortion. Among the operations research projects conducted between 1997 and 2006, two collected information on abortion type. During the first operations research project, conducted in three large hospitals in Dakar between 1997 and 1998, investigators found that 10 percent of women in the first phase and 8 percent in the second phase of the study reported having an induced abortion. During the third operations research project, conducted between 2001 and 2003 in Kaolack and Fatick, investigators estimated that only 6 percent of patients had procured an illegal abortion. However, 33 percent of patients in the first phase and 28 percent of patients in the second phase reported that their pregnancies were unwanted, suggesting that the percentage of induced abortion may have been underestimated.

11. A 2015–2016 survey of the availability, utilization, and quality of EmOC in 120 health facilities estimated that 42.5 percent of maternal deaths in Senegalese health facilities are related to hemorrhage (MSAS, CEFOREP, and UNFPA, 2017).

12. In 2005, 377 abortions were treated, of which only 6 were identified as induced. In 2006, out of a total of 531 treated abortions, 11 were recorded as induced.

13. More recently, a 2015–2016 survey of the availability, utilization, and quality of EmOC in 120 health facilities estimated that abortion complications accounted for 1.7 percent of maternal deaths (MSAS, CEFOREP, and UNFPA 2017).

14. Figure 1.1 in chapter 1 illustrates that abortion as a percentage of admissions was higher at l'Hôpital de Ville than at the other two study hospitals.

15. These concerns are not unique to Senegalese health workers or decision-makers. Before the 1973 legalization of abortion in the United States, anxieties about being known as abortion facilities prompted hospital administrators to introduce quotas to limit the number of legal therapeutic abortions that doctors could perform (Joffe, 1996; Reagan, 1998). In Burkina Faso, while health professionals and health officials support PAC as a form of "life-saving care," most are reluctant to advocate a revision of the abortion law because they do not wish to publicly "support" induced abortion (Storeng and Ouattara, 2014).

16. Examples of survey questions include: Was the woman pregnant when she died? If respondents say "no" or "I don't know," investigators then ask: Did she die during a pregnancy? If the answer is no, investigators ask: Did she die within forty-two days of the termination of a pregnancy or delivery (ANSD and ICF International, 2012)?

17. Mme Camara's reference to menstrual "lateness" (amenorrhea) is intriguing because it resonates with concerns raised by health authorities during the earliest operations research projects that PAC was a de facto form of induced abortion through menstrual regulation in public hospitals. A midwife by profession, Mme Camara was one of very few health officials who stated explicitly that "a very good portion" of PAC cases treated in public hospitals were related to induced abortion.

18. To protect the individual's confidentiality, I have de-identified the name of the region.

19. Health facilities are managed in part by health committees that are composed of health workers and community members. The involvement of health committees is a result of the 1987 Bamako Initiative, which aimed to promote community-based participation in health care.

20. Quasi-experimental research, until recently, has been widely used in public health programming. It is considered inferior to the RCT because it does not involve randomization of study groups. In most of the PAC operations research in Senegal, investigators measured variables such as "percentage of patients treated with MVA" before and after the implementation of PAC.

21. Other experts have refuted the claim that liberalizing abortion laws leads to declines in maternal mortality, pointing to countries like Ireland, Malta, and Poland, which demonstrate low levels of maternal mortality despite the presence of restrictive abortion laws. In Chile,

maternal mortality declined despite a ban on therapeutic abortion implemented in 1989 (Koch et al., 2012). These examples, however, do not account for the role of abortion travel (seeking abortion in places with less restrictive abortion laws) (Singer, 2020) or the increased availability of misoprostol in lowering mortality. Additionally, the notoriously fraught administrative task of classifying abortions (spontaneous and induced) may underestimate mortality and morbidity related to induced abortion (Gerdts, Vohra, and Ahern, 2013; Suh, 2014).

NOTES TO CONCLUSION

1. These countries are Bahrain, Belarus, Brazil, Democratic Republic of the Congo, Egypt, Guatemala, Haiti, Hungary, Iraq, Libya, Mali, Nigeria, Poland, Republic of the Congo, Russia, Saudi Arabia, Sudan, Uganda, United Arab Emirates, United States, and Yemen.
2. Between 2012 and 2019, modern contraceptive prevalence among married women increased from 14.3 to 28.5 percent, and from 10.3 to 20.5 percent among all women (Track20, 2019).
3. PATH is a global health innovation organization. Founded in 1977, the organization was initially known as PIACT, or the Program for the Introduction and Adaptation of Contraceptive Technology. The organization has been known as PATH since 1981.
4. A global reproductive health NGO headquartered in London.
5. I am reminded here of anthropologist Dána-Ain Davis's powerful critique of the neonatal intensive care unit as a racialized "saving technology" in American hospitals. Although such technologies keep Black infants alive and should therefore be available to babies born prematurely, they do not address the epidemiological fact of disproportionately high Black infant mortality as an embodied consequence of obstetric (and other forms of) racism (Davis, 2019).

REFERENCES

Aa, I., Grove, M. A., Haugsjå, A. H., and Hinderaker, S. G. (2011). High maternal mortality estimated by the sisterhood method in a rural area of Mali. *BMC Pregnancy and Childbirth*, *11*(56). https://doi.org/10.1186/1471-2393-11-56

Abbott, A. (1988). *The system of professions: An essay on the division of expert labor*. Chicago: University of Chicago Press.

———. (1995a). Boundaries of social work or social work of boundaries? The social service review lecture. *The Social Service Review*, 545–562.

———. (1995b). Things of boundaries. *Social Research*, *62*(4), 857–882.

Abou-Zahr, C. (2003). Safe motherhood: A brief history of the global movement 1947–2002. *British Medical Bulletin*, *67*, 13–25. https://doi.org/10.1093/bmb/ldg014

Acedo, A. (1995). *History of USAID/Senegal* [Report]. Washington, DC: United States Agency for International Development.

Adams, P. (2018, December 29). How Bangladesh made abortion safer. *The New York Times*. Retrieved from https://www.nytimes.com/2018/12/28/opinion/rohingya-bangladesh-abortion.html

Adams, V. (2005). Saving Tibet? An inquiry into modernity, lies, truths and beliefs. *Medical Anthropology*, *24*(1), 71–110.

———. (2013). Evidence-based global public health: Subjects, profits, erasures. In J. Biehl and A. Petryna (Eds.), *When people come first: Critical studies in global health* (pp. 54–90). Princeton, NJ: Princeton University Press.

———. (2016). *Metrics: What counts in global health*. Durham, NC: Duke University Press.

Adjamagbo, A., Antoine, P., and Delaunay, V. (2004). Naissances prémaritales au Sénégal: Confrontation de modèles urbain et rural. *Cahiers Québécois de Démographie*, *33*(2), 239–272.

African Commission on Human and People's Rights. (2003). Protocol to the African Charter on Human and Peoples' Rights on the Rights of Women in Africa. Retrieved from https://www.un.org/en/africa/osaa/pdf/au/protocol_rights_women_africa_2003.pdf

Agence National de la Statistique et de la Démographie [Sénégal] and ICF International. (2012). *Enquête démographique de la santé à indicateurs multiples au Sénégal (EDS-MICS) 2010–2011* [Report]. Retrieved from the DHS Program. https://dhsprogram.com/pubs/pdf/fr258/fr258.pdf

Agence National de la Statistique et de la Démographie [Sénégal] and ICF. (2016). *Enquête continue sur la prestation des services de soins de santé (ECPSS) 2016* [Report]. Retrieved from the DHS Program. https://dhsprogram.com/pubs/pdf/SPA26/SPA26.T.pdf

Agence Nationale de la Statistique et de la Démographie [Sénégal] and ICF. (2018). *Sénégal: Enquête démographique et de santé continue (EDS-Continue 2017)*. [Report]. Retrieved from the DHS Program. https://www.dhsprogram.com/pubs/pdf/FR345/FR345.pdf

Ahmed, S., Li, Q., Liu, L., and Tsui, A. O. (2012). Maternal deaths averted by contraceptive use: An analysis of 172 countries. *The Lancet*, *380*(9837), 111–125.

Allen, D. (2000). Doing occupational demarcation: The "boundary-work" of nurse managers in a district general hospital. *Journal of Contemporary Ethnography*, *29*(3), 326–356. https://doi.org/10.1177/089124100129023936

Andaya, E. (2014). *Conceiving Cuba: Reproduction, women, and the state in the post-Soviet era*. New Brunswick, NJ: Rutgers University Press.

Archer, N., Finden, A., and Pearson, H. (2018). *Senegal: The law, trials and imprisonment for abortion* [Report]. Retrieved from International Campaign for Women's Right to Safe Abortion. http://www.safeabortionwomensright.org/wp-content/uploads/2018/04/The-law -trials-and-imprisonment-for-abortion-in-Senegal-April-2018.pdf

Arregoces, L., Daly, F., Pitt, C., Hsu, J., Martinez-Alvarez, M., Greco, G., . . . Borghi, J. (2015). Countdown to 2015: Changes in official development assistance to reproductive, maternal, newborn, and child health, and assessment of progress between 2003 and 2012. *The Lancet Global Health, 3*(7), e410–e421. https://doi.org/10.1016/S2214-109X(15)00057-1

Atkinson, P. (1995). *Medical talk and medical work: The liturgy of the clinic*. London, UK: Sage Publications Limited.

Averting Maternal Death and Disability (AMDD). (2020) Evolution. Retrieved from https:// www.mailman.columbia.edu/research/averting-maternal-death-and-disability-amdd /evolution

Avortement. (2011, September 22). *L'Observateur, 2401*, p. 2.

Bâ, M. (2011, March 25). Mme Fatou Kiné Camara demande le recours à l'avortement médicalisé. *Le Populaire, 3450*, p. 5.

Bankole, A. (1995). Desired fertility and fertility behaviour among the Yoruba of Nigeria: A study of couple preferences and subsequent fertility. *Population Studies, 49*(2), 317–328.

Bankole, A., Adewole, I., Hussain, R., Awolude, O., Singh, S., and Akinyemi, J. (2015). The incidence of abortion in Nigeria. *International Perspectives on Sexual and Reproductive Health, 41*(4), 170–181.

Bankole, A., Hussain, R., Sedgh, G., Rossier, C., Kaboré, I., and Guiella, G. (2013). *Unintended pregnancy and induced abortion in Burkina Faso: Causes and consequences* [Report]. Retrieved from the Guttmacher Institute. https://www.guttmacher.org/sites/default/files/report_pdf /unintended-pregnancy-burkina-eng.pdf

Barot, S. (2013). Abortion restrictions in U.S. foreign aid: The history and harms of the Helms Amendment, *Guttmacher Policy Review, 16*(3), 9–13.

———. (2017). When anti-abortion ideology turns into foreign policy: How the Global Gag Rule erodes health, ethics and democracy. *Guttmacher Policy Review, 20*, 73–77.

Barot, S., and Cohen, S. A. (2015). The global gag rule and fights over funding UNFPA: The issues that won't go away. *Guttmacher Policy Review, 18*(2), 27–33.

Barrett, D., and Tsui, A. O. (1999). Policy as symbolic statement: International response to national population policies. *Social Forces, 78*, 213–234.

Basilico, M., Weigel, J., Motgi, A., Bor, S., and Keshavhjee J. (2013). Health for all? Competing theories and geopolitics. In P. Farmer, J. Y. Kim, A. Kleinman, and M. Basilico (Eds.), *Reimagining global health: An introduction* (pp. 74–110). Berkeley: University of California Press.

Becker, H. S. (1998). *Tricks of the trade*. Chicago: University of Chicago Press.

Béhague, D. P., and Storeng, K. T. (2008). Collapsing the vertical–horizontal divide: An ethnographic study of evidence-based policymaking in maternal health. *American Journal of Public Health, 98*(4), 644.

———. (2013). Pragmatic politics and epistemological diversity: The contested and authoritative uses of historical evidence in the Safe Motherhood Initiative. *Evidence & Policy: A Journal of Research, Debate and Practice, 9*(1), 65–85. https://doi.org/10.1332/174426413X663724

Béhague, D., Tawiah, C., Rosato, M., Some, T., and Morrison, J. (2009). Evidence-based policymaking: The implications of globally-applicable research for context-specific problemsolving in developing countries. *Social Science & Medicine, 69*(10), 1539–1546. https://doi .org/10.1016/j.socscimed.2009.08.006

Bendix, D., Foley, E. E., Hendrixson, A., and Schultz, S. (2019). Targets and technologies: Sayana Press and Jadelle in contemporary population policies. *Gender, Place & Culture*, 27(3), 351–369.

Beninguisse, G., and De Brouwere, V. (2004). Tradition and modernity in Cameroon: The confrontation between social demand and biomedical logics of health services. *African Journal of Reproductive Health*, 8(3), 152–175.

Bensonsmith, D. (2005). Jezebels, matriarchs, and welfare queens: The Moynihan Report of 1965 and the social construction of African-American women in welfare policy. In A. Schneider and H. Ingram (Eds.), *Deserving and entitled: Social constructions and public policy* (pp. 243–259). Albany, NY: State University of New York Press.

Berelson, B., and Lieberson, J. (1979). Government efforts to influence fertility: The ethical issues. *Population and Development Review*, 5(4), 581–613.

Berer, M. (2009). Task-shifting: Exposing the cracks in public health systems. *Reproductive Health Matters*, 17(33), 4–8. https://doi.org/DOI: 10.1016/S0968-8080(09)33458-8

Berg, M. (1996). Practices of reading and writing: The constitutive role of the patient record in medical work. *Sociology of Health & Illness*, 18(4), 499–524.

Berg, M., and Bowker, G. (1997). The multiple bodies of the medical record. *The Sociological Quarterly*, 38(3), 513–537.

Berhan, Y., and Berhan, A. (2014). Causes of maternal mortality in Ethiopia: A significant decline in abortion related death. *Ethiopian Journal of Health Sciences*, 24, 15–28.

Bernard, H. R., and Ryan, G. W. (2009). *Analyzing qualitative data: Systematic approaches.* Los Angeles, CA: Sage Publications.

Bhatia, R., Sasser, J. S., Ojeda, D., Hendrixson, A., Nadimpally, S., and Foley, E. E. (2019). A feminist exploration of 'populationism': Engaging contemporary forms of population control. *Gender, Place & Culture*, 27(3), 333–350. https://doi.org/10.1080/0966369X.2018.1553859

Biehl, J. (2007). Pharmaceuticalization: AIDS treatment and global health politics. *Anthropological Quarterly*, 80(4), 1083–1126.

Biehl, J., and Petryna, A. (Eds.) (2013). *When people come first: Critical studies in global health.* Princeton, NJ: Princeton University Press.

Bill & Melinda Gates Foundation. (2007). University of Washington launches new institute to evaluate international health programs. Retrieved from https://www.gatesfoundation.org/Media-Center/Press-Releases/2007/06/GlobalHealthPR070604

———. (2010). Melinda Gates calls for global action to save women's and children's lives. Retrieved from https://www.gatesfoundation.org/Media-Center/Press-Releases/2010/06/Melinda-Gates-Calls-for-Global-Action-to-Save-Womens-and-Childrens-Lives

———. (2017). What we do: Maternal, newborn and child health strategy overview. Retrieved from https://www.gatesfoundation.org/What-We-Do/Global-Development/Maternal-Newborn-and-Child-Health

Billings, D. L., and Benson, J. (2005). Postabortion care in Latin America: Policy and service recommendations from a decade of operations research. *Health Policy and Planning*, 20(3), 158–166.

Billings, D. L., Crane, B. B., Benson, J., Solo, J., and Fetters, T. (2007). Scaling-up a public health innovation: A comparative study of post-abortion care in Bolivia and Mexico. *Social Science & Medicine*, 64(11), 2210–2222.

Biruk, C. (2012). Seeing like a research project: Producing "high-quality data" in AIDS research in Malawi. *Medical Anthropology*, 31(4), 347–366.

———. (2018). *Cooking data: Culture and politics in an African research world.* Durham, NC: Duke University Press.

Bledsoe, C. (2002). *Contingent lives: Fertility, time and aging in West Africa*. Chicago: University of Chicago Press.

Bledsoe, C., Banja, F., and Hill, A. (1998). Reproductive mishaps and Western contraception: An African challenge to fertility theory. *Population and Development Review*, 24(1), 15–57.

Bleek, W. (1981). Avoiding shame: The ethical context of abortion in Ghana. *Anthropological Quarterly*, 54(4), 203–209.

Blystad, A., Haukanes, H., Tadele, G., Haaland, M. E., Sambaiga, R., Zulu, J. M., and Moland, K. M. (2019). The access paradox: Abortion law, policy and practice in Ethiopia, Tanzania and Zambia. *International Journal for Equity in Health*, 18(1), 126. https://doi.org/10.1186/s12939-019-1024-0

Bole, K. 2007. UCSF lands $1.4 million grant to reduce maternal mortality worldwide. Retrieved from https://www.ucsf.edu/news/2007/12/5649/ucsf-lands-14-million-grant-reduce-maternal-mortality-worldwide

Borger, J., and Rourke, A. (2020, May 19). Global report: Trump threatens to pull out of WHO over 'failed response' to pandemic. *The Guardian*. Retrieved from https://www.theguardian.com/world/2020/may/19/global-report-trump-threatens-to-pull-out-of-who-over-failed-response-to-pandemic

Boyle, E., Longhofer, W., and Kim, M. (2015). Abortion liberalization in world society, 1960–2009. *American Journal of Sociology*, 121(3), 882–913.

Bridges, K. M. (2011). *Reproducing race: An ethnography of pregnancy as a site of racialization*. Berkeley: University of California Press.

Briggs, L. (2000). The race of hysteria: "Overcivilization" and the "savage" woman in late nineteenth-century obstetrics and gynecology. *American Quarterly*, 52(2), 246–273.

Briozzo, L., Vidiella, G., Rodríguez, F., Gorgoroso, M., Faúndes, A., and Pons, J. E. (2006). A risk reduction strategy to prevent maternal deaths associated with unsafe abortion. *International Journal of Gynecology & Obstetrics*, 95(2), 221–226.

Brown, W., Druce, N., Bunting, J., Radloff, S., Koroma, D., Gupta, S., . . . Darmstadt, G. L. (2014). Developing the "120 by 20" goal for the global FP 2020 initiative. *Studies in Family Planning*, 45(1), 73–84.

Browner, C., and Sargent, C. (2011). *Reproduction, globalization and the state: New theoretical and ethnographic perspectives*. Durham, NC: Duke University Press.

Brunson, J. (2020). Tool of economic development, metric of global health: Promoting planned families and economized life in Nepal. *Social Science & Medicine*, 254. 112298. https://doi.org/10.1016/j.socscimed.2019.05.003

Brunson, J., and Suh, S. (2020). Behind the measures of maternal and reproductive health: Ethnographic accounts of inventory and intervention. *Social Science & Medicine*, 254. 112730. https://doi.org/10.1016/j.socscimed.2019.112730

Bullough, C., Meda, N., Makowiecka, K., Ronsmans, C., Achadi, E. L., and Hussein, J. (2005). Current strategies for the reduction of maternal mortality. *BJOG: An International Journal of Obstetrics & Gynaecology*, 112(9), 1180–1188.

Burawoy, M., Blum, J., George, S., Gille, Z., and Thayer, M. (2000). *Global ethnography: Forces, connections, and imaginations in a postmodern world*. Berkeley: University of California Press.

Butler, D. (2017). World's foremost institute on death and disease metrics gets massive cash boost. *Nature News*, 542(7639), 19. https://doi.org/10.1038/nature.2017.21373

Campbell, O. M., and Graham, W. J. (2006). Strategies for reducing maternal mortality: Getting on with what works. *The Lancet*, 368(9543), 1284–1299.

Carpenter, L. M., and Casper, M. J. (2009). Global intimacies: Innovating the HPV vaccine for women's health. *WSQ: Women's Studies Quarterly*, 37(1), 80–100.

Casper, M. J., and Morrison, D. (2010). Medical sociology and technology: Critical engagements. *Journal of Health and Social Behavior, 51*(1_suppl) S120–S132.

Castro, A., and Savage, V. (2019). Obstetric violence as reproductive governance in the Dominican Republic. *Medical Anthropology, 38*(2), 123–136. https://doi.org/10.1080/01459 740.2018.1512984

Center for Reproductive Law and Policy. (2001). *Women's reproductive rights in Senegal: A shadow report* [Report]. Retrieved from https://reproductiverights.org/sites/default/files /documents/Senegal%20CESCR%202001_0.pdf

Center for Reproductive Rights. (2003). *Women of the world: Laws and policies affecting their reproductive lives, Francophone Africa* [Report]. Retrieved from http://www.reproductive rights.org/document/women-of-the-world-laws-and-policies-affecting-their-reproductive -lives-francophone-africa

Center for Reproductive Rights and United Nations Population Fund. (2013). *ICPD and human rights: 20 years of advancing reproductive rights through UN treaty bodies and legal reform* [Report]. Retrieved from http://www.unfpa.org/publications/icpd-and-human-rights

Central Intelligence Agency. (2020). *The world factbook.* Retrieved from https://www.cia.gov /library/publications/resources/the-world-factbook/

Centre de Formation et de Recherche en Santé de la Reproduction (CEFOREP). (1998a). *Introduction des soins obstétricaux d'urgence et de la planification familiale pour les patientes présentant des complications liées à un avortement incomplet* [Report]. Dakar, Sénégal: CEFOREP.

———. (1998b). *Revue de la littérature sur les avortements à risque au Sénégal* [Report]. Dakar, Sénégal: CEFOREP.

Chapman, R. R. (2006). Chikotsa—secrets, silence, and hiding: Social risk and reproductive vulnerability in central Mozambique. *Medical Anthropology Quarterly, 20*(4), 487–515.

Chiarello, E. (2013). How organizational context affects bioethical decision-making: Pharmacists' management of gatekeeping processes in retail and hospital settings. *Social Science & Medicine, 98*, 319–329. https://doi.org/10.1016/j.socscimed.2012.11.041

Chimbwete, C., Watkins, S. C., and Zulu, E. M. (2005). The evolution of population policies in Kenya and Malawi. *Population Research and Policy Review, 24*(1), 85–106.

Chinchilla, A. L., Flores, I. F., Morales, A. F., and de Gil, M. P. (2014). Changes in the use of manual vacuum aspiration for post-abortion care within the public healthcare service network in Honduras. *International Journal of Gynecology & Obstetrics, 126*, S24–S27. https:// doi.org/10.1016/j.ijgo.2014.03.006

Cissé, C., Faye, K., and Moreau, J. (2007). Avortement du premier trimestre au CHU de Dakar: Intérêt de l'aspiration manuelle intra-utérine. *Médecine Tropicale, 67*(2), 163–166.

Clarke, A. E., and Fujimura, J. H. (1992). *The right tools for the job: At work in twentieth-century life sciences.* Princeton, NJ: Princeton University Press.

Clarke, A. E., and Montini, T. (1993). The many faces of RU486: Tales of situated knowledges and technological contestations. *Science, Technology, & Human Values, 18*(1), 42–78.

Clarke, A. E., Shim, J. K., Mamo, L., Fosket, J. R., and Fishman, J. R. (2003). Biomedicalization: Technoscientific transformations of health, illness, and US biomedicine. *American Sociological Review, 68*(2), 161–194.

Cleeve, A., Nalwadda, G., Zadik, T., Sterner, K., and Allvin, M. K. (2019). Morality versus duty—A qualitative study exploring midwives' perspectives on post-abortion care in Uganda. *Midwifery, 77*, 71–77.

Cohen, S. A. (2000). Abortion politics and US population aid: Coping with a complex new law. *International Family Planning Perspectives, 26*(3), 137–145.

Collins, P. H. (1989). The social construction of black feminist thought. *Signs: Journal of Women in Culture and Society, 14*(4), 745–773.

Connelly, M. (2006). Population control in India: Prologue to the emergency period. *Population and Development Review*, 32(4), 629–667. https://doi.org/10.1111/j.1728-4457.2006.00145.x

————. (2008). *Fatal misconception: The struggle to control world population*. Cambridge, MA: Harvard University Press.

Conrad, P. (1992). Medicalization and social control. *Annual Review of Sociology*, 1, 209–232.

Cook, S., de Kok, B., and Odland, M. L. (2016). 'It's a very complicated issue here': Understanding the limited and declining use of manual vacuum aspiration for postabortion care in Malawi: A qualitative study. *Health Policy and Planning*, 32(3), 305–313. https://doi.org/10.1093/heapol/czw128

Corbett, M. R., and Turner, K. L. (2003). Essential elements of postabortion care: Origins, evolution and future directions. *International Family Planning Perspectives*, 29(3), 106–111.

Corbin, J. M., and Strauss, A. L. (2008). *Basics of qualitative research: Techniques and procedures for developing grounded theory*. Los Angeles, CA: Sage Publications.

Corrêa, S., and Petchesky, R. (1999). Reproductive and sexual rights: A feminist perspective. In R. Parker and P. Aggleton (Eds.), *Culture, Society and Sexuality: A Reader* (pp. 314–332). London, UK: Routledge.

Crane, B. B. (1994). The transnational politics of abortion. *Population and Development Review*, 20, 241–262.

Crane, B. B., and Dusenberry, J. (2004). Power and politics in international funding for reproductive health: The US global gag rule. *Reproductive Health Matters*, 12(24), 128–137.

Crane, J. (2010). Adverse events and placebo effects: African scientists, HIV, and ethics in the 'global health sciences.' *Social Studies of Science*, 40(6), 843–870.

————. (2013). *Scrambling for Africa: AIDS, expertise, and the rise of American global health science*. Ithaca, NY: Cornell University Press.

Cueto, M. (2013). A return to the magic bullet? Malaria and global health in the twenty-first century. In J. Biehl and A. Petryna (Eds.), *When people come first: Critical studies in global health* (pp. 30–53). Princeton, NJ: Princeton University Press.

Curtis, C. (2007). Meeting health care needs of women experiencing complications of miscarriage and unsafe abortion: USAID's postabortion care program. *Journal of Midwifery & Women's Health*, 52(4), 368–375.

Curtis, C., Faundes, A., Yates, A., Wiklund, I., Bokosi, M., and Lacoste, M. (2019). Postabortion family planning progress: The role of donors and health professional associations. *Global Health: Science and Practice*, 7(Supplement 2), S222–S230.

Daniels, C. R. (2009). *At women's expense: State power and the politics of fetal rights*. Cambridge, MA: Harvard University Press.

Dao, B., Blum, J., Thieba, B., Raghavan, S., Ouedraego, M., Lankoande, J., and Winikoff, B. (2007). Is misoprostol a safe, effective and acceptable alternative to manual vacuum aspiration for post-abortion care? Results from a randomised trial in Burkina Faso, West Africa. *BJOG: An International Journal of Obstetrics & Gynaecology*, 114(11), 1368–1375.

Davis, D. A. (2018). Obstetric racism: The racial politics of pregnancy, labor, and birthing. *Medical Anthropology*, 38(7), 560–573. https://doi.org/10.1080/01459740.2018.1549389

————. (2019). *Reproductive injustice: Racism, pregnancy, and premature birth*. New York: New York University Press.

Davis-Floyd, R. E., and Sargent, C. F. (1997). *Childbirth and authoritative knowledge: Cross-cultural perspectives*. Berkeley: University of California Press.

Dembele, D. M. (2012). Africa's developmental impasse: Some perspectives and recommendations. *Africa Development*, 37(4), 179–196.

Demographic and Health Surveys. (2008, October 6). Macro International awarded MEASURE DHS Phase III contract [Press release]. Retrieved from https://dhsprogram.com

/Who-We-Are/News-Room/Macro-International-awarded-MEASURE-DHS-Phase-III
-contract.cfm

DeVault, M. L. (2006). Introduction: What is institutional ethnography? *Social Problems,* *53*(3), 294–298.

De Zordo, S. (2016). The biomedicalisation of illegal abortion: The double life of misoprostol in Brazil. *História, Ciências, Saúde-Manguinhos, 23*(1), 19–36. https://doi.org/10.1590/S0104 -59702016000100003

Diadhiou, F., Faye, E. O., Sangaré, M., and Diouf, A. (1995). *Mortalité et morbidité liées aux avortements provoqués clandestins dans quatre sites de référence Dakarois au Sénégal* [Report]. Dakar, Sénégal: CHU Le Dantec/UCAD and WHO.

Diadhiou, M., Dieng, T., Ortiz, C., Mall, I., Dione, D., and Sloan, N. L. (2011). Introduction of misoprostol for prevention of postpartum hemorrhage at the community level in Senegal. *International Journal of Gynecology & Obstetrics, 115*(3), 251–255.

Diadhiou, M., Dieng, T., Diop, N., Faye, Y., Moreau, J. C., Thieba, B., . . . and Akpadza, K. (2008). Les soins après avortement en Afrique de l'Ouest Francophone, 10 ans après: Leçons apprises de leur introduction et de leur institutionnalisation. *Journal de la Société Africaine des Gynécologues Obstétriciens (SAGO), 9*(2), 38–46.

Diallo, P.D. (2012, April 26). Avortement clandestin à Tambacounda: Une élève de 1ere condamnée à 3 mois ferme. *L'Observateur, 2580,* 4.

Diedhiou, A. (2011a, October 11). Après des soins intenses pour avorter, la couturière accouche et atterrit aux urgences. *L'Observateur, 2417,* 3.

———. (2011b, October 18). Avortement clandestin qui a failli virée au drame: La sage-femme d'état et l'amant de la victime déférés au parquet. *L'Observateur, 2423,* 5.

Dieng, T., Diadhiou, M., Diop, N., and Faye, Y. (2008). *Evaluation des progrès de l'initiative Africaine Francophone pour les Soins Après Avortement* [Report]. Dakar, Sénégal: CEFOREP and FRONTIERS.

Diop, A., Daff, B., Sow, M., Blum, J., Diagne, M., Sloan, N. L., and Winikoff, B. (2016). Oxytocin via Uniject (a prefilled single-use injection) versus oral misoprostol for prevention of postpartum haemorrhage at the community level: A cluster-randomised controlled trial. *The Lancet Global Health, 4*(1), e37–e44.

Division de la Santé de la Reproduction. (2010). *Rapport de l'analyse de la situation sur les grossesses non désirées et les avortements à risque au Sénégal (en édition)* [Report]. Dakar, Sénégal: DSR/MSAS.

Dixon-Mueller, R. (1993). *Population policy & women's rights: Transforming reproductive choice.* Westport, CT: Praeger Publishers.

DKT International. (2018). DKT International, Inc. monthly sales report 2018 [Report]. Retrieved from https://2umya83uy24b2nu5ug2708w5-wpengine.netdna-ssl.com/wp-content /uploads/2019/03/DKT-2018-Sales-Results.pdf

Doctor, H. V., Findley, S. E., and Afenyadu, G. Y. (2012). Estimating maternal mortality level in rural northern Nigeria by the sisterhood method. *International Journal of Population Research, 2012,* 464657. https://doi.org/10.1155/2012/464657

Dodoo, F., and Frost, A. (2008). Gender in African population research: The fertility/reproductive health example. *Annual Review of Sociology, 34,* 431–452.

d'Oliveira, A. F. P. L., Diniz, S. G., and Schraiber, L. B. (2002). Violence against women in health-care institutions: An emerging problem. *The Lancet, 359*(9318), 1681–1685. https:// doi.org/10.1016/S0140-6736(02)08592-6

Donaldson, P. J. (1990). On the origins of the United States government's international population policy. *Population Studies, 44*(3), 385–399. https://doi.org/10.1080/0032472031000 144816

Drabo, S. (2019). A pill in the lifeworld of women in Burkina Faso: Can misoprostol reframe the meaning of abortion? *International Journal of Environmental Research and Public Health, 16*(22), 4425.

Duclos, D., Cavallaro, F.L., Ndoye, T., Faye, S.L., Diallo, I., Lynch, C.A., Diallo, M., Faye, A. and Penn-Kekana, L. (2019). Critical insights on the demographic concept of "birth spacing": locating Nef in family well-being, bodies, and relationships in Senegal. *Sexual and Reproductive Health Matters, 27*(1), 136–145.

Duclos, D., Ndoye, T., Faye, S. L., Diallo, M., and Penn-Kekana, L. (2019). Why didn't you write this in your diary? Or how nurses (mis)used clinic diaries to (re)claim shared reflexive spaces in Senegal. *Critique of Anthropology, 39*(2), 205–221. https://doi.org/10.1177/0308275X19842913

Duffy-Tumasz, A. (2009). Paying back comes first: Why repayment means more than business in rural Senegal. *Gender and Development, 17*(2), 243–254.

Dumont, A., Gaye, A., de Bernis, L., Chaillet, N., Landry, A., Delage, J., and Bouvier-Colle, M.-H. (2006). Facility-based maternal death reviews: Effects on maternal mortality in a district hospital in Senegal. *Bulletin of the World Health Organization, 84*(3), 218–224.

Durr, B. (2015, January 26). Mozambique loosens anti-abortion laws. *Al Jazeera*. Retrieved from https://www.aljazeera.com/indepth/features/2015/01/mozambique-loosens-anti-abortion-laws-150120081246992.html

Eades, C. A., Brace, C., Osei, L., and LaGuardia, K. D. (1993). Traditional birth attendants and maternal mortality in Ghana. *Social Science & Medicine, 36*(11), 1503–1507.

Eckholm, E. (2015, December 16). Tennessee woman tried coat-hanger abortion, police say. *The New York Times*. Retrieved from https://www.nytimes.com/2015/12/16/us/tennessee-woman-tried-coat-hanger-abortion-police-say.html?searchResultPosition=1

EngenderHealth. (2003). *Taking post-abortion care services where they are needed: An operations research project testing PAC expansion in rural Senegal* [Report]. Washington, DC: EngenderHealth.

Erdman, J. N. (2011). Access to information on safe abortion: A harm reduction and human rights approach. *Harvard Journal of Law & Gender, 34*, 413–462.

Erdman, J. N., Jelinska, K., and Yanow, S. (2018). Understandings of self-managed abortion as health inequity, harm reduction and social change. *Reproductive Health Matters, 26*(54), 13–19.

Erikson, S. L. (2012). Global health business: The production and performativity of statistics in Sierra Leone and Germany. *Medical Anthropology, 31*(4), 367–384. https://doi.org/10.1080/01459740.2011.621908

———. (2015). Secrets from whom? Following the money in global health finance. *Current Anthropology, 56*(S12), S306–S316.

Family Planning (FP) 2020. (2013). *Summaries of commitments* [Report]. Retrieved from https://www.familyplanning2020.org/sites/default/files/London_Summit_Commitments_12-2-2013.pdf

Farmer, P. (2014). Diary. *London Review of Books, 36*(20), 38–39.

Farquharson, R. G., Jauniaux, E., and Exalto, N. (2005). Updated and revised nomenclature for description of early pregnancy events. *Human Reproduction, 20*(11), 3008–3011.

Fathalla, M. F. (2019). Safe abortion: The public health rationale. *Best Practice & Research Clinical Obstetrics & Gynaecology, 63*, 2–12.

Faúndes, A., and Shah, I. H. (2015). Evidence supporting broader access to safe legal abortion. *International Journal of Gynecology & Obstetrics, 131*, S56–S59.

Feierman, S., Kleinman, A., Stewart, K., Farmer, P., and Das, V. (2010). Anthropology, knowledge-flows and global health. *Global Public Health, 5*(2), 122–128.

Fernandez, M. M., Coeytaux, F., Gomez Ponce de León, R., and Harrison, D. L. (2009). Assessing the global availability of misoprostol. *International Journal of Gynecology & Obstetrics, 105*(2), 180–186.

Foley, E. (2007). Overlaps and disconnects in reproductive health care: Global policies, national programs, and the micropolitics of reproduction in Northern Senegal. *Medical Anthropology, 26*(4), 323–354.

———. (2009). *Your pocket is what cures you: The politics of health in Senegal.* New Brunswick, NJ: Rutgers University Press.

Footman, K., Keenan, K., Reiss, K., Reichwein, B., Biswas, P., and Church, K. (2018). Medical abortion provision by pharmacies and drug sellers in low- and middle-income countries: A systematic review. *Studies in Family Planning, 49*(1), 57–70.

Fordyce, L. (2014). When bad mothers lose good babies: Understanding fetal and infant mortality case reviews. *Medical Anthropology, 33*(5), 379–394. https://doi.org/10.1080/01459740.2013.844696

Foucault, M. (1973). *The birth of the clinic: An archaeology of medical perception.* New York: Pantheon Books.

———. (1978). *The history of sexuality.* New York: Vintage Books.

Foucault, M., and Ewald, F. (2003). *"Society must be defended": Lectures at the Collège de France, 1975–1976.* New York: Picador.

Fraser, G. (1995). Modern bodies, modern minds: Midwifery and reproductive change in an African-American community. In F. D. Ginsburg and R. Rapp (Eds.), *Conceiving the new world order: The global politics of reproduction* (pp. 42–58). Berkeley: University of California Press.

Freedman, L. P., Ramsey, K., Abuya, T., Bellows, B., Ndwiga, C., Warren, C. E., . . . Mbaruku, G. (2014). Defining disrespect and abuse of women in childbirth: A research, policy and rights agenda. *Bulletin of the World Health Organization, 92*, 915–917.

Gaestel, A., and Shryock, R. (2017, October 1). The price of Senegal's strict anti-abortion laws. *The New Yorker.* Retrieved from https://www.newyorker.com/news/news-desk/the-price-of-senegals-strict-anti-abortion-laws

Ganatra, B., Gerdts, C., Rossier, C., Johnson, B. R., Tunçalp, Ö., Assifi, A., . . . Alkema, L. (2017). Global, regional, and subregional classification of abortions by safety, 2010–14: Estimates from a Bayesian hierarchical model. *The Lancet, 390*(10110), 2372–2381. https://doi.org/10.1016/S0140-6736(17)31794-4

Garenne, M., and Zwang, J. (2006). Premarital fertility and ethnicity in Africa. *DHS Comparative Reports* [Report]. Retrieved from the DHS Program. https://dhsprogram.com/pubs/pdf/CR13/CR13.pdf

Gaye, A., Diop, A., Shochet, T., and Winikoff, B. (2014). Decentralizing postabortion care in Senegal with misoprostol for incomplete abortion. *International Journal of Gynecology & Obstetrics, 126*(3), 223–226. https://doi.org/10.1016/j.ijgo.2014.03.028

Gebreselassie, H., Gallo, M. F., Monyo, A., and Johnson, B. R. (2005). The magnitude of abortion complications in Kenya. *BJOG: An International Journal of Obstetrics & Gynaecology, 112*(9), 1229–1235.

Geissler, P. W. (2013). Public secrets in public health: Knowing not to know while making scientific knowledge. *American Ethnologist, 40*(1), 13–34. https://doi.org/10.1111/amet.12002

Georgetown University. (2013). USAID awards $19.8M for African, Asian fertility awareness project. *News.* Retrieved from https://www.georgetown.edu/news/usaid-awards-19-8m-for-african-asian-fertility-awareness-project/

Gerdts, C., Vohra, D., and Ahern, J. (2013). Measuring unsafe abortion-related mortality: A systematic review of the existing methods. *PLoS ONE, 8*(1), e53346. https://doi.org/10.1371?journal.pone.0053346

Gerdts, C., Tunçalp, O., Johnston, H., and Ganatra, B. (2015). Measuring abortion-related mortality: Challenges and opportunities. *Reproductive Health*, 12(1), 87. https://doi.org/10.1186/s12978-015-0064-1

Gessessew, A. (2010). Abortion and unwanted pregnancy in Adigrat Zonal Hospital, Tigray, North Ethiopia. *African Journal of Reproductive Health*, 14(3), 183–188.

Geurts, K. (2001). Childbirth and pragmatic midwifery in rural Ghana. *Medical Anthropology*, 20(4), 379–408.

Gieryn, T. F. (1983). Boundary-work and the demarcation of science from non-science: Strains and interests in professional ideologies of scientists. *American Sociological Review*, 48(6), 781. https://doi.org/10.2307/2095325

———. (1999). *Cultural boundaries of science: Credibility on the line.* Chicago: University of Chicago Press.

Gilson, L., Alilio, M., and Heggenhougen, K. (1994). Community satisfaction with primary health care services: An evaluation undertaken in the Morogoro region of Tanzania. *Social Science & Medicine*, 39(6), 767–780.

Ginsburg, F., and Rapp, R. (1991). The politics of reproduction. *Annual Review of Anthropology*, 20(1), 311–343.

Glasier, A., Gülmezoglu, A. M., Schmid, G. P., Moreno, C. G., and Van Look, P. F. A. (2006). Sexual and reproductive health: A matter of life and death. *The Lancet*, 368(9547), 1595–1607.

Goffman, E. (1963). *Stigma: Notes on the management of spoiled identity.* New York: Simon & Schuster.

Goldberg, M. (2009). *The means of reproduction: Sex, power, and the future of the world.* New York: Penguin.

Good, B. J. (1994). *Medicine, rationality and experience: An anthropological perspective.* Cambridge, UK: Cambridge University Press.

Goyaux, N., Alihonou, E., Diadhiou, F., Leke, R., and Thonneau, P. F. (2001). Complications of induced abortion and miscarriage in three African countries: A hospital-based study among WHO collaborating centers. *Acta Obstetricia et Gynecologica Scandinavica*, 80(6), 568–573.

Graham, W. J., and Adjei, S. (2010). A call for responsible estimation of global health. *PLoS Medicine*, 7(11), e1001003.

Graham, W. J., and Campbell, O. M. (1992). Maternal health and the measurement trap. *Social Science & Medicine*, 35(8), 967–977.

Green, W. (2017). *Contraceptive risk: The FDA, Depo-Provera, and the politics of experimental medicine.* New York: New York University Press.

Greenhalgh, S. (1994). Controlling births and bodies in village China. *American Ethnologist*, 21(1), 3–30.

———. (1995). *Situating fertility: Anthropology and demographic inquiry.* Cambridge, UK: Cambridge University Press.

———. (1996). The social construction of population science: An intellectual, institutional, and political history of twentieth-century demography. *Comparative Studies in Society and History*, 38(1), 26–66.

———. (2005). Globalization and population governance in China. In A. Ong and S. Collier (Eds.), *Global assemblages: Technology, politics and ethics as anthropological problems* (pp. 354–372). Cornwall, UK: Blackwell Publishing.

———. (2008). *Just one child: Science and policy in Deng's China.* Berkeley: University of California Press.

———. (2010). *Cultivating global citizens* (Vol. 12). Cambridge, MA: Harvard University Press.

Greenslade, F. C., McKay, H., Wolf, M., and McLaurin, K. (1994). *Post-abortion care: A women's health initiative to combat unsafe abortion* [Report]. Chapel Hill, NC: Ipas.

Grimes, D. A., Benson, J., Singh, S., Romero, M., Ganatra, B., Okonofua, F. E., and Shah, I. H. (2006). Unsafe abortion: The preventable pandemic. *The Lancet, 368*(9550), 1908–1919.

Grollman, C., Cavallaro, F. L., Duclos, D., Bakare, V., Martínez Álvarez, M., and Borghi, J. (2018). Donor funding for family planning: Levels and trends between 2003 and 2013. *Health Policy and Planning, 33*(4), 574–582.

Guilbert, N., and Marazyan, K. (2013). *Being born out of wedlock. Does it affect a child's survival chance? An empirical investigation for Senegal* [Report]. Paris, France: Dauphine Université Paris, Développement, Institutions & Mondialisation, and Institut de Recherche pour le Développement.

Guillaume, A., Rossier, C., and Reeve, P. (2018). Abortion around the world: An overview of legislation, measures, trends, and consequences. *Population, 73*(2), 217–306.

Guttmacher Institute. (2012). *Making abortion services accessible in the wake of legal reforms: A framework and six case studies* [Report]. Retrieved from the Guttmacher Institute. https://www.guttmacher.org/sites/default/files/report_pdf/abortion-services-laws_0.pdf

———. (2015). *Abortion in Senegal*. Retrieved from the Guttmacher Institute. https://www.guttmacher.org/fact-sheet/abortion-senegal

———. (2020). *Medication abortion*. Retrieved from the Guttmacher Institute. https://www.guttmacher.org/state-policy/explore/medication-abortion

Haaland, M. E., Haukanes, H., Zulu, J. M., Moland, K. M., and Blystad, A. (2020). Silent politics and unknown numbers: Rural health bureaucrats and the Zambian abortion policy. *Social Science & Medicine, 251*, 112909. https://doi.org/10.1016/j.socscimed.2020.112909

Halpern, S. A. (1990). Medicalization as professional process: Postwar trends in pediatrics. *Journal of Health and Social Behavior, 31*(1), 28. https://doi.org/10.2307/2137043

Hannaford, D. (2014). Technologies of the spouse: Intimate surveillance in Senegalese transnational marriages. *Global Networks 15*(1), 43–59. https://doi.org/10.1111/glob.12045

Hannaford, D., and Foley, E. E. (2015). Negotiating love and marriage in contemporary Senegal: A good man is hard to find. *African Studies Review, 58*(2), 205–225. https://doi.org/10.1017/asr.2015.44

Haraway, D. (1988). Situated knowledges: The science question in feminism and the privilege of partial perspective. *Feminist Studies, 14*(3), 575–599.

Harding, S. (1992). Rethinking standpoint epistemology: What is "strong objectivity?" *The Centennial Review, 36*(3), 437–470.

———. (2008). *Sciences from below: Feminisms, postcolonialities, and modernities*. Durham, NC: Duke University Press.

Hartmann, B. (1995). *Reproductive rights and wrongs: The global politics of population control*. Boston: South End Press.

Health and Human Services. (2019, September 23). Joint statement on universal health coverage [Text]. Retrieved from https://www.hhs.gov/about/agencies/oga/global-health-diplomacy/protecting-life-global-health-policy/joint-statement-unga/index.html

Heath, C. (1982). Preserving the consultation: Medical record cards and professional conduct. *Sociology of Health & Illness, 4*(1), 56–74.

Heller, A. (2019). *Fistula politics: Birthing injuries and the quest for continence in Niger*. New Brunswick, NJ: Rutgers University Press.

Henshaw, S. K., Adewole, I., Singh, S., Bankole, A., Oye-Adeniran, B., and Hussain, R. (2008). Severity and cost of unsafe abortion complications treated in Nigerian hospitals. *International Family Planning Perspectives, 34*(1), 40–50.

Hernández-Carretero, M. (2015). Renegotiating obligations through migration: Senegalese transnationalism and the quest for the right distance. *Journal of Ethnic and Migration Studies*, 41(12), 2021–2040. DOI: 10.1080/1369183X.2015.1045462

Hodgson, D., and Watkins, S. C. (1997). Feminists and neo-Malthusians: Past and present alliances. *Population and Development Review*, 23(3), 469–523. https://doi.org/10.2307/2137570

Hogan, M. C., Foreman, K. J., Naghavi, M., Ahn, S. Y., Wang, M., Makela, S. M., . . . and Murray, C. J. L. (2010). Maternal mortality for 181 countries, 1980–2008: A systematic analysis of progress towards Millennium Development Goal 5. *The Lancet*, 375(9726), 1609–1623.

Högberg, U., Wall, S., and Broström, G. (1986). The impact of early medical technology on maternal mortality in late 19th century Sweden. *International Journal of Gynecology & Obstetrics*, 24(4), 251–261.

Holcombe, S. J., Berhe, A., and Cherie, A. (2015). Personal beliefs and professional responsibilities: Ethiopian midwives' attitudes toward providing abortion services after legal reform. *Studies in Family Planning*, 46(1), 73–95. https://doi.org/10.1111/j.1728-4465.2015.00016.x

Hsu, J., Berman, P., and Mills, A. (2013). Reproductive health priorities: Evidence from a resource tracking analysis of official development assistance in 2009 and 2010. *The Lancet*, 381(9879), 1772–1782.

Huber, D., Curtis, C., Irani, L., Pappa, S., and Arrington, L. (2016). Postabortion care: 20 years of strong evidence on emergency treatment, family planning, and other programming components. *Global Health: Science and Practice*, 4(3), 481–494.

Hudgins, A. A., and Abernathy, M. 2008. *Stocking facilities with MVA equipment according to caseload* [Report]. Chapel Hill, NC: Ipas.

Hughes, D. (1988). When nurse knows best: Some aspects of nurse/doctor interaction in a casualty department. *Sociology of Health & Illness*, 10(1), 1–22.

Hunsmann, M. (2012). Limits to evidence-based health policymaking: Policy hurdles to structural HIV prevention in Tanzania. *Social Science & Medicine*, 74(10), 1477–1485. https://doi.org/10.1016/j.socscimed.2012.01.023

Hunt, N. R. (1999). *A colonial lexicon of birth ritual, medicalization, and mobility in the Congo.* Durham, NC: Duke University Press.

Hyman, A., Blanchard, K., Coeytaux, F., Grossman, D., and Teixeira, A. (2013). Misoprostol in women's hands: A harm reduction strategy for unsafe abortion. *Contraception*, 87(2), 128–130.

Iaccino, L. (2014, December 2). Senegal: Women "strangle or throw babies in septic tank" as abortion laws too strict. *International Business Times UK*. Retrieved from https://www.ibtimes.co.uk/senegal-women-strangle-throw-babies-septic-tank-abortion-laws-too-strict-1477670

Iliffe, J. (1998). *East African doctors: A history of the modern profession.* Cambridge, UK: Cambridge University Press.

IntraHealth. (2018, March 19). How Senegal rapidly introduced Sayana Press into its family planning method mix. Retrieved from https://www.intrahealth.org/vital/how-senegal-rapidly-introduced-sayana-press-its-family-planning-method-mix

Izugbara, C. O., Egesa, C., and Okelo, R. (2015). 'High profile health facilities can add to your trouble': Women, stigma and un/safe abortion in Kenya. *Social Science & Medicine*, 141, 9–18.

Izugbara, C., Wekesah, F. M., Sebany, M., Echoka, E., Amo-Adjei, J., and Muga, W. (2019). Availability, accessibility and utilization of post-abortion care in sub-Saharan Africa: A systematic review. *Health Care for Women International*. https://doi.org/10.1080/07399332.2019.1703991

Jaffré, Y. (2012). Toward an anthropology of public health priorities: Maternal mortality in four obstetric services in West Africa. *Social Anthropology/Anthropologie Sociale*, 20(1), 3–18.

Jaffré, Y., and Olivier de Sardan, J. P. (2003). *Une médecine inhospitalière: Les difficiles relations entre soignants et soignés dans cinq capitales d'Afrique de l'Ouest.* Paris, France: Karthala.

Jaffré, Y., and Prual, A. (1994). Midwives in Niger: An uncomfortable position between social behaviours and health care constraints. *Social Science & Medicine, 38*(8), 1069–1073.

Jaffré, Y., and Suh, S. (2016). Where the lay and the technical meet: Using an anthropology of interfaces to explain persistent reproductive health disparities in West Africa. *Social Science & Medicine, 156,* 175–183.

Jewkes, R., Abrahams, N., and Mvo, Z. (1998). Why do nurses abuse patients? Reflections from South African obstetric services. *Social Science & Medicine, 47*(11), 1781–1795.

Jewkes, R., Rees, H., Dickson, K., Brown, H., and Levin, J. (2005). The impact of age on the epidemiology of incomplete abortions in South Africa after legislative change. *BJOG: An International Journal of Obstetrics & Gynaecology, 112*(3), 355–359.

Joffe, C. (1996). *Doctors of conscience: The struggle to provide abortion before and after Roe v. Wade.* Boston: Beacon Press.

Joffe, C., and Weitz, T. A. (2003). Normalizing the exceptional: Incorporating the "abortion pill" into mainstream medicine. *Social Science & Medicine, 56*(12), 2353–2366.

Johnson, B. R., Ndhlovu, S., Farr, S. L., and Chipato, T. (2002). Reducing unplanned pregnancy and abortion in Zimbabwe through post-abortion contraception. *Studies in Family Planning, 33*(2), 195–202.

Johnson-Hanks, J. (2002a). On the modernity of traditional contraception: Time and the social context of fertility. *Population and Development Review, 28*(2), 229–249.

———. (2002b). The lesser shame: Abortion among educated women in southern Cameroon. *Social Science & Medicine, 55*(8), 1337–1349.

Jones, E. F., and Forrest, J. D. (1992). Underreporting of abortion in surveys of US women: 1976 to 1998. *Demography, 29*(1), 113–126.

Jones, R. K., and Jerman, J. (2017). Abortion incidence and service availability in the United States, 2014. *Perspectives on Sexual and Reproductive Health, 49*(1), 17–27. https://doi.org/10.1363/psrh.12015

Kagaha, A., and Manderson, L. (2020). Medical technologies and abortion care in Eastern Uganda. *Social Science & Medicine, 247,* 112813. https://doi.org/10.1016/j.socscimed.2020.112813

Kalumbi, C., Farquharson, R., and Quenby, S. (2005). Miscarriage. *Current Obstetrics & Gynaecology, 15*(3), 206–210.

Kanaaneh, R. A. (2002). *Birthing the nation: Strategies of Palestinian women in Israel.* Berkeley: University of California Press.

Kanji, N. (1989). Charging for drugs in Africa: UNICEF'S 'Bamako Initiative.' *Health Policy and Planning, 4*(2), 110–120. https://doi.org/10.1093/heapol/4.2.110

Kassebaum, N., Bertozzi-Villa, A., and Coggeshall, M. (2014). Global, regional, and national levels and causes of maternal mortality during 1990–2013: A systematic analysis for the Global Burden of Disease Study 2013. *The Lancet, 384,* 980–1004.

Kestler, E., Valencia, L., Valle, D. V., and Silva, A. (2006). Scaling up post-abortion care in Guatemala: Initial successes at national level. *Reproductive Health Matters, 14*(27), 138–147.

Khan, K. S., Wojdyla, D., Say, L., Gülmezoglu, A. M., and Van Look, P. F. (2006). WHO analysis of causes of maternal death: A systematic review. *Lancet, 367,* 1066–1074.

Kiemtoré, S., Zamané, H., Sawadogo, Y. A., Ouédraogo, C. M., Kaïn, D. P., Diallo, A. A., . . . Lankoandé, J. (2016). Integration of post abortion care package in the activity of 56 health facilities by the Burkina Faso Society of Obstetricians and Gynecologists (SOGOB). *Open Journal of Obstetrics and Gynecology, 6*(8), 457–462.

Kimport, K., Weitz, T. A., and Freedman, L. (2016). The stratified legitimacy of abortions. *Journal of Health and Social Behavior*, 57(4), 503–516. https://doi.org/10.1177/0022146516669970

Klausen, S. (2016). *Abortion under apartheid: Nationalism, sexuality and women's reproductive rights in South Africa*. New York: Oxford University Press.

Kligman, G. (1998). *The politics of duplicity: Controlling reproduction in Ceauşescu's Romania*. Berkeley: University of California Press.

Knoppers, B. M., Brault, I., and Sloss, E. (1990). Abortion law in francophone countries. *The American Journal of Comparative Law*, 38, 889–922.

Kodio, B., de Bernis, L., Ba, M., Ronsmans, C., Pison, G., and Etard, J. (2002). Levels and causes of maternal mortality in Senegal. *Tropical Medicine & International Health*, 7(6), 499–505.

Koch, E., Thorp, J., Bravo, M., Gatica, S., Romero, C.X, Aguilera, H., and Ahlers, I. (2012). Women's education level, maternal health facilities, abortion legislation and maternal deaths: A natural experiment in Chile from 1957 to 2007. *PLoS ONE*, 7(5): e36613. doi:10.1371/journal.pone.0036613

Kulczycki, A. (2016). The imperative to expand provision, access and use of misoprostol for post-abortion care in sub-Saharan Africa. *African Journal of Reproductive Health*, 20(3), 22–25.

Kumar, A., Hessini, L., and Mitchell, E. M. H. (2009). Conceptualising abortion stigma. *Culture, Health & Sexuality*, 11(6), 625–639.

Kuumba, M. B. (1999). A cross-cultural race/class/gender critique of contemporary population policy: The impact of globalization. *Sociological Forum*, 14, 447–463.

Lambert, H. (2013). Plural forms of evidence in public health: Tolerating epistemological and methodological diversity. *Evidence & Policy: A Journal of Research, Debate and Practice*, 9(1), 43–48.

Lamont, M., and Molnár, V. (2002). The study of boundaries in the social sciences. *Annual Review of Sociology*, 28(1), 167–195. https://doi.org/10.1146/annurev.soc.28.110601.141107

Lane, S. D. (1994). From population control to reproductive health: An emerging policy agenda. *Social Science & Medicine*, 39(9), 1303–1314.

Lange, I. L., Kanhonou, L., Goufodji, S., Ronsmans, C., and Filippi, V. (2016). The costs of 'free': Experiences of facility-based childbirth after Benin's Caesarean-section exemption policy. *Social Science & Medicine*, 168, 53–62.

Langwick, S. (2012). The choreography of global subjection: The traditional birth attendant in contemporary configurations of world health. In K. Dilger, A. Kane, and S. Langwick (Eds.), *Medicine, mobility and power in global Africa: Transnational health and healing* (pp. 31–59). Bloomington: Indiana University Press.

Layne, L. L. (2010). Introduction. In L. L. Layne, S. L. Vostral, and K. Boyer (Eds.), *Feminist technology* (pp. 1–35). Urbana: University of Illinois Press.

Layne, L. L., Vostral, S. L., and Boyer, K. (Eds.). (2010). *Feminist technology*. Urbana: University of Illinois Press.

Levandowski, B. A., Kalilani-Phiri, L., Kachale, F., Awah, P., Kangaude, G., and Mhango, C. (2012). Investigating social consequences of unwanted pregnancy and unsafe abortion in Malawi: The role of stigma. *International Journal of Gynecology & Obstetrics*, 118, S167–S171. https://doi.org/10.1016/S0020-7292(12)60017-4

Levandowski, B. A., Mhango, C., Kuchingale, E., Lunguzi, J., Katengeza, H., Gebreselassie, . . . Singh, S. (2013). The incidence of induced abortion in Malawi. *International Perspectives on Sexual and Reproductive Health*, 39(2), 88–96.

Liljestrand, J., and Pathmanathan, I. (2004). Reducing maternal mortality: Can we derive policy guidance from developing country experiences? Critical elements in reducing maternal mortality. *Journal of Public Health Policy*, 25(3/4), 299–314.

Lince-Deroche, N., Sène, I., Pliskin, E., Owolabi, O. O., and Bankole, A. (2020). The health system costs of post-abortion care in Senegal. *International Perspectives on Sexual and Reproductive Health, 46*, 99–111. https://doi.org/10.1363/46e9220

Lince-Deroche, N., Kayembe, P., Blades, N., Williams, P., London, S., Mabika, C., . . . and Bankole, A. (2019). *Unintended pregnancy and abortion in Kinshasa, Democratic Republic of Congo: Challenges and progress* [Report]. Retrieved from the Guttmacher Institute. https://www.guttmacher.org/report/unintended-pregnancy-abortion-kinshasa-drc

Livingston, J. (2012). *Improvising medicine: An African oncology ward in an emerging cancer epidemic.* Durham, NC: Duke University Press.

Lofland, J., and Lofland, L. H. (2006). *Analyzing social settings.* Belmont, CA: Wadsworth.

Løkeland, M. (2004). Abortion: The legal right has been won, but not the moral right. *Reproductive Health Matters, 12*(24), 167–173.

Loudon, I. (1992). The transformation of maternal mortality. *British Medical Journal, 305*(6868), 1557–1560.

———. (2000). Maternal mortality in the past and its relevance to developing countries today. *The American Journal of Clinical Nutrition, 72*(1), 241s–246s.

Lubiano, W. (1992). Black ladies, welfare queens, and state minstrels: Ideological war by narrative means. In T. Morrison (Ed.), *Race-ing justice, en-gendering power: Essays on Anita Hill, Clarence Thomas and the construction of social reality* (pp. 65–87). New York: Pantheon Books.

Luna, Z., and Luker, K. (2013). Reproductive justice. *Annual Review of Law and Social Science, 9*, 327–352.

MacDonald, M. (2019). The image world of maternal mortality: Visual economies of hope and aspiration in the global campaigns to reduce maternal mortality. *Humanity: An International Journal of Human Rights, Humanitarianism, and Development, 10*, 263–285. https://doi.org/10.1353/hum.2019.0013

Maimbolwa, M. C., Yamba, B., Diwan, V., and Ransjö-Arvidson, A. (2003). Cultural childbirth practices and beliefs in Zambia. *Journal of Advanced Nursing, 43*(3), 263–274.

Maine, D., and Rosenfield, A. (1999). The Safe Motherhood Initiative: Why has it stalled? *American Journal of Public Health, 89*(4), 480–482.

Mamdani, M. (1972). *The myth of population control: Family, caste and class in an Indian village.* New York: Monthly Review Press.

Management Sciences for Health. (2006). *Senegal Maternal Mortality and Morbidity Reduction (PREMOMA) Project: End-of-project report, August 2006* [Report]. Cambridge, MA: Management Sciences for Health.

Mann Global Health. (2019). *Landscape assessment: Leveraging the role of national distributors to increase access to MA combi-packs in Africa* [Report]. Retrieved from https://www.rhsupplies.org/uploads/tx_rhscpublications/Landscape_Assessment_Combi-Packs_RHSC_01.pdf

Mbembe, J. A., and Meintjes, L. (2003). Necropolitics. *Public Culture, 15*(1), 11–30.

McCann, C. R. (2017). *Figuring the population bomb: Gender and demography in the mid-twentieth century.* Seattle: University of Washington Press.

McKay, R. (2012). Documentary disorders: Managing medical multiplicity in Maputo, Mozambique. *American Ethnologist, 39*(3), 545–561. https://doi.org/10.1111/j.1548-1425.2012.01380.x

McLean, E., Desalegn, D. N., Blystad, A., and Miljeteig, I. (2019). When the law makes doors slightly open: Ethical dilemmas among abortion service providers in Addis Ababa, Ethiopia. *BMC Medical Ethics, 20*(1), 1–10.

McPake, B., Hanson, K., and Mills, A. (1993). Community financing of health care in Africa: An evaluation of the Bamako initiative. *Social Science & Medicine, 36*(11), 1383–1395. https://doi.org/10.1016/0277-9536(93)90381-D

Médecins Sans Frontières. (2019). *Essential obstetric and newborn care: Practical guide for midwives, doctors with obstetrics training and health care personnel who deal with obstetric emergencies*. Retrieved from MSF. https://medicalguidelines.msf.org/viewport/ONC/english/essential-obstetric-and-newborn-care-51415817.html

Merry, S. E. (2016). *The seductions of quantification: Measuring human rights, gender violence and sex trafficking*. Chicago: University of Chicago Press.

MSAS, CEFOREP, and UNFPA. (2017). *Evaluation rapide de la disponibilité, de l'utilisation, et de la qualité des soins obstétricaux et néonataux d'urgence au Sénégal, 2015 à 2016* [Report]. Dakar, Sénégal: MSAS, CEFOREP, and UNFPA.

Mizrachi, N., Shuval, J. T., and Gross, S. (2005). Boundary at work: Alternative medicine in biomedical settings. *Sociology of Health & Illness, 27*(1), 20–43.

Mol, A. (2002). *The body multiple: Ontology in medical practice*. Durham, NC: Duke University Press.

Mol, A., and Berg, M. (1994). Principles and practices of medicine. *Culture, Medicine and Psychiatry, 18*(2), 247–265.

Morgan, L. M. (2019). Reproductive governance, redux. *Medical Anthropology, 38*(2), 113–117. https://doi.org/10.1080/01459740.2018.1555829

Morgan, L. M., and Roberts, E. (2012). Reproductive governance in Latin America. *Anthropology & Medicine, 19*, 241–254.

Morsy, S. (1995). Deadly reproduction among Egyptian women: Maternal mortality and the medicalization of population control. In F. D. Ginsburg and R. Rapp (Eds.), *Conceiving the new world order: The global politics of reproduction* (pp. 162–176). Berkeley: University of California Press.

Moseson, H., Ouedraogo, R., Diallo, S., and Sakho, A. (2019). Infanticide in Senegal: Results from an exploratory mixed-methods study. *Sexual and Reproductive Health Matters, 27*(1), 203–214. https://doi.org/10.1080/26410397.2019.1624116

Murphy, M. (2012). *Seizing the means of reproduction: Entanglements of feminism, health, and technoscience*. Durham, NC: Duke University Press.

———. (2017). *The economization of life*. Durham, NC: Duke University Press.

Mutua, M. M., Manderson, L., Musenge, E., and Achia, T. N. O. (2018). Policy, law and post-abortion care services in Kenya. *PLoS ONE, 13*(9), e0204240. https://doi.org/10.1371/journal.pone.0204240

Ndembi, A. P. N., Mekui, J., Pheterson, G., and Alblas, M. (2019). Midwives and post-abortion care in Gabon: "Things have really changed." *Health and Human Rights, 21*(2), 145–155.

N'Diaye, S., and Ayad, M. (2006). *Enquête démographique et de santé, Sénégal 2005* [Report]. Retrieved from the DHS Program. https://dhsprogram.com/pubs/pdf/FR177/FR177.pdf

Norris, A., Bessett, D., Steinberg, J. R., Kavanaugh, M. L., De Zordo, S., and Becker, D. (2011). Abortion stigma: A reconceptualization of constituents, causes, and consequences. *Women's Health Issues, 21*(3), S49–S54.

Oberman, M. (2018). *Her body, our laws: On the frontlines of the abortion wars from El Salvador to Oklahoma*. Boston: Beacon Press.

Odland, M. L., Rasmussen, H., Jacobsen, G. W., Kafulafula, U. K., Chamanga, P., and Odland, J. Ø. (2014). Decrease in use of manual vacuum aspiration in postabortion care in Malawi: A cross-sectional study from three public hospitals, 2008–2012. *PLoS ONE, 9*(6), e100728. https://doi.org/10.1371/journal.pone.0100728

Ogden, J. (2003). The politics of branding in policy transfer: The case of DOTS for tuberculosis control. *Social Science & Medicine, 57*, 179–188.

Olsen, B. E., Hinderaker, S. G., Kazaura, M., Lie, R. T., Bergsjø, P., Gasheka, P., and Kvåle, G. (2000). Estimates of maternal mortality by the sisterhood method in rural northern Tanzania: A household sample and an antenatal clinic sample. *BJOG: An International Journal of Obstetrics & Gynaecology, 107*(10), 1290–1297.

Ong, A., and Collier, S. J. (Eds.). (2005). *Global assemblages: Technology, politics, and ethics as anthropological problems*. Malden, MA: Wiley.

Oni-Orisan, A. (2016). The obligation to count: The politics of monitoring maternal mortality in Nigeria. In V. Adams (Ed.), *Metrics: What counts in global health* (pp. 82–104). Durham, NC: Duke University Press.

Oudshoorn, N. (2003). *Beyond the natural body: An archaeology of sex hormones*. New York: Routledge.

Owens, D.C. (2017). *Medical bondage: Race, gender, and the origins of American gynecology*. Athens, GA: University of Georgia Press

Owolabi, O. O., Biddlecom, A., and Whitehead, H. S. (2018). Health systems' capacity to provide post-abortion care: A multicountry analysis using signal functions. *The Lancet Global Health, 7*(1), e110–e118. https://doi.org/10.1016/S2214-109X(18)30404-2

PAC Consortium. (2012). Fact sheet: Results from the 2012 PAC Consortium Mapping Exercise. Retrieved from http://www.pac-consortium.org/index.php/where-work/28-where-we-work/49-results-of-mapping

———. (2016). Updates from the PAC Consortium. Retrieved from https://www.postabortioncare.org/sites/pac/files/6%20Japheth%20Ominde.pdf

Packard, R. M. (2007). *The making of a tropical disease: A short history of malaria*. Baltimore, MD: Johns Hopkins University Press.

———. (2016). *A history of global health: Interventions into the lives of other peoples*. Baltimore, MD: Johns Hopkins University Press.

Påfs, J., Rulisa, S., Klingberg-Allvin, M., Binder-Finnema, P., Musafili, A., and Essén, B. (2020). Implementing the liberalized abortion law in Kigali, Rwanda: Ambiguities of rights and responsibilities among health care providers. *Midwifery, 80*, 102568. https://doi.org/10.1016/j.midw.2019.102568

Paganini, A. (2004). The Bamako Initiative was not about money. *Health Policy and Development, 2*(1), 11–13.

PAI (2018, February 23). The Abortion and Post-Abortion Care Consortium and the Global Gag Rule. Retrieved from https://trumpglobalgagrule.pai.org/the-abortion-and-post-abortion-care-consortium-and-the-global-gag-rule/

Paltrow, L., and Flavin, J. (2013). Arrests of and forced interventions on pregnant women in the United States, 1973–2005: Implications for women's legal status and public health. *Journal of Health Politics Policy and Law, 38*(2), 299–343. https://doi.org/10.1215/03616878-1966324

Parkhurst, J., Ettelt, S., and Hawkins, B. (2018). Studying evidence use for health policymaking from a policy perspective. In J. Parkhurst, S. Ettelt, and B. Hawkins (Eds.), *Evidence Use in Health Policy Making* (pp. 1–20). Cham, Switzerland: Palgrave Macmillan.

Parmar, D., Leone, T., Coast, E., Murray, S. F., Hukin, E., and Vwalika, B. (2017). Cost of abortions in Zambia: A comparison of safe abortion and post abortion care. *Global Public Health, 12*(2), 236–249. https://doi.org/10.1080/17441692.2015.1123747

Parsons, T. (1951). *The social system*. Glencoe, IL: Free Press.

Partenariat de Ouagadougou. (2015). Le Partenariat de Ouagadougou. Retrieved from https://partenariatouaga.org/a-propos/le-partenariat/

PATH. (2018). *How to introduce and scale up DMPA-SC (Sayana Press)* [Report]. Retrieved from https://path.azureedge.net/media/documents/PATH_DMPA-SC_practical_guidance_rev_2018.pdf

Paul, M., Gemzell-Danielsson, K., Kiggundu, C., Namugenyi, R., and Klingberg-Allvin, M. (2014). Barriers and facilitators in the provision of post-abortion care at district level in central Uganda—a qualitative study focusing on task sharing between physicians and mid-wives. *BMC Health Services Research, 14*(1), 1–12. https://doi.org/10.1186/1472-6963-14-28

Paxton, A., Maine, D., Freedman, L., Fry, D., and Lobis, S. (2005). The evidence for emergency obstetric care. *International Journal of Gynecology & Obstetrics, 88*(2), 181–193.

Payne, C. M., Debbink, M. P., Steele, E. A., Buck, C. T., Hassinger, J. A., and Harris, L. H. (2013). Why women are dying from unsafe abortion: Narratives of Ghanaian abortion providers. *African Journal of Reproductive Health, 17*(2), 118–128.

Petchesky, R. (1995). From population control to reproductive rights: Feminist fault lines. *Reproductive Health Matters, 3*(6), 152–161.

Pfeiffer, J. (2013). The struggle for a public sector: Pepfar in Mozambique. In J. Biehl and A. Petryna (Eds.), *When people come first: Critical studies in global health* (pp. 166–181). Princeton, NJ: Princeton University Press.

———. (2019). Austerity in Africa: Audit cultures and the weakening of public sector health systems. *Focaal, 2019*(83), 51–61.

Pfeiffer, J., and Chapman, R. (2010). Anthropological perspectives on structural adjustment and public health. *Annual Review of Anthropology, 39*, 149–165.

Pfeiffer, J., and Nichter, M. (2008). What can critical medical anthropology contribute to global health? *Medical Anthropology Quarterly, 22*(4), 410–415.

Pigg, S. L. (1997). Authority in translation: Finding, knowing, naming and training "traditional birth attendants" in Nepal. In R. Davis-Floyd and C. Sargent (Eds.), *Childbirth and authoritative knowledge: Cross-cultural perspectives* (pp. 233–262). Berkeley: University of California Press.

Population Council. (2007). *Assessment of the extension of post-abortion care services in Senegal* [Report]. Washington, DC: Population Council.

Population Reference Bureau (PRB). (2020). Expanding access to safe abortion in the Democratic Republic of Congo. Retrieved from https://www.prb.org/expanding-access-to-safe-abortion-in-the-democratic-republic-of-congo/

Prada, E., Mirembe, F., Ahmed, F., Nalwadda, R., and Kiggundu, C. (2005). *Abortion and postabortion care in Uganda: A report from health care professionals and health facilities* [Report]. Retrieved from the Guttmacher Institute. https://www.guttmacher.org/sites/default/files/pdfs/pubs/2005/05/28/or17.pdf

PRWEB. (2017, May 10). Ipas and DKT International Partnership expands access to safe abortion and reduces associated maternal deaths for millions in 100+ countries worldwide. Retrieved from https://www.prweb.com/releases/2017/05/prweb14321090.htm

Rance, S. (1997). Safe motherhood, unsafe abortion: A reflection on the impact of discourse. *Reproductive Health Matters, 5*(9), 10–19.

———. (2005). Abortion discourse in Bolivian hospital contexts: Doctors' repertoire conflicts and the Saving Women device: Abortion discourse in Bolivian hospital contexts. *Sociology of Health & Illness, 27*(2), 188–214. https://doi.org/10.1111/j.1467-9566.2005.00439.x

Ray, C. E. (2015). *Crossing the color line: Race, sex, and the contested politics of colonialism in Ghana.* Athens: Ohio University Press.

Reagan, L. J. (1998). *When abortion was a crime: Women, medicine, and law in the United States, 1867–1973.* Berkeley: University of California Press.

Reiss, K., Footman, K., Burke, E., Diop, N., Ndao, R., Mane, B., . . . Ngo, T. (2017). Knowledge and provision of misoprostol among pharmacy workers in Senegal: A cross sectional study. *BMC Pregnancy and Childbirth, 17*, 211. https://doi.org/10.1186/s12884-017-1394-5

Renne, E. (2016). Interpreting population policy in Nigeria. In R. Solinger and M. Nakachi (Eds.), *Reproductive states: Global perspectives on the invention and implementation of population policy* (pp. 260–289). New York: Oxford University Press.

Ridde, V. (2003). Fees-for-services, cost recovery, and equity in a district of Burkina Faso operating the Bamako initiative. *Bulletin of the World Health Organization, 81*(7), 532–538.

Roberts, D. E. (1997). *Killing the black body: Race, reproduction, and the meaning of liberty.* New York: Pantheon Books.

Robinson, R. S. (2012). Negotiating development prescriptions: The case of population policy in Nigeria. *Population Research and Policy Review, 31*(2), 267–296. https://doi.org/10.1007/s11113-011-9222-5

———. (2015). Population policy in sub-Saharan Africa: A case of both normative and coercive ties to the world polity. *Population Research and Policy Review, 34*(2), 201–221. https://doi.org/10.1007/s11113-014-9338-5

———. (2016). Population policy adoption in sub-Saharan Africa: An interplay of global and local forces. *Population Horizons, 13*(1), 9–18. https://doi.org/10.1515/pophzn-2016-0001

———. (2017). *Intimate interventions in global health: Family planning and HIV prevention in sub-Saharan Africa.* Cambridge, UK: Cambridge University Press.

Roe, G. (2005). Harm reduction as paradigm: Is better than bad good enough? The origins of harm reduction. *Critical Public Health, 15*(3), 243–250.

Rosenfield, A., and Maine, D. (1985). Maternal mortality—a neglected tragedy: Where is the M in MCH? *The Lancet, 326*(8446), 83–85.

Ross, L., and Solinger, R. (2017). *Reproductive justice: An introduction.* Oakland: University of California Press.

Rossier, C. (2007). Abortion: An open secret? Abortion and social network involvement in Burkina Faso. *Reproductive Health Matters, 15*(30), 230–238.

Rossier, C., Guiella, G., Ouédraogo, A., and Thiéba, B. (2006). Estimating clandestine abortion with the confidants method—results from Ouagadougou, Burkina Faso. *Social Science & Medicine, 62*(1), 254–266.

Rwirahira, R. (2018, January 22). Rwanda's proposed abortion amendment takes procedure out of the courts. *News Deeply.* Retrieved from https://www.newsdeeply.com/womenand girls/articles/2018/01/22/rwandas-proposed-abortion-amendment-takes-procedure-out -of-the-courts

Sadler, M., Santos, M. J., Ruiz-Berdún, D., Rojas, G. L., Skoko, E., Gillen, P., and Clausen, J. A. (2016). Moving beyond disrespect and abuse: Addressing the structural dimensions of obstetric violence. *Reproductive Health Matters, 24*(47), 47–55. https://doi.org/10.1016/j .rhm.2016.04.002

Sasser, J. S. (2018). *On infertile ground: Population control and women's rights in the era of climate change.* New York: New York University Press.

Say, L., Chou, D., Gemmill, A., Tunçalp, Ö., Moller, A.-B., Daniels, J., . . . and Alkema, L. (2014). Global causes of maternal death: A WHO systematic analysis. *The Lancet Global Health, 2*(6), e323–e333. https://doi.org/10.1016/S2214-109X(14)70227-X

Schuster, S. (2005). Abortion in the moral world of the Cameroon grassfields. *Reproductive Health Matters, 13*(26), 130–138.

Seamark, C. J. (1998). The demise of the D&C. *Journal of the Royal Society of Medicine, 91*(2), 76–79.

Sedgh, G., Bearak, J., Singh, S., Bankole, A., Popinchalk, A., Ganatra, B., . . . Alkema, L. (2016). Abortion incidence between 1990 and 2014: Global, regional, and subregional levels and trends. *The Lancet, 388*(10041), 258–267. https://doi.org/10.1016/S0140-6736 (16)30380-4

Sedgh, G., Sylla, A. H., Philbin, J., Keogh, S., and Ndiaye, S. (2015). Estimates of the incidence of induced abortion and consequences of unsafe abortion in Senegal. *International Perspectives on Sexual and Reproductive Health, 41*(1), 11. https://doi.org/10.1363/4101115

Segall, A. (1976). The sick role concept: Understanding illness behavior. *Journal of Health and Social Behavior*, 17(2), 162–169.

Senderowicz, L. (2019). "I was obligated to accept": A qualitative exploration of contraceptive coercion. *Social Science & Medicine*, 239, 112531. https://doi.org/10.1016/j.socscimed.2019 .112531

Sherris, J., Bingham, A., Burns, M. A., Girvin, S., Westley, E., and Gomez, P. I. (2005). Misoprostol use in developing countries: Results from a multicountry study. *International Journal of Gynecology & Obstetrics*, 88(1), 76–81.

Shiffman, J., and Smith, S. (2007). Generation of political priority for global health initiatives: A framework and case study of maternal mortality. *The Lancet*, 370(9595), 1370–1379.

Shochet, T., Diop, A., Gaye, A., Nayama, M., Bal Sall, A., Bukola, F., . . . Winikoff, B. (2012). Sublingual misoprostol versus standard surgical care for treatment of incomplete abortion in 5 sub-Saharan African countries. *BMC Pregnancy and Childbirth*, 12, 127–134.

Singer, E.O. (2020). Abortion exile: navigating Mexico's fractured abortion landscape. *Culture, Health & Sexuality*, 22(8), 855–870. https://doi.org/10.1080/13691058.2019.1631963

Singh, J. A., and Karim, S. S. A. (2017). Trump's "global gag rule": Implications for human rights and global health. *The Lancet Global Health*, 5(4), e387–e389. https://doi.org/10.1016 /S2214-109X(17)30084-0

Singh, S., and Maddow-Zimet, I. (2016). Facility-based treatment for medical complications resulting from unsafe pregnancy termination in the developing world, 2012: A review of evidence from 26 countries. *BJOG: An International Journal of Obstetrics & Gynaecology*, 123(9), 1489–1498. https://doi.org/10.1111/1471-0528.13552

Singh, S., Prada, E., Mirembe, F., and Kiggundu, C. (2005). The incidence of induced abortion in Uganda. *International Family Planning Perspectives*, 31(4), 183–191.

Singh, S., Remez, L., Sedgh, G., Kwokand, L., and Onda, T. (2018). *Abortion worldwide 2017: Uneven progress and unequal access* [Report]. Retrieved from the Guttmacher Institute. https://www.guttmacher.org/sites/default/files/report_pdf/abortion-worldwide-2017 .pdf

Singh, S., Remez, L., and Tartaglione, A. (Eds.). (2010). *Methodologies for estimating abortion incidence and abortion related morbidity: A review* [Report]. Retrieved from the Guttmacher Institute. https://www.guttmacher.org/sites/default/files/pdfs/pubs/compilations/IUSSP /abortion-methodologies.pdf

Smith, A. D. (2014, April 4). Senegalese law bans raped 10-year-old from aborting twins. Retrieved from *The Guardian*. https://www.theguardian.com/global-development/2014 /apr/04/sengalese-law-bans-rape-survivor-aborting-twins

Smith, D. E. (1993). *Texts, facts and femininity: Exploring the relations of ruling*. London, UK: Routledge.

Smith, S. L., and Shiffman, J. (2016). Setting the global health agenda: The influence of advocates and ideas on political priority for maternal and newborn survival. *Social Science & Medicine*, 166, 86–93.

Solheim, I., Moland, K., Kahabuka, C., Pembe, A., and Blystad, A. (2020). Beyond the law: Misoprostol and medical abortion in Dar es Salaam, Tanzania. *Social Science & Medicine*, 245, 112676. https://doi.org/10.1016/j.socscimed.2019.112676

Sommer, J. M., Shandra, J. M., Restivo, M., and Reed, H. E. (2019). The African Development Bank, organized hypocrisy, and maternal mortality: A cross-national analysis of sub-Saharan Africa. *Sociology of Development*, 5(1), 31–49.

Specia, M. (2018, May 27). How Savita Halappanavar's death spurred Ireland's abortion rights campaign. *The New York Times*. Retrieved from https://www.nytimes.com/2018/05/27 /world/europe/savita-halappanavar-ireland-abortion.html

Ssuunal, I. (2018, October 19). Rwanda unveils gender-balanced cabinet with 50% women. *The Independent*. Retrieved from https://www.independent.co.uk/news/world/africa/rwanda -cabinet-women-gender-balance-government-africa-ethiopia-a8592461.html

Starrs, A. M. (2017). The Trump global gag rule: An attack on US family planning and global health aid. *The Lancet, 389*(10068), 485–486. https://doi.org/10.1016/S0140-6736(17)30270-2

Stoler, A. (2002). *Carnal knowledge and imperial power: Race and the intimate in colonial rule*. Berkeley: University of California Press.

Storeng, K. T., Baggaley, R. F., Ganaba, R., Ouattara, F., Akoum, M. S., and Filippi, V. (2008). Paying the price: The cost and consequences of emergency obstetric care in Burkina Faso. *Social Science & Medicine, 66*(3), 545–557.

Storeng, K. T., and Béhague, D. P. (2014). "Playing the numbers game": Evidence-based advocacy and the technocratic narrowing of the Safe Motherhood Initiative. *Medical Anthropology Quarterly, 28*(2), 260–279.

———. (2017). "Guilty until proven innocent": The contested use of maternal mortality indicators in global health. *Critical Public Health, 27*(2), 163–176. https://doi.org/10.1080/09581596 .2016.1259459

Storeng, K. T., Murray, S. F., Akoum, M. S., Ouattara, F., and Filippi, V. (2010). Beyond body counts: A qualitative study of lives and loss in Burkina Faso after 'near-miss' obstetric complications. *Social Science & Medicine, 71*(10), 1749–1756. https://doi.org/10.1016/j.socscimed .2010.03.056

Storeng, K. T., and Ouattara, F. (2014). The politics of unsafe abortion in Burkina Faso: The interface of local norms and global public health practice. *Global Public Health, 9*(8), 946–959.

Suh, S. (2014). Rewriting abortion: Deploying medical records in jurisdictional negotiation over a forbidden practice in Senegal. *Social Science & Medicine, 108*, 20–33.

———. (2015). "Right tool," wrong "job": Manual vacuum aspiration, post-abortion care and transnational population politics in Senegal. *Social Science & Medicine, 135*, 55–66.

———. (2018). Accounting for abortion: Accomplishing transnational reproductive governance through post-abortion care in Senegal. *Global Public Health, 13*(6), 662–679, https:// doi.org/10.1080/17441692.2017.1301513

———. (2019). Post-abortion care in Senegal: A promising terrain for medical sociology research on global abortion politics. *Advances in Medical Sociology, 20 (Reproduction, Health, and Medicine), 19–43.* https://doi.org/10.1108/S1057-629020190000020007

———. (2020). What post-abortion care indicators don't measure: Global abortion politics and obstetric practice in Senegal. *Social Science & Medicine, 254*, 112248. https://doi.org/10.1016 /j.socscimed.2019.03.044

Sullivan, N. (2017). Multiple accountabilities: Development cooperation, transparency, and the politics of unknowing in Tanzania's health sector. *Critical Public Health, 27*(2), 193–204. https://doi.org/10.1080/09581596.2016.1264572

Sully, E., Dibaba, Y., Fetters, T., Blades, N., and Bankole, A. (2018). Playing it safe: Legal and clandestine abortions among adolescents in Ethiopia. *Journal of Adolescent Health, 62*(6), 729–736.

Sundaram, A., Vlassoff, M., Mugisha, F., Bankole, A., Singh, S., Amanya, L., and Onda, T. (2013). Documenting the individual- and household-level cost of unsafe abortion in Uganda. *International Perspectives on Sexual and Reproductive Health, 39*(4), 174.

Tagoe-Darko, E. (2013). "Fear, shame and embarrassment": The stigma factor in post abortion care at Komfo Anokye Teaching Hospital, Kumasi, Ghana. *Asian Social Science, 9*(10), 134–141. https://doi.org/10.5539/ass.v9n10p134

Takeshita, C. (2012). *The global biopolitics of the IUD: How science constructs contraceptive users and women's bodies*. Cambridge, MA: MIT Press.

Taussig, M. T. (1999). *Defacement: Public secrecy and the labor of the negative.* Stanford, CA: Stanford University Press.

Taylor, J., Diop, A., Blum, J., Dolo, O., and Winikoff, B. (2011). Oral misoprostol as an alternative to surgical management for incomplete abortion in Ghana. *International Journal of Gynecology & Obstetrics, 112*(1), 40–44.

Temmerman, M. (2018). Missed opportunities in women's health: Post-abortion care. *The Lancet Global Health, 7*(1), e12–e13. https://doi.org/10.1016/S2214-109X(18)30542-4

Tessema, G. A., Laurence, C. O., Melaku, Y. A., Misganaw, A., Woldie, S. A., Hiruye, A., . . . and Deribew, A. (2017). Trends and causes of maternal mortality in Ethiopia during 1990–2013: Findings from the Global Burden of Diseases study 2013. *BMC Public Health, 17*(1), 160.

Thiam, F., Suh, S., and Moreira, P. (2006). *Scaling up postabortion care services: Results from Senegal* [Report]. Retrieved from Management Sciences for Health. https://www.msh.org/sites/default/files/scaling-up-postabortion-care-services-results-from-senegal.pdf

Thomas, L. (2003). *Politics of the womb: Women, reproduction, and the state in Kenya.* Berkeley: University of California Press.

Thomson, M., Kentikelenis, A., and Stubbs, T. (2017). Structural adjustment programmes adversely affect vulnerable populations: A systematic-narrative review of their effect on child and maternal health. *Public Health Reviews, 38*(13). https://doi.org/10.1186/s40985-017-0059-2

Tichenor, M. (2016). The power of data: Global malaria governance and the Senegalese data retention strike. In V. Adams (Ed.), *Metrics: What counts in global health* (pp. 105–124). Durham, NC: Duke University Press.

Timmermans, S., and Berg, M. (2003). *The practice of medical technology. Sociology of Health & Illness, 25*(3), 97–114.

Touré, T. (1997). *Contribution à l'étude de l'avortement thérapeutique au Sénégal* (Thesis). Dakar, Sénégal: UCAD.

Track20. (2019). Track20 Senegal. Retrieved from http://www.track20.org/Senegal

Tunc, T. (2008). Designs of devices: The vacuum aspirator and American abortion technology. *Dynamis, 28,* 353–376.

Turner, K. L., Senderowicz, L., and Marlow, H. (2016). *Comprehensive abortion care needs and opportunities in Francophone West Africa: Situational assessment results* [Report]. Retrieved from https://www.ipas.org/wp-content/uploads/2020/06/FWSSARE16-SituationalAssessmentResultsFrancophoneWestAfrica.pdf

Udry, J. R., Gaughan, M., Schwingl, P. J., and van den Berg, B. J. (1996). A medical record linkage analysis of abortion underreporting. *Family Planning Perspectives, 28*(5), 228. https://doi.org/10.2307/2135842

United Nations. (2018). Goal 3: Sustainable Development Knowledge Platform. Retrieved from https://sustainabledevelopment.un.org/sdg3

United Nations Population Fund. (2014). Programme of Action adopted at the International Conference on Population and Development Cairo, 5–13 September 1994. (20th Anniversary Edition). Retrieved from https://www.unfpa.org/sites/default/files/pub-pdf/programme_of_action_Web%20ENGLISH.pdf

United States Agency for International Development. (2019). Financial Aid Explorer—Senegal. Retrieved from https://explorer.usaid.gov/cd/SEN?fiscal_year=2018&implementing_agency_id=1&measure=Obligations

United States Agency for International Development. (2020, May 18). Acting Administrator John Barsa letter to UN Secretary General Guterres [Press release]. Retrieved from https://www.usaid.gov/news-information/press-releases/may-18-2020-acting-administrator-john-barsa-un-secretary-general-antonio-guterres

Uzochukwu, B. S., Onwujekwe, O. E., and Akpala, C. O. (2002). Effect of the Bamako-Initiative drug revolving fund on availability and rational use of essential drugs in primary health care facilities in south-east Nigeria. *Health Policy and Planning, 17*(4), 378–383.

van der Meulen Rodgers, Y. (2018). *The Global Gag Rule and women's reproductive health: Rhetoric versus reality.* New York: Oxford University Press.

Vlassoff, M., Fetters, T., Kumbi, S., and Singh, S. (2012). The health system cost of postabortion care in Ethiopia. *International Journal of Gynecology & Obstetrics, 118*(S2), S127–S133.

Vlassoff, M., Shearer, J., Walker, D., and Lucas, H. (2008). *Economic impact of unsafe abortion-related morbidity and mortality: Evidence and estimation challenges* [Report]. Institute of Development Studies, University of Sussex. Retrieved from: http://www.abortionresearch consortium.org/reports/Rr59.pdf

Warriner, I., and Shah, I. H. (Eds.). (2006). *Preventing unsafe abortion and its consequences: Priorities for research and action* [Report]. Retrieved from the Guttmacher Institute. https://www.guttmacher.org/sites/default/files/pdfs/pubs/2006/07/10/Preventing UnsafeAbortion.pdf

Watkins, S. C. (1987). The fertility transition: Europe and the Third World compared. *Sociological Forum, 2*(4), 645–673.

———. (1990). From local to national communities: The transformation of demographic regimes in Western Europe, 1870–1960. *Population and Development Review, 16*(2), 241–272.

———. (1993). If all we knew about women was what we read in Demography, what would we know? *Demography, 30*(4), 551–577.

Weeks, A. D., Fiala, C., and Safar, P. (2005). Misoprostol and the debate over off-label drug use. *BJOG: An International Journal of Obstetrics & Gynaecology, 112*(3), 269–272.

Wendland, C. (2016). Estimating death: A close reading of maternal mortality metrics in Malawi. In V. Adams (Ed.), *Metrics: What counts in global health* (pp. 57–81). Durham, NC: Duke University Press.

Wertz, R., and Wertz, D. (2019). Notes on the decline of midwives and the rise of medical obstetricians. In P. Conrad and V. Leiter (Eds.), *The sociology of health and illness: Critical perspectives* (10th ed.) (pp. 279–292). Thousand Oaks, CA: Sage Publications, Inc.

Whyte, S. R., van der Geest, S., and Hardon, A. (2002). *Social lives of medicines.* New York: Cambridge University Press.

Wood, M., Ottolenghi, E., and Marin, C. (2007). *What works: A policy and program guide to the evidence on postabortion care* [Report]. Retrieved from https://www.postabortioncare .org/sites/pac/files/Compendium.pdf

World Health Organization. (2004). *Beyond the numbers: Reviewing maternal deaths and complications to make pregnancy safer* [Report]. Retrieved from WHO. https://apps.who.int /iris/bitstream/handle/10665/42984/9241591838.pdf?sequence=1&isAllowed=y

———. (2007). Managing complications in pregnancy and childbirth: A guideline for midwives and doctors, Figure P36. Retrieved from WHO. https://apps.who.int/iris/bitstream /handle/10665/43972/9241545879_eng.pdf;sequence=1

——— (2008). Managing incomplete abortion. In *Educational material for teachers of midwifery: Midwifery education modules* (2nd ed.). Retrieved from WHO. https://apps.who.int/iris /bitstream/handle/10665/44145/9789241546669_3_eng.pdf?sequence=3

———. (2011). *Unsafe abortion: Global and regional estimates of the incidence of unsafe abortion and associated mortality in 2008* [Report]. Retrieved from WHO. https://apps.who.int/iris /bitstream/handle/10665/44529/9789241501118_eng.pdf?sequence=1

———. (2012). *Safe abortion: Technical and policy guidance for health systems* (2nd ed.) [Report]. Retrieved from WHO. https://apps.who.int/iris/bitstream/handle/10665/70914/9789241 548434_eng.pdf?sequence=1

————. (2015). MDG 5: Improve maternal health. Retrieved from WHO. https://www.who
.int/topics/millennium_development_goals/maternal_health/en/

————. (2018). *Medical management of abortion* [Report]. Retrieved from WHO. https://
apps.who.int/iris/bitstream/handle/10665/278968/9789241550406-eng.pdf?ua=1

————. (2019). Trends in maternal mortality 2000 to 2017: Estimates by WHO, UNICEF,
UNFPA, World Bank Group, and the United Nations Population Division [Report].
Retrieved from WHO. https://apps.who.int/iris/bitstream/handle/10665/327596/WHO
-RHR-19.23-eng.pdf?ua=1

Zacher Dixon, L. (2015). Obstetrics in a time of violence: Mexican midwives critique routine
hospital practices. *Medical Anthropology Quarterly, 29*(4), 437–454. https://doi.org/10.1111
/maq.12174

Zaidi, S., Yasmin, H., Hassan, L., Khakwani, M., Sami, S., and Abbas, T. (2014). Replacement
of dilation and curettage/evacuation by manual vacuum aspiration and medical abortion,
and the introduction of postabortion contraception in Pakistan. *International Journal of
Gynecology & Obstetrics, 126*(S1), S40–S44. https://doi.org/10.1016/j.ijgo.2014.03.016

INDEX

abdominal expression, 49

abortion: in Bangladesh, 59, 167n3; criminalization of, 4, 13, 30, 34, 87, 143, 150; declines in mortality related to, 12, 144, 173n21; decriminalization of, 57; de-identified complications of in Senegal, 124–126; in Democratic Republic of Congo, 36, 137; in El Salvador, 167n4; in Ethiopia, 39, 137, 144, 150, 167n3; in Guyana, 144; hostility to, 7, 142–143; measurement of abortion-related death, 122, 130, 133–134, 138; measurement of incidence in Senegal, 22, 100–101, 108, 119–124, 130; in Mozambique, 39, 137; in Nepal, 144; nonphysiological signs of, 95, 97, 142, 154; physiological signs of, 94–95, 102; prevalence paradox of, 107–108; and record keeping, 4, 27, 33, 45–46, 83, 107, 131; in Romania, 16, 144; in Rwanda, 39, 137, 150; science in Senegal, 119–124; seeking illegal, 94–100; in South Africa, 16, 44, 144, 149; stigma, 10, 78, 104, 133, 149–151, 170n15; in Sweden, 144; in Zambia, 144. *See also* Senegal

Abortion Incidence Complications Methodology (AICM), 167n3

abortionist/avorteur, 66, 71, 151

abortion laws, 8–9, 12–14, 22–23, 27–29, 33, 52, 54–55, 57–58, 60–61, 73, 86, 95, 100–101, 104, 110, 133, 144, 149, 167n3, 171n4, 173n21

Adams, V., 9, 10, 15, 18–19, 27, 107, 109–110, 113–114, 125, 135–136, 139, 144

l'Association des Juristes Sénégalaises (AJS), 6, 38, 92, 150–151, 156–157

Alma Ata Declaration, 18, 112–113

amenorrhea, 56, 173n17

anemia, 130, 132

antenatal care/prenatal care, 84, 113

anti-abortion policies, 7–8, 60, 69, 151

antibiotics, 1, 78, 167–168n9, 172n3

Averting Maternal Death and Disability (AMDD), 37, 65, 170n6

Azar II, A. M., 142

Bamako Initiative, 48, 50, 69, 173n19

Banda, J., 118

Behague, D. *See* Storeng, K. and D. Behague

Biruk, C., 9, 20, 138, 144–145

boundary work, 55, 83, 101; in Senegal, 65, 70

Brazil, misoprostol in, 148

Bridges, K., 84

Briggs, L., 71, 167–168n9

Bush, G. W., 25

Camara, F. K., 151

Camara, M. I. B. A., 136

catheter, 92, 105, 121

Centre Hospitalier Universitaire Le Dantec, 39, 42, 63–64, 120–123

Centre Régionale de Formation, de Recherche, et de Plaidoyer en Santé de la Reproduction / Regional Center for Training, Research, and Advocacy in Reproductive Health (CEFOREP), 39, 63–68, 122, 148, 156, 172n9

cervix, 77, 79, 94–95, 104, 171n19

Child Fund, 38, 40, 71, 163

China, 15–16, 57, 167n7, 171n6

Cissé, C, 123, 131

clandestine abortion, 2–3, 12, 14, 16, 33, 38, 40, 58, 61–63, 68–69, 83, 87, 92, 98, 100, 102, 106, 108, 121, 123, 131, 139, 143, 149, 150, 170n15

Cold War, 21, 24, 169n17

colonial, 15, 23–24, 26, 34, 65, 143, 151, 167–168n9

Columbia University, 32, 37, 65

Comité National d'Ethique pour la Recherche en Santé (National Ethics Committee for Health Research), 157, 163

confidentiality: patient, 6, 88; professional ethics, 6; research participants, xvii, 30, 33–34; violations of, 79

Conrad, P., 4, 16, 41, 119

contraception/family planning: global goals related to, 14, 22, 146, 148; training in family planning counseling, 32, 39–40, 66, 102, 124, 157, 172n4

Convention on the Elimination of all Forms of Discrimination Against Women (CEDAW), 38, 150

COVID-19, 142
Crane, J., 30, 170n5
Cytotec, 41, 146

Dakar, city of, 100; regional tribunal of, 29, 35, 91, 156–157, 164; region of, 2, 67, 89, 120, 123, 156, 172n1
Davis, D., 84, 174n5
Depo Provera, 169n18
Diadhiou, F., 63, 120–122, 131
digital evacuation, 6–7, 10, 12, 27, 39, 45–47, 56, 64, 66, 69, 72–78, 80, 124, 128, 140–141, 143, 145, 153, 160–161, 167n1; absence of digital evacuation, 145; *curage digitale*, 2; training in, 56, 66, 80
dilation and curettage, 4–8, 12, 27, 39, 42, 45–46, 56–57, 60–61, 64, 72–73, 75–77, 80, 115, 124, 127, 160, 161, 167n6
Diouf, A., 63, 102, 120–121
Diouf, P. D., 120
DKT International, 61, 141, 145–147, 171n3
doctors, 1, 5, 44, 49, 52, 54, 76–77, 112–113, 151, 155, 167n1, 167–168n9, 173n15
dysmenorrhea, 56

eclampsia, 19, 114, 116
electric vacuum aspiration (EVA), 4, 8, 22, 27, 30, 45–46; in America, 57; in China, 57; mainstreaming of, 57; in Russia, 57; in Senegal, 72–73, 76–77, 128
emergency obstetric care (EmOC), 5, 8, 22, 25, 37, 63, 65, 113–115, 118, 121, 126, 139, 170n6, 173n11, 173n13; basic, 172n3; comprehensive, 172n3
EngenderHealth, 38–39, 60, 63, 66
epidemiological: abortion data, 3, 6, 8, 37, 100, 102, 119; accounts, 28, 143; maternal mortality data, 39, 63, 174n5; PAC data, 10, 27; truths, 107
Erikson, S., 9, 18–19, 146
evidence-based policymaking, 10, 18, 109–110, 115, 144

Family Planning 2020 Initiative (FP 2020), 13, 18–20, 117, 146, 148–149; sale and social marketing of contraceptive technologies, 146
Faye, E. O., 102, 120
Faye, K., 123
Federal Drug Administration (FDA), 169n18, 171n4

feminist technology, 54–55, 58
fetus, 46, 69, 84, 91, 98, 103–104, 122, 149, 161, 167–168n9
Ford Foundation, in Senegal, 120
Foucault, M., 12, 14, 101
France, colonial abortion law in Senegal, 28, 34
Futures Group, 36

Georgetown University, 169n2, 171n1
Ghana, unsafe abortion in, 95; PAC in, 104
Ghebreyesus, T. A., 142
Global Gag Rule, 7, 168n12, 171n6. *See also* Mexico City Policy
Global Health: Science and Practice, 141
global reproductive governance, 4, 11, 13, 20–22, 28, 83, 149
gold standard, 109, 111, 144–145
Green, W., 169n18
Guatemala, MVA in, 61, 80
Guinea, MVA in, 63
Guterres, A., 142
Guttmacher Institute, 3, 39, 137, 144, 167n3, 171n4
Gynuity Health Projects, 41

Halavanappar, S., 149
harm reduction: as misoprostol, 146–148; PAC as, 4–9, 139–143, 149; public health approaches, 12, 38, 41
health workers: authorization for MVA, 68, 73; male nurses, 30, 71; moral character of, 66; PAC training, 30, 41, 43, 61, 146; withholding care, 78, 172n3. *See also* manual vacuum aspiration (MVA); post-abortion care (PAC)
Healthy Newborn Partnership, 115
Helms Amendment, 7, 26, 28–29, 59–61, 69, 80, 114, 120, 146
hemorrhage, postpartum, 19, 41, 114, 146–147, 172n3
HIV/AIDS, 4, 111, 115–117, 122, 142, 144, 169n19, 170, 172n7
l'Hôpital Roi Baudouin, 91
hospitals/health care facilities: interventions in, 10, 21, 109, 113, 115, 118, 136, 138, 140, 143; MVA authorization in, 68, 73; referrals to for MVA, 56, 67, 77–78, 80, 143; technical environment/capacity, 46, 69, 71, 117. *See also* manual vacuum aspiration (MVA); post-abortion care (PAC)

illegal abortion, 2–3, 6, 8, 10, 12, 24, 26, 28–34, 43–44, 56–57, 62, 64, 68, 70–72, 76, 78, 82–83, 87–91, 93–99, 102–104, 128, 143, 156, 164, 172n1, 173n10

induced abortion, 7, 9–11, 24, 27–28, 33, 38, 41, 43–44, 48, 55, 60, 62–65, 71, 78, 82, 86–107, 119–121, 123–124, 128, 130–131, 133, 145, 157, 159–161, 167n3, 170n12, 170n15, 171n18, 173n10, 173n12, 173n15, 173n17, 173–174n21

Inner City Fund (ICF), 8, 19, 86, 99, 132–133, 141, 145, 168n14, 173n16

Institute for Health Metrics and Evaluation (IHME), 19, 118, 168n15

Institute for Reproductive Health (IRH), 169n2, 171n1

International Federation of Gynecology and Obstetrics (FIGO), 62, 72

International Fertility Research Program, 59

International Monetary Fund (IMF), 35–36, 113

International Planned Parenthood Federation (IPPF), 36, 59–60, 168n10, 172n2

International Pregnancy Advisory Committee, 59. See also Ipas

interrogation, xvii, 2, 12, 46, 47, 90, 94–99, 102–103, 105–107, 140

intrauterine device (IUD), 54, 58, 146

Ipas, 40, 59–62, 67, 72, 135, 148, 154, 157, 163, 171n7

Jaffré, Y., 33, 50, 79–80, 84–85, 99, 101, 134, 138

Jamra, 3

Johns Hopkins Program for International Education in Gynecology and Obstetrics (JHPIEGO), 38–39, 60, 63–65, 122

Johnson, L. B., 35

Karman, H., 57–58

Kemp-Kasten Amendment, 69, 167n7, 171n6

Kenya, quality of PAC care, 78; misoprostol in, 148

kinship, 86–87, 97

Koly, F., 121

labor induction, 41, 146–147

laminaria, 42

Lancet Global Health, 117, 141

law enforcement/police, 10, 33, 43, 83–84, 87–89, 101, 104, 164

List of Essential Medications (LEM), 41, 63, 66, 147

Livingston, J., 172n7

long-acting reversible contraceptives (LARCs), 13, 16, 19–20, 149

magic bullet, 19, 21, 55, 149

magnesium sulfate, 19, 114

Maine, D., 37, 65, 112–113, 114, 117

malaria, 111, 115, 130, 132, 142

Malthus, T., 19–20, 168n16

Management Sciences for Health (MSH), 25–26, 28, 31, 38, 40–41, 45, 63, 66, 115, 171n7

manual vacuum aspiration (MVA): authorization for health facilities, 63, 67–68, 73, 77, 80, 141; authorization for health workers, 68, 147; cost of, 65, 75; decentralization of, 28, 42, 66, 69, 88; delays in care, 42, 56, 75, 77–78, 140, 143, 145; donations of by NGOs, 61–62, 67, 72; in Guatemala, 61, 80; in Guinea, 63; health workers' perceptions in Bolivia, 62; in Honduras, 54, 62, 72, 80; institutionalization of, 62; life span/shelf life, 67–68; under lock and key, 52, 75; as magic bullet, 55; in Malawi, 62, 72, 75; in Mexico, 62; misuse of, 52, 70, 74; national supply in Bolivia, 62; in Pakistan, 75; preferred PAC technology, 10, 24, 55, 72, 75; procurement of, 67–69, 72, 80; safety of, 10, 65, 75, 80; in Senegal, 30, 63–69, 73, 75, 145; sterilization of, 73, 75; in study hospitals, 70–78; training of health workers in, 30, 56, 60–63, 66, 72–73, 76–77, 89, 157, 171n7; trustworthiness of health workers, 64; in Uganda, 75

Maputo Protocol, 38, 150

Marie Stopes International (MSI), 146–147, 163

Marsa, J., 142

maternal death audits, 119, 123

maternal mortality: direct causes of, 60, 110, 116, 123; global estimates of, 118; indirect causes of, 116; measurement problems related to, 12, 14, 22, 111, 125. See also reduction of maternal mortality

maternal mortality ratio, 8–9, 15, 17–18, 22, 115, 117–118, 119, 130, 133, 137–138, 144

matron, 35, 56

Mbembe, A., 13, 148

measurement trap, 111. See also maternal mortality

Médecins Sans Frontières (MSF), 2, 4, 167n1, 167n6
medicalization, 4, 11, 16, 41, 51, 112, 119, 120, 150
menstruation, 56, 91; menstrual period, 94–95; menstrual regulation, 58–59, 61, 173n17; menstrual suppression, 54
Mexico City Policy, 7–9, 18, 22–23, 25–26, 28, 29, 34, 60–61, 69, 114, 120, 142–143, 145, 151, 167n7, 168n12, 171n6; advocacy and USAID, 7, 26, 61, 146; reinstatement of, 23, 25, 142
midwives, 1, 4–5, 30–33, 39–40, 45–46, 49, 55–56, 66, 69–74, 76–77, 84–85, 88–89, 91, 96–98, 101, 106, 112, 113, 124, 141, 155–156, 167n1, 167n9, 171n7, 172n1
mifepristone, 147, 171n4; and misoprostol, 147
Millennium Development Goals (MDGs), 38, 117, 125
miscarriage, 2–3, 9–10, 12, 24, 78, 82–83, 85, 87, 94–95, 98–101, 104, 111, 118, 125, 127, 139–140, 143, 145; frequency of, 132–133; medical management of, 106–109, 131. See also spontaneous abortion
Misoclear, 147
misoprostol: for abortion, 41, 147–148; in Brazil, 148; in Burkina Faso, 148; as form of harm reduction, 146, 148–149; in Kenya, 148; and PAC, 148; for PPH, 19, 41, 114, 146–157; recent studies in Tanzania, 148; as reproductive health care, 141
moral regimes, 14
Moreau, J. C., 123
Morgan, L. and E. Roberts, 3, 12, 14, 27, 83, 116
Morocco, maternal mortality in, 18
motherhood: desirability of, 86; health workers' perception of, 83–86, 107; ideal of, 83; within marriage, 86; and sexuality, 86, 99. See also reproductive subject
Murphy, M., 7, 9–10, 16–17, 19–21, 35, 54–59, 116, 168n10

necropower, 13–14, 23, 148
neocolonial, 26, 28
neoliberalism, 18–20, 34–35, 48, 85, 113, 116, 118, 138
New Yorker, The, 136
Niger, MVA in, 54, 63, 74, 80
Nimbona, P. C., 120–121, 123, 131

Obama, B., 26, 69
L'Observateur, 130

obstetric racism, 84
obstetric violence, 11–12, 30, 34, 49–50, 56, 78–79, 81, 96, 108, 140
Oni-Orisan, A., 9, 18, 22, 110, 118, 127
operating theater, 43, 86
Ouagadougou Partnership, 13, 18, 146
Owens, D. C., 167–168n9

Pap smear, 54
Parsons, T., 85
Partnership for Maternal, Child and Newborn Health, 115
PATH, 146, 174n3
Pathfinder International (previously Pathfinder Fund), 36, 59–60
Pfizer, 146
Pharmacie Nationale d'Approvisionnement / National Pharmacy Supply (PNA), 66–69, 73, 141, 147–148
Platform of Action/ICPD, 5, 17, 20–21, 37, 61, 112, 119
polygamy, 86
population control, in relation to development, 20, 28, 34–36, 80; as reproductive governance, 16–17, 21, 23–24, 55; role in family planning/ contraception, 17, 54, 112, 116; USAID role in, 20, 28, 36
Population Council, 38–39, 59, 63–64, 66, 75, 122, 172n2
population policies: in China, 15–16; in India, 15, 35; in Malawi, 15, 36; in Nigeria, 15, 36; in Senegal, 28, 34, 36–38; USAID role in, 29, 36
post-abortion care (PAC): acceptance of, 109, 143; clinical protocols, 70, 72, 141; cost of, 39, 143–144; data in Senegal, 126–137; decentralization of, 28, 42, 88; global model of, 4, 6, 8, 13, 24–25, 31, 41, 43, 48, 51, 55–56, 61, 72–73, 82, 89, 96, 107, 110, 138, 146, 148; medical jurisdiction over, 87, 108; philosophy of, 63; public health impact of, 134, 143, 144; record keeping practices, 4, 27, 33, 45, 46, 83, 107, 131; research in Senegal, 39–41, 63–66, 124–126; technologies, 9, 22–24, 127, 145; treatment ethic of, 6, 82, 87, 96, 107; women's affect during, 99–100. See also Senegal

Post-Abortion Care Consortium, 4, 60–61, 171nn1–2
pre-eclampsia, 19, 114, 116, 123
preferred account, 101, 107, 131. *See also* boundary work
pregnancy: premarital, 100; unwanted, 3, 33, 40, 44, 86, 98, 108, 154, 157
Prevention of Maternal Mortality and Morbidity Project (PREMOMA), 115
process indicators, 114, 124–125, 128, 130
professional jurisdiction, 70, 101

quasi-experimental research, 173n20

randomized controlled trials (RCTs), 10, 19, 110, 114, 136, 138
rape, 6, 38–39, 88, 92–93, 150, 151, 170n15
Ravenholt, R., 58–59
Reagan, R., 7, 60
reduction of maternal mortality: in England, 144; in Malaysia, 112; in Sri Lanka, 112; Sweden, 112, 144
reproductive autonomy, 17, 55, 80
reproductive governance, 1, 3–4, 9, 11, 13–14, 16, 19–24, 27–28, 33, 54, 56, 80, 83, 108, 110–111, 118, 127, 136–137, 140, 145, 149, 151
Reproductive Health Supplies Coalition, 147–148
reproductive justice, 23–24, 33, 116, 141, 143, 149–150
reproductive subject, 83, 116
rétention des données/data strike, 71, 129, 135
Rosenfield, A., 112–113, 117

safe abortion, 11, 12, 18, 38, 61, 80, 139, 143–144, 149, 151, 171n2
safe motherhood, 21, 23–24, 62, 69, 108, 110, 113–114, 118, 119, 121, 124–127, 131, 136–137
Safe Motherhood Initiative (SMI), 5, 10, 21, 60, 110, 112–113, 115–117, 119, 138–139
Safe Motherhood Interagency Group, 115
Sangaré, E., 63, 102, 120–121
Sanger, M., 168n10
Sayana Press, 20, 146, 169n18
science and technology studies, 9, 54, 55
Seko, M. S., 37
Senderowicz, L., 3, 16, 149
Senegal: abortion law, xiii, 3, 12, 28–29, 35, 48, 93, 128, 131, 133, 136–137, 145, 148, 150; FP

2020 in, 146; maternal mortality in, 111, 130; population policy in, 28; structural adjustment in, 37, 65, 120; USAID in, 13, 25–26, 29, 35, 38–39, 69, 120, 122, 124–126, 128, 134, 136, 146. *See also* manual vacuum aspiration (MVA); post-abortion care (PAC)
sepsis, 116, 122–123
sick role, 85
sisterhood method, 133
speculum, 46, 49, 94–95
spontaneous abortion, xvii, 38, 44, 82, 84, 94–95, 97, 100–107, 120–121, 127–128, 130–131, 161, 170nn12–13, 171n18
sterilization, 73, 75, 147
Storeng, K. and D. Béhague, 9, 15, 18–21, 33, 111, 113–116, 118, 138, 139
structural adjustment, 35–37, 48, 50, 65, 120. *See also* neoliberalism
Sustainable Development Goals (SDGs), 38, 117, 144
Swedish International Development Cooperation, 136

Takeshita, C., 7, 12, 20, 54, 58–59, 120
task shifting, 77–78
theoretical sampling, 154
total fertility rate (TFR), 15; in Senegal, 25, 86
Touré, T., 122
transportation, 40, 77–79, 89, 99, 134, 143, 172n4
Trump, D., 23, 142
tuberculosis (TB), 111, 115, 122, 142

ultrasound, 2, 46, 69–70, 78, 92, 94–95, 97–98, 102
unmet contraceptive need, 17, 170n13
unsafe abortion, 4–6, 8, 13–14, 23, 29, 38–41, 44, 55, 60–61, 63, 96, 108, 110, 116–117, 119, 123–126, 130, 135, 138, 147–148, 150–151, 154, 157, 167n2, 170n15
unwanted pregnancy, 33, 40, 44, 86, 98, 108, 139, 154, 157, 170n13, 173n10
uterine aspiration technologies. *See* manual vacuum aspiration (MVA); EVA; or misoprostol
uterus, 5, 46, 49, 69, 91, 94, 104–105, 121, 167–168n9

vaginal exam, 46, 79, 83, 94, 102

Wendland, C., 9, 15, 18, 22, 110, 117–118, 127
William and Flora Hewlett Foundation,
    169n1
Wolof, xvii, 1, 156–157
Woman Care Global, 61
Women Deliver, 115–116, 118
World Bank, 28, 35–37, 65, 113, 168n13, 172n2

World Health Organization (WHO), 5, 7, 17,
    40, 56, 60, 73, 103–104, 111, 116–118, 120–121,
    135, 142, 147, 163, 172n1

Xylocaine, 48, 50, 64

Yocca, A., 149

Zika, 142

ABOUT THE AUTHOR

SIRI SUH is an assistant professor of sociology at Brandeis University. Her research bridges the fields of global health, population and development, science and technology studies, and African studies. Born to Cameroonian and Dutch parents, she has lived in Burkina Faso, Kenya, Nigeria, and Ghana. Suh first became interested in post-abortion care while working with an NGO in Senegal during the mid-2000s. Her research has been funded by the National Institute of Child Health and Human Development, the Social Science Research Council, the American Council of Learned Societies, and the American Association of University Women. She has worked with health organizations such as the Guttmacher Institute, Management Sciences for Health, Global Doctors for Choice, and the United Nations Population Fund.

Cocoa®
Programming
FOR
DUMMIES®

by Erick Tejkowski

WILEY

Wiley Publishing, Inc.

Cocoa® Programming For Dummies®

Published by
Wiley Publishing, Inc.
909 Third Avenue
New York, NY 10022

www.wiley.com

For general information on our other products and services or to obtain technical support, please contact our Customer Care Department within the U.S. at 800-762-2974, outside the U.S. at 317-572-3993, or fax 317-572-4002.

Wiley also publishes its books in a variety of electronic formats. Some content that appears in print may not be available in electronic books.

Library of Congress Control Number: 2002114835

ISBN: 0-7645-2613-8

Manufactured in the United States of America

10 9 8 7 6 5 4 3 2 1

1O/QW/QT/QT/IN

Cocoa® Programming For Dummies®

Cheat Sheet

Useful Cocoa Internet Resources

Apple Developer

developer.apple.com/techpubs/macosx/macosx.html

Your Cocoa adventure online should begin at Apple's Developer site. This is the mothership of all Cocoa programming, where you can find the full Cocoa documentation, dozens of code samples, tips, tricks, and advice from the creators of Cocoa.

CocoaDev

www.cocoadev.com

Offering a large collection of Cocoa source code, links, threaded Cocoa discussion groups, and book reviews, CocoaDev is a useful reference site for Cocoa development. You'll find yourself visiting this site frequently.

CocoaDev Central

www.cocoadevcentral.com

CocoaDev Central has a lot to offer the budding Cocoa programmer. Staffed by some of the most well-versed Cocoa developers around, CocoaDev offers a wide range of tutorials representing all aspects of Cocoa programming. It's a good reference site when you need to know how to perform a task quickly.

Vermont Recipes

www.vermontrecipes.com

A longtime bastion of Cocoa (and previously NEXT) programming, the Vermont Recipes site consist of a series of tutorials to get you started on the road to Cocoa development. Although some of this information is available elsewhere, this site is considered a classic among Cocoa aficionados and shouldn't be missed.

Stepwise

www.stepwise.com

Stepwise is one of the more professional-looking Cocoa development sites that you'll encounter. Offering tutorials, source code, and reviews, StepWise is near the top of the list of sites that all Cocoa geeks frequent. There's a reason that Stepwise has such a comprehensive site. They've been at it a long time. More than a decade ago, Stepwise provided Objective-C development tools for MPW (Macintosh Programmers Workshop).

Cocoa® Programming For Dummies®

Project Builder Keyboard Shortcuts

Shortcut	Action
Cmd-Q	Quit Project Builder
Cmd-Shift-N	Create a new project
Cmd-N	Create a new file
Cmd-F	Run a single-window Find
Cmd-Shift-F	Run a batch Find
Cmd-B	Build
Cmd-R	Build and run
Option-double click	Look up any definition by Option-double-clicking its keyword in the code
Cmd-?	Display Project Builder Help

Interface Builder Keyboard Shortcuts

Shortcut	Action
Cmd-Q	Quit Interface Builder
Cmd-N	Create a new nib file
Cmd-R	Test the interface
Cmd-Opt-O	Add an outlet
Cmd-Opt-A	Add an action
Cmd-Opt-F	Create files for a class
Cmd-Shift-I	Display the Info window
Cmd-?	Display Interface Builder Help

Data Types

Type	Represents
NSString	String of Unicode text
NSAttributedString	Stylized text string
NSCalendarDate	Date
NSColor	Color
NSNumber	Number
NSRange	Beginning and endpoint of a numeric range
NSImage	Graphics image
NSArray	Array
NSDictionary	Collection of key-value pairs

Components of a Cocoa Project

Group Name	Contains
Classes	Source code files for user-defined classes
Other Sources	main.m; additional source code files
Resources	nib file, InfoPlist.strings file, icon files, documentation files, image files, and audio files
Frameworks	Cocoa Frameworks; libraries that define how Cocoa works
Products	Application you're building

For Dummies: Bestselling Book Series for Beginners

About the Author

Erick Tejkowski is a freelance author and programmer. He is the author of *REALbasic For Dummies* and a contributing author of *Mac OS X All-in-One Desk Reference For Dummies*. He serves in editorial and writing roles for popular Macintosh publications such as *MacTech*, *MacWorld*, *RB Developer*, and ResExcellence.com. When not computing, he enjoys spending free time with his wife, Maria, and their children, Mercedes and Leopold.

Dedication

To Maria Paredes — my fiercest advocate, my fairest critic, my best friend, and my wife. Without her, this book would not have been possible.

Author's Acknowledgments

To Greg Croy, Dennis Cohen, and especially Susan Pink for editing this book. The quality of the final transcript is a direct result of their suggestions, recommendations, and sharp editing skills.

To Mixi and Bubbers for inspiration.

Publisher's Acknowledgments

We're proud of this book; please send us your comments through our online registration form located at www.dummies.com/register/.

Some of the people who helped bring this book to market include the following:

Acquisitions, Editorial, and Media Development

Project Editor: Susan Pink

Acquisitions Editor: Gregory S. Croy

Technical Editor: Dennis R. Cohen

Editorial Manager: Carol Sheehan

Permissions Editor: Laura Moss

Media Development Specialist: Greg Stafford

Media Development Manager: Laura Carpenter

Media Development Supervisor: Richard Graves

Editorial Assistant: Amanda Foxworth

Cartoons: Rich Tennant (www.the5thwave.com)

Production

Project Coordinator: Maridee Ennis

Layout and Graphics: Seth Conley, Carrie Foster, Joyce Haughey, Tiffany Muth, Jacque Schneider, Jeremey Unger

Proofreaders: John Bitter, John Tyler Connoley, John Greenough, Andy Hollandbeck, Carl William Pierce, TECHBOOKS Production Services

Indexer: TECHBOOKS Production Services

Special Help
Sarah Cummings, Bonnie Mikkelson, Greg Stafford

Publishing and Editorial for Technology Dummies

Richard Swadley, Vice President and Executive Group Publisher

Andy Cummings, Vice President and Publisher

Mary C. Corder, Editorial Director

Publishing for Consumer Dummies

Diane Graves Steele, Vice President and Publisher

Joyce Pepple, Acquisitions Director

Composition Services

Gerry Fahey, Vice President of Production Services

Debbie Stailey, Director of Composition Services

Contents at a Glance

Introduction *1*

Part 1: Developer Tools *7*
Chapter 1: A Brief Tour of Cocoa Development 9
Chapter 2: Creating Your First Cocoa Application 21
Chapter 3: Project Builder 43
Chapter 4: Interface Builder 69
Chapter 5: More Utilities for Cocoa Development 93

Part 11: Instant Cocoa and the Objective-C Language *113*
Chapter 6: Cocoa's Flavor of Object-Oriented Programming 115
Chapter 7: The Basics of Objective-C 131
Chapter 8: A Window with a View 147
Chapter 9: Working with Interface Controls 161
Chapter 10: Cocoa Data Types 181

Part 111: Putting 1t All Together: Cocoa Programming in Depth *189*
Chapter 11: Text 191
Chapter 12: Graphics 211
Chapter 13: Managing Your Files 237
Chapter 14: Printing with Cocoa 255
Chapter 15: Cocoa on the Internet 265
Chapter 16: Multimedia 281

Part 1V: Advanced Cocoa Topics *301*
Chapter 17: Document-Based Applications 303
Chapter 18: Cocoa and the Command Line 313
Chapter 19: Cocoa and AppleScript 323

Part V: The Part of Tens 333

Chapter 20: Ten Tips to Make Cocoa Programming Easier 335
Chapter 21: Ten Great Web Sites for Cocoa Developers 341

Appendix: Installing Mac OS X Developer Tools 345

Index 347

Table of Contents

Introduction 1

About This Book 1
Conventions Used in This Book 2
Foolish Assumptions 2
How This Book Is Organized 3
   Part I: Developer Tools 3
   Part II: Instant Cocoa and the Objective-C Language 3
   Part III: Putting It All Together: Cocoa Programming in Depth 3
   Part IV: Advanced Cocoa Topics 4
   Part V: The Part of Tens 4
Icons Used in This Book 4
Where to Go from Here 5

Part 1: Developer Tools 7

Chapter 1: A Brief Tour of Cocoa Development 9

Mac OS X Is a Programmer's Dream 9
Why Program with Cocoa? 10
The Cocoa Development Process 11
The Tools You Need 12
   Project Builder 13
   Interface Builder 17

Chapter 2: Creating Your First Cocoa Application 21

Creating a Cocoa Application in Six Simple Steps 21
Beginning a Project 23
   Think of an idea 23
   Create a Cocoa project 24
Building an Interface 25
   Add controls to the interface 28
   Wiring the interface 30
   Making connections 32
Adding Code to Make Your App Work 37
Debugging and Building the Application 39

Chapter 3: Project Builder 43

Project Builder: The Core of Apple's Development Tools 43
Finding Your Way around Project Builder 44
   Customizing Project Builder Preferences 45
   Hitting the target 48
   Working with project files 51

Browsing Classes 53
Debugging Your Project 55
Use Bookmarks to Simplify Development 62
Where to Go for Help 64
Building the Final Application 66

Chapter 4: Interface Builder **69**

A Tour of Interface Builder 69
The nib file window 72
Design window 74
Palettes window 75
Info window 77
Menu editor window 79
The Interface Building Process 81
Using an Interface in Project Builder 88

Chapter 5: More Utilities for Cocoa Development **93**

FileMerge 93
IconComposer and the icns Browser 102
IconComposer 103
icns Browser 108
PackageMaker 109
Property List Editor 111

**Part II: Instant Cocoa and the Objective-C
Language** *113*

Chapter 6: Cocoa's Flavor of Object-Oriented Programming **115**

Why Use Object-Oriented Programming? 116
Cocoa Is Classy 117
Designing Your Own Class 117
Using an Object 121
How Objects Work Together 128

Chapter 7: The Basics of Objective-C **131**

Objective-C: The Best Language for the Job 131
Working with Your Own Classes 133
Creating Instances without a Fuss 142
Working with Cocoa's Built-in Objects 144

Chapter 8: A Window with a View **147**

Working with Windows 147
Opening and closing a window 148
Hiding and showing a window 148
Positioning windows 149

Keeping track of windows 149
Putting windows to work for you 150
Changing the Appearance of Windows 152
Different windows for different tasks 152
Sizing up your windows 154
Setting a window's title 154
Windows that you can see through 154
Beneath the Sheets 156

Chapter 9: Working with Interface Controls **161**

Button Controls 161
Push button 162
Round button 165
Check box 166
Square and rounded bevel buttons 167
Radio Control 168
Slider Control 170
Tab Views 172
Making Progress at the Bar 174
Table Control 175

Chapter 10: Cocoa Data Types **181**

Working with Numbers 181
Working with Arrays 182
Working with Boolean Data Types 185
Working with Dates 185

Part III: Putting It All Together: Cocoa Programming in Depth **189**

Chapter 11: Text **191**

Working with Text 191
Build an interface 192
Add a controller class 193
Wire the interface 194
Add the code 196
Doing Style the Easy Way! 197
Manipulating Text 199
Pasteboard manipulations 199
Manual editing 200
Saving Text for a Rainy Day 202
Retrieving Text 206

Chapter 12: Graphics **211**

Cocoa and the Art of Graphics 211
Points 212
Rects and sizes 212
Colors 213
Building a Graphics Interface 217
Painting with Lines and Shapes 221
Bezier paths 221
Fill a path 222
Draw a path 226
Fancy-pants paths 228
Drawing Text 231
Displaying an Image 234

Chapter 13: Managing Your Files **237**

About Files and Folders in Mac OS X 237
Opening Files and Using Them 239
Building the interface 239
Open sesame . . . er, panel 243
Finding a file's path, name, and more .245
Viewing a file's icon 247
Reading from and writing to documents 250
Working with Files and Folders 250
Copying files and folders 251
Moving files and folders 252
Deleting files and folders 253
Creating folders 253

Chapter 14: Printing with Cocoa **255**

How Printing Works in Cocoa 255
Tweaking the Page Settings 257
Setting Up the Print Job and Printing the View 260
Printing to Places Other Than a Printer 261

Chapter 15: Cocoa on the Internet **265**

Interacting with the Web 265
Loading a Web page in a browser 266
Downloading files 267
Displaying HTML 268
Putting it all together 269
Sending E-mail from a Cocoa Application 272
Sending e-mail from your favorite client 272
Sending e-mail from your own apps 274
Adding e-mail functions to the project .276

Chapter 16: Multimedia **281**

Listening to Audio 281
Playing system sounds 282
Loading and playing sound files 283
Building a simple audio player .284
Watching Movies with Cocoa 289
NSMovie 290
NSMovieView 290
Building a simple movie player .294
When a movie is not a movie 298

Part IV: Advanced Cocoa Topics **301**

Chapter 17: Document-Based Applications **303**

Creating the Project 303
Building the Interface 307
Adding the Code 309

Chapter 18: Cocoa and the Command Line **313**

Wrapping Command-line Utilities 313
Creating the Project and Building the Interface 315
Adding the Code 319

Chapter 19: Cocoa and AppleScript **323**

What's So Great about AppleScript Anyway? 323
Creating the Project and Building the Interface 324
Adding the Code 326

Part V: The Part of Tens **333**

Chapter 20: Ten Tips to Make Cocoa Programming Easier **335**

Use Keyboard Shortcuts 335
Read the Documentation 336
Use Class Browser 337
Adjust the Window Count 337
Use Drag and Drop 337
Initialize and Awaken! 338
Don't Forget the Superclass 338
Position Items with Cocoa Coordinates 339
Use Guidelines in Interface Builder 339
Reuse Your Code 339

Chapter 21: Ten Great Web Sites for Cocoa Developers **341**

MacTech Magazine 341
CocoaDev 342
CocoaDev Central 342
MacTelligence 342
Cocoa Mailing List Archive 342
Vermont Recipes 343
Scotland Software 343
iDevGames 343
HyperJeff Network 344
Stepwise 344

Appendix: Installing Mac OS X Developer Tools *345*

System Requirements 345
Installing the Developer Tools 345
What to Do If You Don't Have the Developer Tools CD 346

Index *347*

Introduction

· ·

Welcome to *Cocoa Programming For Dummies*. This book shows you how to create applications for Mac OS X, complete with beautiful Aqua interfaces and advanced functionality. The best part is that Cocoa provides you with programming skills that you could only dream of a few short years ago.

About This Book

Cocoa Programming For Dummies is a newcomer's guide to Cocoa programming for Mac OS X. It guides you through the basics of Cocoa application development, so you can finally realize the full potential of your Macintosh. Although Cocoa isn't the easiest thing on earth to learn, it is easy enough that beginners can create applications. Furthermore, even beginner projects can have features that rival professional applications. You'll be surprised at how easy it is to add complex features — features that would have taken an army of engineers to build in the past.

This book will not make you a certified Cocoa expert, but it will give you a good start on your way to becoming proficient with Cocoa. From the beginning of the book to the very end, you'll explore Cocoa programming by using it. Each chapter guides you through the process of creating at least one simple application that illustrates the features presented in that chapter. The examples are purposely simple, so you aren't encumbered with the book-long application common in many other programming books. This helps you see the task at hand more clearly and makes it easier to use the book as a quick reference later.

Cocoa Programming For Dummies covers the fundamentals of Cocoa programming as well as advanced features. The weird thing about Cocoa is that you sometimes can't tell which is which. In Cocoa, the simple is complex, and the complex simple. You'll gasp in awe as you add full PDF support, sophisticated graphics, multimedia, and professional typography to your application in minutes. Then you'll turn around and bang your head against the wall trying to remember how to create a simple list of items in Cocoa. The great part about Cocoa is that after you get the hang of the basics, you can build applications with high-quality features that would have been near impossible for a beginner to achieve in the past.

Conventions Used in This Book

This book guides you through the process of building Cocoa applications. Throughout, you create interfaces and make them functional with the use of Objective-C code. The code examples in this book appear in a monospaced font. For instance:

```
#import <Cocoa/Cocoa.h>
```

Objective-C is intimately connected to the C language, which is a case-sensitive language. Therefore, it's a good idea to enter the code that appears in this book *exactly* as it appears in the text. Some capitalization may not be mandatory (for example, the capitalization of variable names), but until you're familiar with the rules, it's best not to stray from the text. If you're ever uncertain about case sensitivity, you can always use the source code on the *For Dummies* Web site, at www.dummies.com/extras. All URLs in this book appear in a monospaced font as well:

```
www.apple.com
```

Foolish Assumptions

To begin programming Cocoa applications, you need a Macintosh computer, a copy of Mac OS X (preferably 10.2 or higher), and the Developer Tools that accompany the operating system discs. If you're not sure how to install the Developer Tools, the appendix can lead you through the steps necessary to prepare your Mac for Cocoa development.

In addition to the computer and software, you'll also need some computing skills. For starters, you should be familiar with using the Macintosh operating system. You should know how to launch applications, save files, work with Finder, and use the Internet.

You should also have at least a passing knowledge of some computer language. Ideally, you would have basic skills in the C programming language and at least some experience with an object-oriented language such as C++, Java, or REALbasic. This isn't to say that you will be completely lost without these skills. Different computer languages tend to share many features in common. Whether you have a Pascal, a JavaScript, or an AppleScript background, you'll find that Objective-C, although strange looking at first, is easy to learn.

The examples in this book stay focused on the Cocoa aspects of programming. Although some accessory C code is necessary to make this happen, the examples are not obfuscated code that an average beginning programmer can't grasp. If you're still not sure that you're ready for Cocoa, jump on in anyway. There's a good chance that you'll understand what's going on. When you get lost, you can always refer to one of the many C language references on the Internet for extra help.

How This Book Is Organized

Cocoa Programming For Dummies has five main parts. As you proceed through the book, each part increases in complexity. Each chapter covers a specific topic and provides code examples, explanations, and sample projects for you to complete. As you complete each chapter, you will have completed one or more projects that demonstrate the main ideas discussed in that chapter.

Part 1: Developer Tools

Part I introduces you to the world of Cocoa programming. You explore the tools that you need to write Cocoa software and in the process build your first Cocoa application.

Part II: Instant Cocoa and the Objective-C Language

In Part II, you continue your quest for Cocoa enlightenment by examining the basics of the Objective-C language, the elements of a Cocoa interface, and object-oriented programming. These chapters give you the fundamental background knowledge that you need to use the features presented throughout the rest of the book.

Part III: Putting It All Together: Cocoa Programming in Depth

Now that you have the basics behind you, it's time to dive into the fun features of Cocoa. In Part III, you add some glitz and glamour to your applications using graphics, audio, video, Internet features, and stylized text. It's the stuff that applications are made of!

Part IV: Advanced Cocoa Topics

Part IV takes you into the realm of advanced Cocoa programming topics. Until now, applications remained simple one-window affairs. With Cocoa, you can easily create applications with multiple documents or even other executables that aren't traditional Mac applications at all. In this part, you discover some of the more advanced features of Cocoa and find out how to use them in your own projects.

Part V: The Part of Tens

Part V consists of useful Cocoa tips, tricks, and pointers. Whether its advice about how to make the most of Cocoa or help for what to do when things go wrong, Part V covers some common issues you'll encounter when using Cocoa.

Icons Used in This Book

When you see this icon, you can be sure that the code on the *For Dummies* Web site applies to the current example. The Web site contains the code for all projects in this book for those who don't feel like typing the code. Just go to www.dummies.com/extras and click <u>Cocoa Programming For Dummies</u>.

This icon indicates a useful pointer that you shouldn't skip.

This icon represents a friendly reminder. It describes a vital point that you should keep in mind while proceeding through a particular section of the chapter.

This icon signifies that the accompanying explanation might be informative (dare we say, interesting?), but it isn't essential to understanding Cocoa. Feel free to skip past these tidbits if you're a technophobe.

This icon alerts you to potential problems that you may encounter along the way. Read and obey these blurbs to avoid trouble.

Where to Go from Here

It's time to explore Cocoa! If you're apprehensive about embarking upon this journey, relax in the knowledge that anyone can program in Cocoa. This book will show you how to get started.

Part I
Developer Tools

The 5th Wave   By Rich Tennant

AT THE REAL PROGRAMMERS DATING BAR

WHOA! LOOK AT THE POCKET PROTECTORS ON THIS ONE!

In this part . . .

Your first sip of Cocoa begins with an introduction to the Cocoa development process. Next, it's on to Apple's Developer Tools, where you'll put that process into practice.

Part I guides you through the basics of Cocoa development using Project Builder and Interface Builder. These two applications form the foundation of your Cocoa experience, and you'll use them throughout the book. To help you understand how they work, you'll build your own working Cocoa application. As you progress through Part I, you'll continue to improve that application, adding features and improving functionality as you go. After you're happy with the results, the end of Part I shows you how to prepare the final application for public consumption.

Chapter 1

A Brief Tour of Cocoa Development

• •

In This Chapter

▶ Programming for Mac OS X

▶ Discovering the Cocoa development process

▶ Exploring the tools for programming Cocoa applications

• •

*T*hese are exciting times for Macintosh users. When Apple unleashed Mac OS X upon the world, they ushered in a new era of computing for the Mac faithful. Besides the rock-solid stability of UNIX, Mac OS X offers functionality and features that Mac users could only dream of a few short years ago. Along with this great new operating system, Apple saw fit to remember Macintosh developers. Principal among Apple's achievements is Cocoa, the subject of this book. This chapter introduces you to the world of Mac OS X programming and, in particular, Cocoa programming.

Mac OS X Is a Programmer's Dream

Macintosh programming has never been as easy and accessible as it is with Mac OS X. For starters, Apple, the friendly company that it is, thought it would be a great idea to give away their development tools. Each copy of Mac OS X comes bundled with a Developer Tools CD. By installing this disc, you instantly gain access to a complete collection of tools, utilities, documentation, and source code to get you started programming for the Mac OS. In the past, a developer bundle this comprehensive would have cost hundreds of dollars. Apple includes it with Mac OS X for no additional charge.

Some versions of Mac OS X ship with a Developer Tools CD; others do not. If you're searching for the disc and can't find it, you may have an installation of Mac OS X that does not include the Developer Tools CD. You needn't worry, though, because you can still download the Developer Tools by signing up for a free user account at Apple's developer site (developer.apple.com). In fact, even if you already have the Developer Tools CD, it's a good idea to check Apple's developer site for updates. Apple seems to release one each time they update Mac OS X. Note that some installations of the Developer Tools CD can total in the hundreds of megabytes, so you'll probably need a fast Internet connection to download them.

Just because the Developer Tools CD accompanies your copy of Mac OS X or is a free download doesn't mean the software is second rate. On the contrary, Mac OS X Developer Tools are world class. When developing software for the Macintosh with these tools, you are able to gain the following benefits:

- ✔ Write code in a variety of programming and scripting languages: C, Objective-C, Java, or even AppleScript

- ✔ Create beautiful interfaces that follow Apple's Human Interface Guidelines

- ✔ Develop applications rich with features, some of which you can add to your project without one line of code

Furthermore, because Mac OS X has a flavor of UNIX at its core, you can take advantage of the work of the decades of UNIX users. For example, most open-source software runs on different varieties of UNIX, so you can leverage thousands of compatible source-code examples for use in your own Mac OS X applications.

Why Program with Cocoa?

Cocoa is one kind of programming that you can perform with Apple's Developer Tools. Cocoa is a collection of tools and libraries that allows you to get the most out of Mac OS X programming. Many features make Cocoa great; the primary ones follow:

- ✔ Modular object-oriented design

- ✔ Use of frameworks

- ✔ Visual interface design

Object-oriented programming is all the rage these days, and for good reason. By programming with an object-oriented design, your code can more closely model items in the real world. This book isn't an object-oriented text; in fact, you should be coming to Cocoa with at least an idea of how to program in an object-oriented fashion. This book does, however, discuss the object-oriented nature of Cocoa and examines its foremost programming language: Objective-C. Objective-C, as you can tell from its name, is an object-oriented derivative of the C language. It permits you to program in an object-oriented fashion without all the messy baggage that C++ has.

The use of frameworks is another great aspect of Cocoa development. Experienced programmers may be tempted to call them by another name — libraries. Frameworks are collections of classes that provide you, the Cocoa developer, with a specific type of functionality. Mac OS X ships with several frameworks for you to choose from, but two stand out: AppKit and Foundation. The AppKit Framework provides you with scores of classes and functions for working with interfaces, and the Foundation Framework gives you utilitarian functions relating to data manipulation and program execution.

The object-oriented nature of Cocoa, combined with a large collection of frameworks to perform all sorts of tasks, forms an unbeatable code-reuse duo. Computer programmers can be a lazy bunch, not wanting to repeat a single task. To aid developers in their pursuit of reusable code, Cocoa offers a wide array of classes, tools, and code. After you've completed some programming tasks, you can even store the results in your own framework for use in other projects. Thus, Apple gives you reusable code out of the box, and you can reuse your own code as well. The object-oriented design of Cocoa makes this reuse possible.

Reusable code is good for a variety of reasons. It lets you create software quickly, it reduces the number of bugs in your code, and it prevents you from having to reinvent the wheel each time you sit down to program. Just remember, no one ever said that you had to reuse your own code. By reusing the frameworks that Apple provides with the Developer Tools, you gain all sorts of great functionality without having to know how it works under the hood.

Besides the geekier benefits, you'll love many other aspects of Cocoa programming. For starters, the frameworks that accompany Mac OS X provide a rich set of interface elements that you can use to build sophisticated interfaces that rival professional software. Furthermore, Cocoa programming gives you instant access to a wide range of freebies. Whether you need an About box, a spell-checker, or QuickTime movies in your application, Cocoa has a solution for you.

The Cocoa Development Process

Cocoa is not an easy hurdle to jump. It takes some time and perseverance to familiarize yourself with Cocoa but, after you do, you'll feel like your applications are super powered. Despite its hefty learning curve, most Cocoa projects follow the same five steps.

1. **Create a Cocoa project.**

   This is probably the easiest part of the process. If you've ever pressed Cmd-N, you're already a pro at this step.

2. **Build an interface and add it to the project.**

   With the tools that Apple provides, you can create stunning Aqua interfaces in minutes. Furthermore, you don't have to write a single line of code, because you can often perform this step by only dragging and dropping.

3. **Add some code to the project.**

   Now that your project has an interface, you need to write some code to make it functional. Using the easy-to- understand Objective-C language, you'll be on your way to Cocoa stardom before you know it.

4. **Test the code.**

   Because you'll write computer code that requires strict attention to detail, it's easy to make a mistake. That's where testing comes into play. Cocoa development requires the use of a variety of C that may be foreign to you. The best way to overcome its intricacies is to thoroughly test your code. Then when you've tested it to your satisfaction, test it some more! You want to iron out any problems you encounter early in the process, before they become large issues.

5. **Build an application.**

   This is where your Cocoa development journey ends — a Cocoa application. The main purpose (beyond fame and fortune) behind writing software is to create full-fledged applications. Using the tools that Apple provides, you'll have your Cocoa projects running as applications in minutes.

As you progress through this book, you'll discover that each part of the Cocoa development process is really a collection of steps. Whenever you feel like you're getting lost, consult this list. It will also help you get your bearings during particularly grueling Cocoa projects.

The Tools You Need

To help facilitate your Cocoa development, Apple was nice enough to provide you with a large selection of tools and utilities. With these tools, you can begin creating Cocoa software from the ground up. When you're finished programming, the tools will even build the application, prepare it for distribution, and put together an installer.

To begin programming with Cocoa, you need to find the development tools. They reside in the following directory on your hard drive.

```
/Developer/Applications/
```

If you discover that you don't have the development tools on your system, consult the appendix to find out how to install them.

You won't need all the applications that Apple provides in the /Developer/ Applications directory. In fact, you can probably get away with using only two: Project Builder and Interface Builder. If we start with the Cocoa development process outlined in the preceding section, and then update it to include the Project Builder and Interface Builder applications, it might look like this:

1. **Create a Cocoa project.**

   Most Cocoa projects begin their lives in Project Builder. Project Builder is the heart of your Cocoa development. This is where you store the various elements that make up your Cocoa projects.

2. **Build an interface and add it to the project.**

   Joined at the hip, Interface Builder forms the other half of the conjoined twins that are Apple's Developer Tools. Interface Builder is a WYSIWYG (what you see is what you get) editor for creating attractive Mac OS X interfaces that conform to Apple's Aqua standards. Interface Builder does other tricks too, including writing some of your code for you in Project Builder.

3. **Add some code to the project.**

   You've built an interface, and now it's time to make it do something. You use Project Builder again for this task, because it puts a suite of code-editing tools in your hands. You get built-in documentation, plus code that's colored to make it easier to perform your programming tasks.

4. **Test the code.**

   Again, Project Builder interfaces with the included debugging tools to help you produce bug-free code. There's also nothing wrong with trial-and-error testing, where you use your application, looking for mistakes or errors in its operation.

5. **Build an application.**

   Finally, the part you've been waiting for: building an application. Project Builder compiles, links, and builds your final executable application.

Project Builder

Project Builder is the main application that you use for all your Cocoa projects. Project Builder (sometimes called PB) serves a number of roles in the Cocoa development process.

First, Project Builder acts as the central repository for all the files in your Cocoa projects. Using a familiar document approach, Project Builder lets you organize the components of a Cocoa project in one easy-to-use document. Figure 1-1 shows a Cocoa project opened in Project Builder.

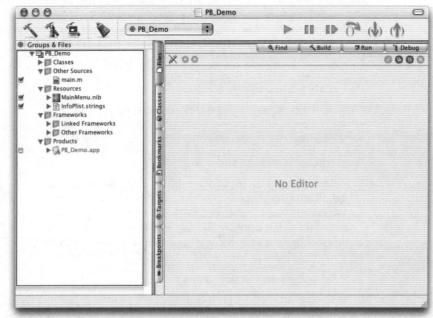

Figure 1-1: Project Builder acts as your primary tool for writing Cocoa software.

You use Project Builder also to write and edit Cocoa source code. As you write code for a project, Project Builder guides you by coloring the syntax. It also offers convenient one-click access to all the functions in your code, as shown in Figure 1-2.

Your Cocoa project may have other types of files beyond code, and Project Builder is prepared to help you work with them. For example, if you want to include images in your project, Project Builder lets you view them in the main project window without skipping a beat. There's no need to use another application to view those images. Project Builder displays them right in the code editor, as shown in Figure 1-3.

When you get stuck, Project Builder gives you access to the complete collection of Cocoa documentation. You can view and navigate the documentation with Project Builder in much the same way as you would a Web browser. Figure 1-4 shows what the screen looks like when documentation is loaded into Project Builder.

Figure 1-2:
Edit your
code in
Project
Builder.

Figure 1-3:
You can
view other
types of files
in Project
Builder.

Figure 1-4:
You can
view the
Cocoa
documen-
tation in
Project
Builder.

After you complete your Cocoa project, you use Project Builder to compile, link, and build a final application. You can then distribute the application to friends, co-workers, and even the world (as long as they use Mac OS X).

Project Builder wears many hats. If you're accustomed to other development environments, you may be surprised to discover that Project Builder performs tasks that require multiple tools in other environments. For example, Project Builder functions as a

- ✔ Project organizer, managing files and resources in your Cocoa projects

- ✔ Code editor, allowing you to write and edit Cocoa code

- ✔ Browser, displaying built-in documentation or other kinds of resources in your Cocoa projects

- ✔ Compiler and linker, spitting out a complete Cocoa application at the end of the development process.

Interface Builder

Interface Builder is a constant companion to Project Builder. As you can probably guess, Interface Builder's main purpose is to create interfaces. With it, you can build Aqua interfaces that adhere to Apple's Human Interface Guidelines.

Interface Builder provides a complete set of controls that you can add to your application. From windows and drawers to buttons and sliders, Interface Builder gives you drag-and-drop access to a full suite of interface elements to make your software the best it can be. Don't forget that Interface Builder is an Apple product. No one knows the Macintosh user interface better than Apple, so you can be certain that the controls in Interface Builder follow the strictest Apple guidelines.

Figure 1-5 shows an example interface with many different types of controls available to you in Interface Builder. The interface won't win any design awards, but it does show you the range of elements that you can use in your own Cocoa software.

Figure 1-5: Interface Builder has a complete set of interface controls for you to use in your Cocoa projects.

Interface Builder's features aren't limited to WYSIWYG interface editing. You can also create classes that have no visual representation. Although you don't actually write the code in Interface Builder for your classes, you do define the basic structures and methods for them there. You can also connect the interface to your classes using simple drag-and-drop techniques, as shown in Figure 1-6.

Do you speak the language?

Cocoa programming (like any kind of computer programming) requires the use of a computer language. To create Cocoa applications, you need to know Objective-C, Java, or AppleScript. This book uses Objective-C because it is the "native language" of Cocoa. Objective-C is a superset of the traditional C programming language. If you have experience with C, you're well on your way to understanding Objective-C. All the C functions you know and love are available to you in Cocoa. Objective-C, however, goes one step further and enhances C by adding object-oriented features to the language.

Objective-C has a syntax that may look a little foreign to you at first. But after you get the hang of it, you'll find that it isn't hard to understand at all. Chapter 7 goes into the details of Objective-C, but you start using it in Chapter 2 to build your first Cocoa project.

Figure 1-6: Connecting an interface element to a class is a simple drag-and-drop operation.

After you complete an interface, Interface Builder goes the extra mile and creates the header and implementation files for you and then inserts them into the desired Project Builder project. Although Interface Builder's strongest features pertain to designing and creating great-looking interfaces, many other features make it much more than an interface-building tool. It plays a big part in the Cocoa programming experience.

Chapter 2

Creating Your First Cocoa Application

In This Chapter

▶ Attaining fame and fortune with Cocoa in six simple steps

▶ Creating a project

▶ Building an interface

▶ Adding code to the project

▶ Testing and building a completed application

*P*rogramming computers can be grueling. Apple tries to simplify that task by offering a complete set of tools, an easy-to-understand programming language, and a sophisticated object-oriented framework to help you produce great software. The complete package is so well honed that you can create an application in one sitting with only a small amount of code.

This chapter shows you how to create your first Cocoa application from scratch. In the process, you work with Apple's Developer Tools. Whether you're building an interface, adding code to make the interface functional, or building the finished product, you'll see that Developer Tools offers a professional development environment that lets you work quickly to produce amazing applications.

Creating a Cocoa Application in Six Simple Steps

Writing your own software is a process. Much like following a recipe, you proceed through a sequence of steps until you end up with a working application. Fortunately, the series of tasks for programming Cocoa applications is short. To create a Cocoa application, you should follow this six-step process.

1. **Think of an application.**

   For some people, this can be the toughest step in the programming process. For others, it's the simplest. The idea here is that you want to build an application that carries out a task. Consider a task that you want your computer to perform. Then think of a computer program that would do it. What would it look like? How would it operate? What behaviors must it possess?

2. **Create a Cocoa project in Project Builder.**

   Cocoa development usually begins in the Project Builder application. Project Builder is at the center of Cocoa programming. It's where you create and work with the various parts of your Cocoa projects.

3. **Build an interface in Interface Builder.**

   After you create a project in Project Builder, you launch Interface Builder to work on your application's interface. In traditional Mac fashion, creating an interface is as easy as drag and drop. Using only the tools in Interface Builder, you can quickly build attractive interfaces in minutes.

4. **Return to Project Builder and add some code.**

   After you create an interface, you go back to Project Builder to add code. This step of the programming process gives functionality to the interface you just created. Luckily, Interface Builder helps with the process by laying out a shell in Project Builder where you can enter your code.

5. **Test your work.**

   No one gets everything right the first time; especially not with something as technical as computer programming. To help you out, Project Builder gives you a complete set of tools for testing your application before you unleash it on the world.

6. **Build an application.**

   You've built an interface, added code, and tested your project. Now it's time to build an application. With one click, you can build an application that you can run on almost any Mac OS X computer.

If you're using a version of Mac OS X prior to 10.2 (nicknamed Jaguar), you may not be able to run your application on later versions of Mac OS X. To remedy this problem, upgrade to the most recent version of Mac OS X and its corresponding Developer Tools. This ensures that you have the necessary frameworks to target the newer versions of Mac OS X.

Now that you have a basic understanding of the series of steps that you must perform to create a Cocoa application, it's time to create your own! The remainder of this chapter guides you through the process of building, coding, and creating your first Cocoa application.

Beginning a Project

To begin creating your first piece of Cocoa software, you need to come up with an idea of what you want to create. After you establish the type of software you want to build, you'll create a new project using Project Builder to commence programming.

Think of an idea

Instead of putting you through the sometimes-arduous task of dreaming up your own idea, I'll give you one to get you started.

Everyone needs a calculator. Whether you want to add your earnings from selling great Cocoa software or figure out how soon you can retire from said earnings, a calculator is a handy tool for the task. Sure, the Mac OS has a suitable calculator, but no one said you aren't allowed to build a better one.

One troublesome aspect of traditional calculator applications rears its head when you press an operator key (+, -, *, /) and enter another number. You can't see the first number that you entered. Your application will solve this problem by always displaying the two numbers you are working with.

Unlike a traditional calculator interface, your calculator will look more like a form. You enter numbers in the various fields of the interface and press a button to calculate the result. Figure 2-1 shows what the completed application will look like.

Figure 2-1:
When thinking of an idea for an application, try to imagine what it will look like.

As you can see, I thought of an idea (build a better calculator), thought of how to do it (using a form-like interface), and constructed a mental image of what it would look like. Of course, in this example, the mental image is an image of the finished product (see Figure 2-1). But because you can't read my mind, I provided an actual image.

Create a Cocoa project

Now that you have an idea in mind, you can begin the Cocoa development process:

1. **Launch Project Builder by double-clicking its icon.**

    The icon is on your hard drive at the following location:

    ```
    /Developer/Applications/Project Builder
    ```

2. **Chose File⇨New Project.**

    The New Project dialog box appears, asking you what kind of project you want to create.

3. **Select Cocoa Application from the list of choices, as shown in Figure 2-2.**

Figure 2-2:
Choose
the Cocoa
Application
option.

4. **Click the Next button.**

5. **Type a name for your project. Then click the Choose button and select a location for the project.**

    In this example, the name of the project is MyFirstProject, as shown in Figure 2-3. If you're a newcomer to UNIX, you may be wondering about that weird looking ~ character in the Location field in Figure 2-3. That character is called a *tilde*, and UNIX uses it to denote a user's Home directory.

Figure 2-3:
Give your
project a
descriptive
name.

6. **Click the Finish button.**

   Your hard drive buzzes and whirs for a few seconds, and then Project Builder displays a project window. On the left side of this window are the components that make up your project. These components include interface files and source code files, among other items.

7. **In the Resources folder, double-click the MainMenu.nib file to open it in Interface Builder, as shown in Figure 2-4.**

   This is the interface file for your project.

Files in your project reside in one of a handful of folders. You can read all about these folders in Chapter 3, which covers the operation of Project Builder. For now, the only folder you need concern yourself with is the Resources folder.

Building an Interface

When you double-click the MainMenu.nib file in Project Builder, the Interface Builder application is launched. If you're an old pro when it comes to Macintosh programming, you may remember ResEdit from the old days. You may be tempted to make a comparison between it and Interface Builder. In some respects, you're correct in making this leap.

Figure 2-4:
The Main-
Menu.nib
file contains
the inter-
face for
your
project.

Like ResEdit, Interface Builder lets you create interfaces using simple drag-
and-drop operations. However, Interface Builder can do much more. In addition to generating source code files for your Cocoa projects, Interface Builder
is tightly integrated with Project Builder. You've already seen this when you
double-clicked the MainMenu.nib file to open it in Interface Builder.

Figure 2-5 shows the MainMenu.nib file opened in Interface Builder. If you
don't see an open window in Interface Builder, double-click the Window
object in the Instances tab of the MainMenu.nib file.

This window is the starting point for your application's interface. Because
other people may use this application, it's a good idea to make it look as nice
as possible. Begin by changing the window's title:

1. **Open the Info window by choosing the Tools⇨Show Info menu.**

   A tall and narrow window appears, showing you a selection of properties that pertain to the window.

2. **In the Info window, change the Window Title property.**

   To follow along with the example, change the title to Simple Calculator,
   as shown in Figure 2-6.

3. **Change the title's size from the default settings.**

   To do so, simply click and drag the resize widget at the bottom-right
   corner of the Window window, as you would resize a window in Finder.

Figure 2-5:
Interface
Builder is
where you
design and
create your
application's
interface.

Figure 2-6:
The Info
window lets
you change
many
aspects of
a window,
including
its title.

4. **To prevent users from resizing the window while they use your application, uncheck the Resize option in the Controls section of the window's Info window.**

To continue constructing the interface, you must drag controls from the Palettes window, which displays a variety of controls for you to use in your Cocoa interfaces.

5. **In the top row of the Palettes window, click the second button from the left.**

You see the controls shown in Figure 2-7, and the title of the Palettes window changes to read Cocoa-Views.

Cocoa Views button

Add controls to the interface

For your first project, you'll use a handful of controls in your interface. Perform the following steps to add the controls you'll need for this project:

1. **Drag a button control from the Palettes window to your application's interface window.**

2. **Give the button a new label.**

To do so, double-click the button and type the text. To follow along with the example, type Calculate, as shown in Figure 2-8.

3. **Drag three large text field controls to the window.**

   The large text field control is the widest text field displayed in the Palettes window. It resides directly above the Field1 and Field2 text fields (as displayed in Figure 2-7).

   The user will type numbers (the operand) in the first two text fields that you add to the window. The result of the mathematical operation is displayed in the third text field. You need not change the properties for the first two text fields, but the third one needs a minor adjustment.

4. **The answer to the calculation will appear in the third text field in your window, so make its contents unalterable.**

   Select the text field, and then choose Tools⇨Show Info to display the Info window. From the list of properties, uncheck the Editable option (see Figure 2-9). This makes the text field uneditable, as you may have guessed.

Figure 2-9:
Uncheck the Editable property of a text field so your users can't change its contents.

5. **Add two text fields to serve as visual cues in the interface.**

   Despite being the same type of control (a text field) as those you added earlier, their appearance is quite a bit different. Rather than serving as a place for entering numbers in your application, these text fields serve strictly as visual cues in the interface. Because you're laying out this interface to look like a traditional math problem, change the title of one text field to + and the other to =. Figure 2-10 shows the completed interface with the new text field controls.

Table 2-1 lists the controls that make up your interface. Before you go on, now is a good time to double-check that everything is as you want it.

Table 2-1		Controls in Your First Interface	
Control Type	*Quantity*	*Identifying It in the Palettes Window*	*Other Info*
Button	1	Icon labeled *Button*	Title is *Simple Calculator*
Large text field	2	The large text field directly above the one labeled *Field1*	
Large text field	1	The large text field directly above the one labeled *Field1*	Uncheck the Editable option
Text field label	1	Icon labeled *System Font Text*	Title is +
Text field label	1	Icon labeled System Font Text	Title is =

Wiring the interface

Now that you've constructed your interface, it's time to wire it. After all, a light switch in your house can't turn on a lamp without a wire that connects the two; your interface is no different. At the center of a typical home's electrical system is a fuse box, or circuit breaker box. All wires in the home lead back to the centrally located fuse box. Cocoa interfaces follow a similar pattern. Instead of a fuse box, however, you use a class. You then add outlets to connect the main fuse box to the elements of your interface.

To create a class:

1. **In the MainMenu.nib file of Interface Builder, click the Classes tab.**

2. **Move the horizontal slider at the bottom all the way to the left until you see the leftmost column.**

   You'll see a class named NSObject.

3. **Select NSObject.**

   To do so, click it and then press Return on your keyboard. This creates a new class based on the NSObject class.

4. **Name your class and press Return.**

   To follow along with the example, name the class Fusebox. Figure 2-11 shows the newly created Fusebox class.

Figure 2-11:
The
Fusebox
class con-
nects the
interface
elements
to your
application.

Now you can finally add some outlets to this new class. *Outlets* are where you plug interface elements into a class.

In the simple calculator project, users will enter numbers for a calculation in two text fields. The third text field displays the result of the calculation. Therefore, you need to make three outlets — one for each text field. To add outlets to a class, perform the following steps:

1. **Select the class in the MainMenu.nib file.**

2. **Open the Info window.**

   Choose Tools➪Show Info.

3. **Select the Outlets tab in the Info window.**

4. **Add three new outlets.**

   To do so, click the Add button three times.

5. **Rename the three outlets.**

To rename an outlet, simply double-click its name in the Info window. Edit the text and press Return to make the name change take effect. To follow along with the example, use these names: `numberField1`, `numberField2`, `numberField3`. Figure 2-12 shows the `Fusebox` class with its three new outlets.

Figure 2-12:
The
`Fusebox`
class has
three
outlets.

6. **Click the Actions tab, and then click the Add button again.**

7. **Name this new action.**

   To follow along with the example, name the action calculateAnswer.

   An *action* is like a relay for your interface's electrical system. Flick a switch and big things happen. Later, you connect your button to this action. Then when a user clicks the button, the `calculateAnswer` action fires. You can then use some simple code to decide what action will take place. Figure 2-13 illustrates the new action that is now part of the `Fusebox` class.

Making connections

Now that you've created a `Fusebox` class and added three outlets and an action, it's time to make connections between `Fusebox` and your interface. You won't connect your interface to the `Fusebox` class, though. Instead, you'll connect the elements of your interface to an instance of the class.

When you create an instance (also known as an object) from a class, programmers say that you have *instantiated* it. Instantiate the `Fusebox` class by performing these steps:

Figure 2-13:
The
Fusebox
class has
one action.

1. **Select the** Fusebox **class.**

   You can find it in the Classes tab of MainMenu.nib.

2. **Create a new object based on your** Fusebox **class.**

   To do so, choose Classes⇨Instantiate Fusebox.

3. **Behold your new instance!**

   Interface Builder automatically clicks the Instances tab for you, revealing the new Fusebox instance, as shown in Figure 2-14.

Figure 2-14:
The Fuse-
box icon
appears
in the
Instances
tab of
MainMenu.
nib.

You've just created a new `Fusebox` object based on the `Fusebox` class. You'll make connections between this new instance and your interface using the outlets and action you added earlier. For starters, connect the three outlets to the three corresponding text fields in the interface. To get you started, here's how to connect the `numberField1` outlet to the interface:

1. **Select the `Fusebox` instance in MainMenu.nib.**

2. **Control-drag from the `Fusebox` instance to the leftmost text field in the interface.**

   Figure 2-15 shows what this drag operation looks like in action.

Figure 2-15: To make a connection to an outlet, Control-drag from an instance to an interface element.

3. **Select an outlet from the list.**

   When you Control-drag to text field and let go of the mouse, the Info window appears with the list of outlets available in your instance. Select the one you want. To follow along with the example, select `numberField1`.

4. **Connect the text field to the `Fusebox` instance.**

   To do so, simply click Connect. A small dot appears to the right of the outlet's name in the Info window, as shown in Figure 2-16.

5. **Repeat Steps 2 through 4 for the other two outlets, `numberField2` and `answerField`.**

   Make sure to Control-drag from the instance to the appropriate control in the interface before selecting the outlet to connect.

Figure 2-16:
A
connected
outlet
displays a
dot next to
its name in
the Info
window.

The process for wiring your action works in a similar fashion, except for one important point: It's in reverse! Instead of Control-dragging from the instance to the interface, you drag from the interface to the instance. To connect your action to the interface, follow these steps:

1. **Control-drag from the button in your interface to the** Fusebox **instance in MainMenu.nib.**

   Figure 2-17 shows this process.

Figure 2-17:
Control-drag
from the
button to the
Fusebox
instance to
connect the
instance's
action.

2. Select an action from the list.

To follow along with the example, select the `calculateAnswer` action in the Info window.

3. Connect the action to the button.

To do so, simply click Connect. You can see the completed connection in Figure 2-18.

Figure 2-18:
A connected action has a dot next to its name in the Info window.

You've finally finished creating and wiring your interface! To wrap up this step of the programming process, save your MainMenu.nib file:

1. Press Cmd-S.

2. Double-click the `Fusebox` **instance and choose Classes⇨Create Files for Fusebox.**

A window appears asking which files you want to include and where.

3. Use the default settings, and then click Choose.

Interface Builder creates new source code files named Fusebox.m and Fusebox.h and adds them to your project in Project Builder.

4. Return to Project Builder.

In the next section, you begin adding code to your application.

Adding Code to Make Your App Work

Back in Project Builder, you can see two files that weren't there before: Fusebox.m and Fusebox.h. They're probably in the Other Sources folder. If so, drag them to the Classes folder, because that's where Cocoa geeks put them — and you're well on your way to Cocoa geekdom.

Click the Fusebox.h file to see its contents. This header file contains the declarations for your Fusebox instance. Don't worry if you don't understand everything in the header file right now. You don't have to change anything here just yet.

Cocoa programmers are a special breed. Instead of using the term *header files*, they speak of *interface files*. Likewise, *source code files* are called *implementation files*.

Next, click the Fusebox.m file to reveal its contents. This is your main source code file and the place where you add commands to make this application do something. The file isn't empty. Interface Builder was kind enough to add some code to get you started:

```
#import "Fusebox.h"

@implementation Fusebox

- (IBAction)calculateAnswer:(id)sender
{
}

@end
```

Again, don't worry if you don't understand everything just yet. This code is a shell for you to use as you begin coding the project. It uses the header file with this line:

```
#import "Fusebox.h"
```

If you're a seasoned C programmer, just remember that #import in Cocoa is like #include in standard C. The directive lets you code know where the definition of your class is.

Next, the source code lists the implementation of the Fusebox class by means of the remaining code. One part of that class is an action called calculateAnswer. By adding code to calculateAnswer, you can make your application functional. All code that appears between the two empty braces of the calculateAnswer method executes whenever a user clicks the button in your interface.

The user clicks the button, which in turn fires the `calculateAnswer` action, which then executes your code. Add to Fusebox.m the following code between the curly brackets:

```
{
  //this is where your code begins
  int num1, num2, answer;

  num1 = [numberField1 intValue];
  num2 = [numberField2 intValue];
  answer = num1 + num2;

  [answerField setIntValue:answer];
  //this is where your code ends
}
```

If you have any programming experience, you'll probably recognize the first line of code in `calculateAnswer`:

```
int num1, num2, answer;
```

This line creates three integer variables for temporarily storing three integer numbers in memory. Next, the code assigns values to the `num1` and `num2` variables. The values it uses are ones that it pulls from the corresponding interface elements `numberField1` and `numberField2`. These two elements are text fields. To get the integer value from a text field, you send it the `intValue` message, which replies with the correct value. To send a message to an object, such as an interface element, enclose the object name and message name in square brackets:

```
num1 = [numberField1 intValue];
num2 = [numberField2 intValue];
```

Next, the code adds the two numbers and sticks the result in the `answer` variable. Finally, you display the answer by sending `answerField` a `setIntValue` message. This particular message requires a parameter: an integer value. You use the `answer` variable for that:

```
answer = num1 + num2;
[answerField setIntValue:answer];
```

The completed Fusebox.m file looks like this:

```
#import "Fusebox.h"

@implementation Fusebox

- (IBAction)calculateAnswer:(id)sender
{
  //this is where your code begins
  int num1, num2, answer;
```

```
num1 = [numberField1 intValue];
num2 = [numberField2 intValue];
answer = num1 + num2;

[answerField setIntValue:answer];
//this is where your code ends
}

@end
```

Save the Fusebox.m file with its new source code by choosing File➪Save.

Debugging and Building the Application

You've constructed an interface, wired it to your Fusebox instance, and added the code. Now it's time to see the results of your hard work. To test the project, choose Build➪Build and Run or click the Build and Run button in Project Builder, which is labeled in Figure 2-19.

As Project Builder builds your application, the Debugger window appears with lots of text flying by at a rapid rate. This is normal. If anything goes wrong during the build (such as an error in your code), the Debugger is the first place you'll want to look for clues as to what exactly did go wrong. When the build is finished, the Debugger tells you so (see Figure 2-20).

Build and Run

Figure 2-19: Click the Build and Run button to see the fruit of your efforts.

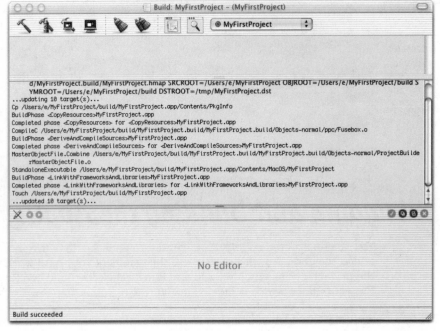

Figure 2-20:
If a build
goes off
without a
hitch, the
Debugger
displays
*Build
Succeeded.*

After your build succeeds, Project Builder launches the completed application, as shown in Figure 2-21. Your next step in the programming process is to test the functionality of the application. Enter numbers in the first two text fields and then click the button. Does it display the answer you expect?

Figure 2-21:
The
completed
application
in action.

000	Simple Calculator			
113	+	513	=	626
				Calculate

Keep in mind that because you're working with only integers, as shown in Figure 2-22, you won't get correct results if you enter numbers with fractional values. If you use a number with a decimal in it, you'll get a result without the fractional part. Clearly, the calculator isn't as robust as you might need.

Figure 2-22:
Oops! Your
calculator
works
only with
integers.

In Chapter 3, you expand on this project to account for decimal numbers. For now, bask in the glory of having built your first Cocoa application. The resulting executable file resides in your project's folder in Finder. Open the MyFirstProject folder and locate the Build folder within it. Open the Build folder to reveal your MyFirstProject application. You built that application, and it can run on any Mac OS X computer. Good job!

Chapter 3

Project Builder

In This Chapter

▶ Jumping headfirst into Project Builder

▶ Customizing the Project Builder window

▶ Adjusting the settings for your project

▶ Editing source code with Project Builder

▶ Debugging your Cocoa projects to remove errors

▶ Using the built-in help features of Project Builder

▶ Building an application from your project

C ocoa programming requires the use of some sophisticated development tools. Chief among these is Project Builder. Using Project Builder, you can manage your Cocoa projects. It is here that you write code, test your project, and finally build an application that you can run on any Mac OS X computer.

Project Builder is the main component of Apple's *integrated development environment* (a.k.a. the *IDE*). It has elaborate faculties for managing Cocoa projects, editing source code, debugging builds, and creating applications. This chapter gives you a tour of these features by demonstrating them in use. As you discover the different features of Project Builder, you'll continue to improve on the calculator project you create in Chapter 2. By the end of the chapter, you'll have a calculator application that has improved functionality and is free of bugs. These two goals are what all professional programmers want from their software and Project Builder can help you achieve them.

Project Builder: The Core of Apple's Development Tools

Because Project Builder is a first-class development tool, its array of windows, menus, and settings can look daunting to a budding Cocoa programmer. You're in the big leagues now, so expect a bit of a learning curve. Apple created the Mac OS for the average Joe (and Jane), but it made Project Builder for, you guessed it, developers. A typical Macintosh interface is here, but the subject matter is technical, so don't feel too bad if you don't understand everything at once.

With Project Builder, you can do many types of programming. Because of this fact, Project Builder offers tools, documentation, and settings for doing all these different kinds of programming.

As a Cocoa programmer, you're focusing on only one aspect of Project Builder's total capabilities. Thus, you'll need to use only the tools, documentation, and settings that pertain to Cocoa programming. Don't be surprised if you find that you use items in Project Builder only occasionally, rarely, or never at all.

Think of Project Builder as a hardware store. You might customarily go to the hardware store to buy nails, screws, or wood glue. Once in a while, you pick up a hammer, screwdriver, or even a tape measure. Every so many years, you even buy paint for the exterior of your house. You dare not go into the roofing aisle, though. You're afraid of heights and always leave that work to the professionals.

You use Project Builder in the same way you use the local hardware store. You perform some kinds of tasks all the time (writing code for your application), some tasks less frequently (assigning an icon to your application), and some rarely (adjusting the preferences for a Project Builder setting). Others you may never approach at all (creating drivers for a CD burner). This isn't to say that adjusting preferences in Project Builder is a task you'll seldom perform and that CD drivers are only for professionals. It's that Project Builder is a tool for many kinds of development. Like a hardware store, everyone uses Project Builder for specific needs. Maybe your neighbor likes to do plumbing and CD driver development. You, on the other hand, stick to furniture repair and Cocoa application development. The hardware store and Project Builder can assist both you and your neighbor in your endeavors even if neither of you understands what the other does.

Finding Your Way around Project Builder

To begin your tour of Project Builder, you can use a copy of the project you create in Chapter 2 as a starting point for this chapter's examples. Activate the Finder, select the Chapter 2 project folder (named MyFirstProject if you're using the code from the www.dummies.com/extras Web site) by clicking it, and choose File⇨Duplicate. Rename the duplicate CalculatorProject and the project within it CalculatorProject.pbproj. In this chapter, you upgrade the previous calculator project.

Instead of duplicating the project in Chapter 2, you can find the project files for this chapter on the *For Dummies* Web site at www.dummies.com/extras. The files reside in the following directory:

```
/Book Examples/Chapter 3
```

After you have a fresh copy of the calculator code ready to go, open its project file by double-clicking it in Finder. Project Builder launches, displaying the project and its components. The default Project Builder settings appear in Figure 3-1. If you've read Chapter 2, this window should look familiar because you used it to create your first project.

Customizing Project Builder Preferences

Project Builder displays the code and other components of your project in its main window. When you compile the project, Project Builder opens a new window that displays first the building process and then your application. Next, you quit the test run of the application and return to yet another window in Project Builder. If your project executed without a hitch, the window might display a message like this:

```
MyFirstProject has exited with status 0.
```

The status 0 message indicates that Project Builder encountered no errors during execution of the application. This is a good thing and means that your project is free from certain kinds of errors.

Project Builder displays these multiple windows by default, but you aren't limited to this setup. Display the Project Builder Preferences window by choosing Project Builder⇨Preferences. Across the top of this window is a row of buttons. Click the Task Templates button to make its settings appear, as shown in Figure 3-2.

The Task Templates preferences consist of three tabs:

- ✔ **Basic Settings:** Click to choose from preset Task Templates preferences.
- ✔ **Expert Configuration:** Click to configure your own Task Templates preset.
- ✔ **Manage Templates:** Click to edit Window templates.

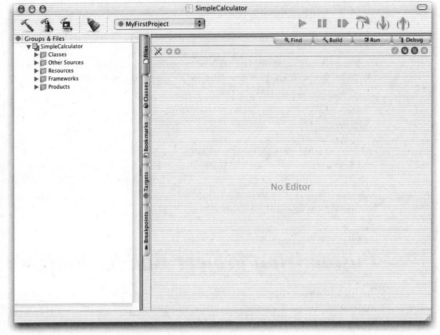

Figure 3-1:
Project Builder displays the main window when you first open a project.

Figure 3-2:
You can choose how many windows Project Builder displays during development.

For now, you should concern yourself with only the first tab, Basic Settings. As you can see in Figure 3-2, four large buttons make up the Basic Settings tab. The buttons have the labels and functions listed in Table 3-1.

Table 3-1	Basic Settings of the Task Templates Preferences
Button	*Function*
Single Window	Displays all development tasks in one window
Some Windows	Displays a new window for the Find, Build, and Debug tasks
Many Windows	Displays a new window for each development task
Custom Settings	Displays windows based on settings in the Expert Configuration tab

By default, Project Builder uses the Some Windows preset. To reduce clutter, you can go with the Single Window preset. Neat freaks love this preset. If you have a large monitor or a multiple-monitor configuration, you may prefer the Many Windows approach to spread out your work. Apple was nice enough to let you choose.

To adjust the Basic Settings of the Task Templates Preferences, perform the following steps.

1. **Make sure the Basic Settings tab is displayed.**

   If necessary, choose Project Builder⇨Preferences, click the Task Templates button, and then click the Basic Settings tab.

2. **Click the Single Window button to display all tasks in one window.**

   In the Basic Settings tab, click the Single Window button. The Single Window format appears throughout this book.

3. **Click OK to apply the setting and dismiss the Preferences window.**

4. **Back in the Project window, choose Build⇨Build and Run.**

   Your application runs as usual.

5. **Quit the application to return to Project Builder.**

   This time, note that your screen displays not three different windows but one solitary window. This window has some new horizontal tabs that weren't there before: Find, Build, Run, and Debug. The last three tabs represent the various windows that Project Builder displayed when the Some Windows settings were active in the Task Templates preferences window.

6. **Click the Run tab to display the status of the last run.**

You should recognize the status 0 message, which was displayed earlier. Figure 3-3 shows the project window with the Run tab displayed.

Figure 3-3:
The Single Window setting compacts the various development windows into one tidy window.

Hitting the target

Besides the horizontal tabs that you activated in your project window in the last section, the project window also hides several panes of settings that you can access using a column of vertical tabs (see Figure 3-4). Click any of the tabs to display that group of settings for your project.

If you've read Chapter 2, you're probably familiar with the Files tab, because you used it when working on your code in that chapter. This tab displays the files in your project along the left side of the project window. The other important one for the Cocoa newbie is the Targets tab. By clicking it, you'll see the settings for your project's target.

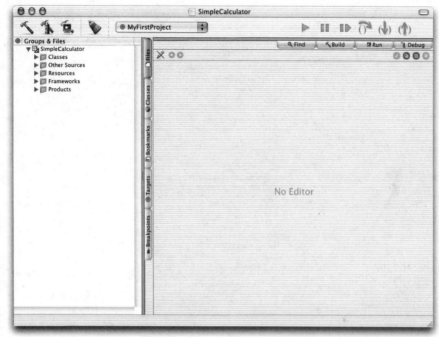

Perform the following steps to change the name of your target from
MyFirstProject to SimpleCalculator.

1. **Click the Targets tab.**

   The Target settings appear on the right side of the project window in the
   Target pane.

2. **In the Target pane, select Summary.**

   Summary appears first in the list. The Target Summary settings appear
   to the right of the list, as shown in Figure 3-5.

3. **Change the name of the product.**

   The *product* is your final executable application. Type a new name in the
   Base product name box. For example, you might call the final application SimpleCalculator, which is more descriptive than MyFirstProject.
   Now, when you build your project, Project Builder creates an application
   with the new target name and places it in the build directory, which
   resides in your project's development directory.

4. **Change the name of the target.**

   In the list on the far-left side of the project window, choose MyFirstProject
   from the Target submenu. Then choose Project➪Show Info to display the
   Target Info window. Change the Name box to SimpleCalculator (see Figure
   3-6). Close the Target Info window to make the setting take effect.

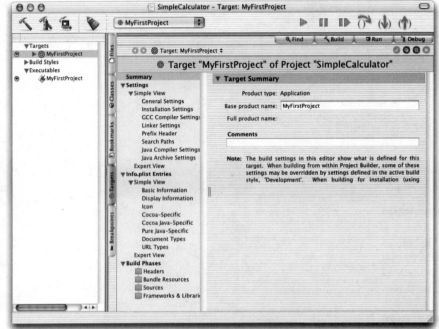

Figure 3-5:
You can change the name of your product in the Target Summary settings.

Figure 3-6:
You can change the name of the target in the Target Info window.

You can avoid all these steps by recreating the project in Chapter 2 by hand and replacing MyFirstProject with SimpleCalculator, but what fun would that be? This way, you can see how Project Builder works and tweak the settings later if you want.

Working with project files

In the last chapter, you discovered that the calculator could add integers but not numbers with decimals. To change the way the application operates, you need to alter the code in the project:

1. **In your main project window of Project Builder, click the Files tab from the selection of vertical tabs.**

   The files in your project are displayed.

2. **In the list on the left side of the project window, find and expand the SimpleCalculator group.**

   What you'll probably recognize as a folder, Project Builder calls a *group*. The small folder icons that appear to the left side of the project window are groups. Clicking the disclosure triangle located on the left side of each group displays the files in that group.

3. **Click the Fusebox.m file to display its code, as shown in Figure 3-7.**

4. **Change the code in the Fusebox.m file to read like this:**

```
#import "Fusebox.h"

@implementation Fusebox

- (IBAction)calculateAnswer:(id)sender
{
    //this is where your code begins
    float num1,num2,answer;

    num1 = [numberField1 floatValue];
    num2 = [numberField2 floatValue];
    answer = num1 + num2;

    [answerField setFloatValue:answer];
    //this is where your code ends
}

@end
```

You need to make three changes:

   a. **First, change the three variables from an** int **type to a** float **type. The float data type supports numbers with decimals.**

```
float num1,num2,answer;
```

```
#import "Fusebox.h"

@implementation Fusebox

- (IBAction)calculateAnswer:(id)sender
{
    //this is where your code begins
    int num1,num2,answer;

    num1 = [numberField1 intValue];
    num2 = [numberField2 intValue];
    answer = num1 + num2;

    [answerField setIntValue:answer];
    //this is where your code ends
}

@end
```

Figure 3-7:
The vertical
Files tab
displays the
code in a
project.

> **b. Second, because you're working with** float **variables now, use
> the** floatValue **function to retrieve decimal data from the two
> number fields.**

```
num1 = [numberField1 floatValue];
num2 = [numberField2 floatValue];
```

> **c. Third, you must to use the** setFloatvalue **function instead of
> the** setIntValue **function to display the result in** answerField.

```
[answerField setFloatValue:answer];
```

**5. Now that you've edited the source code in Fusebox.m, select
Fusebox.h in the Groups & Files list by expanding the Classes group
in the SimpleCalculator folder.**

As you may recall from Chapter 2, Fusebox.h holds the definitions for
your interface. You can also put the usual header stuff here, including
function prototypes, defines, and global variables you may need.

**6. In the Groups & Files list, navigate to the Other Sources folder and
select the main.m file.**

In this file, you'll see code that looks like this:

```
#import <Cocoa/Cocoa.h>

int main(int argc, const char *argv[])
{
    return NSApplicationMain(argc, argv);
}
```

This code appears in every Cocoa application project that you create. It is responsible for making your application go, much like a set of keys makes an automobile run. The nice part is that Project Builder automatically adds it to the project for you, and you don't need to make any changes to it.

7. **To see your handiwork in action, choose the Build➪Build and Run menu.**

8. **After Project Builder compiles the project for you, test the SimpleCalculator application, using decimal numbers (see Figure 3-8).**

Figure 3-8:
The calculator supports decimals!

Browsing Classes

Your next stop on the Project Builder tour is Class Browser. To open Class Browser, click the vertical tab labeled Classes in your project's main window. Project Builder displays a complete list of available classes on the left side of the project window.

For example, the first class in the list is the Fusebox class, the only class you implemented in this project. The name of the Fusebox class appears in blue lettering. Select the Fusebox class to display its member functions in the list below the list of classes. In this class, you implemented only one function — calculateAnswer — as shown in Figure 3-9.

Next, in the popup menu that appears at the bottom of the project window below Class Browser, choose Flat, project classes. Class Browser displays only the classes specific to your project. As usual, Class Browser also displays the member functions of the selected class below the list of classes (see Figure 3-10).

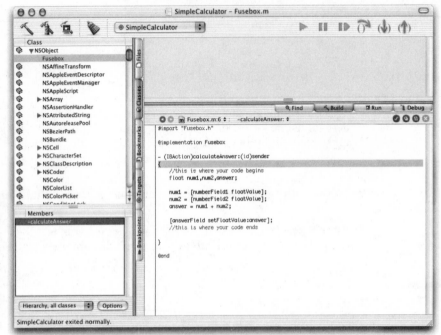

Figure 3-9:
Class
Browser
displays
the classes
available to
your project.

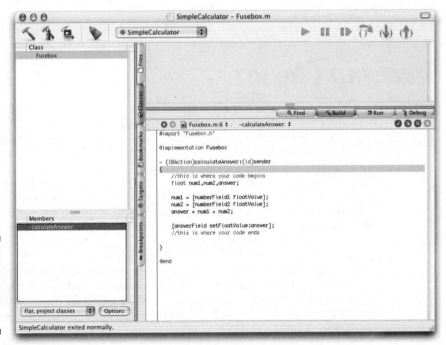

Figure 3-10:
You can
view just the
classes in
your project.

When you select a class, Project Builder displays the member functions for that class. Select any one of those function names to instantly jump to that function in the code editor.

Debugging Your Project

Because computer programming is a complex process, it's easy to make mistakes. You can introduce errors to your code in a number of ways. For example, typographical mistakes in your code may lead to syntax errors in your project. A *syntax error* is an error in the grammar of your code that makes Project Builder unable to interpret the code.

Other mistakes might be syntactically correct and allow Project Builder to compile and link your code into an application, yet produce unexpected or incorrect results. These are *runtime errors* and have nothing to do with the syntax of your code. Rather, the logic of your code contains errors that produce an application that doesn't function properly. The application may run and even work somewhat as expected, but at some point your application will do something wrong. A purple apple might be displayed instead of a red one in your graphics application, an enemy invader won't die when shot in your video game, or a miscalculation yields an incorrect numerical result in your spreadsheet application.

The only way to know if you have any bugs in your code is to thoroughly test your projects. When you debug a project, you build, run, and test your application until you're convinced that it's bug free.

To begin debugging:

1. **Build and run the project you've been working with throughout this chapter.**

2. **Type values in the two number fields and then click the Calculate button.**

3. **Change the numbers and click the button again.**

4. **Repeat Step 3 until you're convinced that the project operates as it should.**

For example, three consecutive tests of the project yields the following results:

$$1 + 2 = 3$$
$$3.25 + 4.75 = 8$$
$$3.2 + 4.75 = 7.949999809265137$$

Uh oh! That last test didn't produce results that you might expect. What's going on here?

First, it appears that the code is calculating the sum of the two numbers incorrectly in some situations. Second, the problem seems to occur only when using decimal numbers. Further, it happens only when the count of digits in the decimal portion doesn't match between the two numbers. In this example, 3.2 has only one decimal digit (2), but 4.75 has two (7 and 5).

To help you figure out where things are going wrong, Project Builder includes a powerful debugger. Using the debugger, you can follow along as your project's code executes and watch for any indication of a problem.

To begin debugging this code, you'll first need to set some breakpoints. *Breakpoints* are small markers that appear in the column to the left of the code. To insert a breakpoint, simply click in that leftmost column next to the line of code that you'd like to check with the debugger, as shown in Figure 3-11.

For this example, it's a good idea to set three breakpoints: one for each time you assign a value to a variable (that is, `num1`, `num2`, and `answer`).

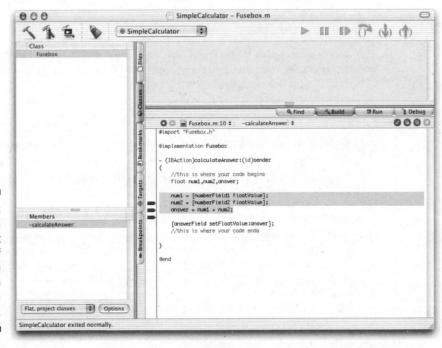

Figure 3-11:
Click in the leftmost column of the code editor to set a breakpoint.

Notice that the breakpoints in Figure 3-11 come after the line of code in question. The line of code that sets a variable has to execute before you can check the variable's value to see its result.

Now that you've set some breakpoints, it's time to debug the project. Choose Build⇨Build and Debug. When you do, Project Builder begins building your project just as it always has, but then something happens. Project Builder opens the Debug tab. As your built application runs, various kinds of data appear in the Debug tab, based on where you set the breakpoints.

For now, you won't see any information in the Debugger. Rather, your project's main window will come to the foreground and look like it always has. Enter the same numbers in your application's interface (3.2 and 4.75) and click the OK button.

After you click OK, the Debugger comes to the foreground and displays all sorts of data in the Debug tab. In the left side of the Debugger, you see the name of the class and method that the code is currently executing. In this case, it's the Fusebox class and the calculateAnswer method. The bottom section of the Debugger displays the code for the calculateAnswer method.

Because you set breakpoints, the Debugger stops at the first one it encounters. This indicates the *next* line of code that the Debugger will execute. In the upper-right section of the Debugger, you can view the current state of all variables in your code. So far, only this code has executed:

```
float num1,num2,answer;
num1 = [numberField1 floatValue];
```

Therefore, you might expect that the Debugger displays only a value for the num1 variable. Figure 3-12 shows the debugging process thus far.

As you can see in Figure 3-12, we already have a problem. The value of num1 isn't 3.2 as you might expect. Instead, it has a value of 3.20000005. Continue executing the code by choosing Debug⇨Continue. The Debugger then displays the value of num2, 4.75. Click Debug⇨Continue again to make the Debugger jump to the third breakpoint and display the value of answer, 7.94999981. When you choose Debug⇨Continue again, the variables in the Debugger disappear and the application sits and waits for you to press the Calculate button again. Click the project window and choose Debug⇨Stop Debugging to cease the debugging process.

Although the numbers that your code displays are very close to the actual values, they aren't the exact values that you want. Clearly, you need a solution that formats numbers according to some guidelines. For example, you may only care about two decimal points of precision.

Figure 3-12:
As the
Debugger
executes
code, it
displays
the values
of variables.

Without getting into a bunch of technicalities just yet, a float variable can have many digits in the decimal portion of its value. When you set num1 and num2 to values that share the same count of decimal digits, your compiler spits out a like number. When the number of decimal digits doesn't match in both num1 and num2, the code yields a number with a whole bunch of digits.

To get around this problem, one solution is to format the answer variable before displaying it. A few lines of code will take of the problem:

```
NSNumberFormatter *answerFormatter =
        [[[NSNumberFormatter alloc] init] autorelease];

    [answerFormatter setFormat:@"#,###.00;0.00;(#,##0.00)"];
    [[answerField cell] setFormatter:answerFormatter];
```

Don't be frightened if you don't understand this intimidating blurb of code. This chapter is about Project Builder, not Objective-C code, so we'll only brush over it for now.

The first two lines of code (which incidentally are just one function that appears on two lines) create an NSNumberFormatter object. The purpose behind an NSNumberFormatter object is to regulate the format of numbers.

Next, the code sends the setFormat message to the answerFormatter object, passing it a long string of text. This string designates what formats are allowed for this NSNumberFormatter object. The string is a series of three formats, each separated by a semicolon. You don't have to worry about the precise format of these three strings but, to give you a hint, the first one defines the format of positive numbers, the second one accounts for cases when the number is 0, and the last bit formats negative numbers.

Finally, the code applies the NSNumberFormatter object to answerField in the interface. To help you understand where this bit of code fits into the big picture, here's the listing of the completed source code for Fusebox.m. Note that when you add the code, the last breakpoint moves accordingly.

```
#import "Fusebox.h"

@implementation Fusebox

- (IBAction)calculateAnswer:(id)sender
{
    //this is where your code begins
    float num1,num2,answer;

    num1 = [numberField1 floatValue];
    num2 = [numberField2 floatValue];
    answer = num1 + num2;

    NSNumberFormatter *answerFormatter =
        [[[NSNumberFormatter alloc] init] autorelease];

    [answerFormatter setFormat:@"#,###.00;0.00;(#,##0.00)"];
    [[answerField cell] setFormatter:answerFormatter];

    [answerField setFloatValue:answer];
    //this is where your code ends
}

@end
```

Now that you've formatted answerField properly, choose Build➪Build and Run to see your changes in action. If you entered the code correctly, you should see results like that show in Figure 3-13.

Figure 3-13:
Using the
NSNumber-
Format-
ter object
in your
code, you
can dictate
how your
application
displays
floating-
point
numbers.

Before you leave the debugging section of this chapter, let's look at one more kind of error that you may come across when using Project Builder to program Cocoa applications. Change the last line of your code in Fusebox.m to this:

```
[answerField setFloatValue:answer]
```

This time you are intentionally leaving off the trailing semicolon (a common mistake that even pros make). Choose Build⇨Run and Build to see what happens. The result is that the horizontal Build tab appears, displaying two errors and one warning, as shown in Figure 3-14.

Yes, one simple mistake can cause the compiler to report more than one error. The first error that Project Builder reports is the real cause of the aborted build: the missing semicolon. The remaining error and warning stems from the first error. Because the compiler couldn't parse the line with the missing semicolon, it can't figure out what to do with the rest of the code either, so it starts spitting out errors and warnings wherever it continues to have problems.

Double-click the first error that the horizontal Build tab displays, to place your cursor at that line of troubled code in the code editor. Add the semicolon again to the end of the line to repair the code. Press Cmd-S to save the correction.

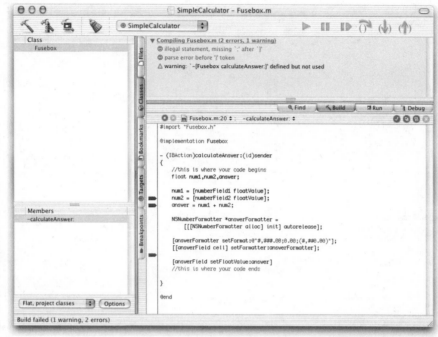

Figure 3-14:
One mistake can cause Project Builder to display multiple errors.

The point behind this demonstration is to show you that you may encounter different kinds of errors when programming with Project Builder. Some errors, like this last one, occur during the build process and Project Builder shows you where they are. Other bugs are trickier to track down, such as the earlier example. For those, it never hurts to use the built-in Debugger to solve the problem.

Now that you're finished debugging your project, you may want to remove the breakpoints that you added earlier in this chapter. In Project Builder, click the vertical tab labeled Breakpoints. You see all your breakpoints in a list on the left side of the project window. Select a breakpoint from the list and press Delete on your keyboard to remove that breakpoint. Do the same for the remaining breakpoints. Figure 3-15 shows the list of breakpoints in your project prior to deletion.

Nothing prevents you from keeping the breakpoints set in the project. You can safely leave them in place without causing any problems for yourself.

Figure 3-15:
Manage
your break-
points in the
Breakpoints
tab.

Use Bookmarks to Simplify Development

As your projects grow, you'll find that locating code can sometimes become problematic. For large projects, it's not uncommon to jump between dozens of source code files. To help you out, Project Builder has bookmarks, much like a Web browser does. Instead of pointing to URLs on the Web, though, Project Builder *bookmarks* point to specific places in your source code. This is useful when you want to quickly jump to certain spots in your code without the hassle of surfing through the numerous files that might make up your project.

To begin working with bookmarks in Project Builder, follow these steps:

1. **Click the vertical Bookmarks tab.**

   The list of bookmarks for your project appears, as shown in Figure 3-16.

2. **Select any file from your project and click anywhere in the code editor for that file.**

   Choose a spot that you'd like to return to quickly.

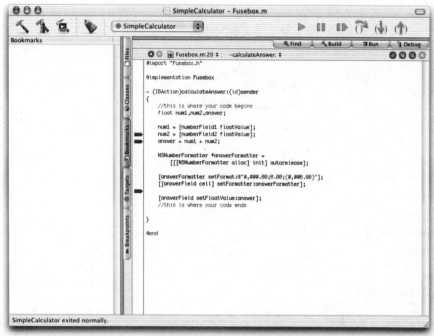

Figure 3-16:
Click the
Bookmarks
tab to
view the
bookmarks
for your
project.

3. **Choose View⇨Add to Bookmarks to create a new bookmark to this location in the code editor.**

   By default, Project Builder names the bookmark according to its location in the source code. You are free to change the name of any bookmark to whatever you want.

4. **To rename a bookmark:**

   a. **Control-click it in the Bookmarks list and then choose Rename, as shown in Figure 3-17.**

   The highlighted name of the bookmark appears in the Bookmarks list.

   b. **Type any name you want, and then press Enter to make the name change permanent.**

5. **To delete a bookmark from your project, select that bookmark and press Delete on your keyboard.**

   The bookmark instantly vanishes.

Figure 3-17:
Control-
click a
bookmark to
rename it.

Where to Go for Help

At some point, you're going to want more information about how the Mac OS X Developer Tools operate. Fortunately, Apple has you covered with its built-in documentation. Choose Help⇨Developer Tools Help to view documents about the following Developer Tools:

- **Project Builder:** The application you've been using throughout this chapter

- **Interface Builder:** The tool you use to create interfaces for your Cocoa code

- **AppleScript Studio:** A set of tools for developing AppleScript-based applications using Project Builder and Interface Builder

- **GNU C:** The open source compiler that's part of Project Builder

- **GDB:** The GNU source-level debugger

The built-in Help offers documentation on each aspect of Mac OS X development in HTML and PDF formats. It also includes a few helpful tutorials for getting started with Project Builder.

Besides the standard Help, Project Builder offers one-click access to information about Cocoa classes and frameworks in the code editor. To test this feature, do the following:

1. Click the vertical Files tab.

The source code in your project appears on the left side of the Project Builder window.

2. Select the Fusebox.m source code file.

Project Builder displays the file in the code editor.

3. Locate a keyword in the source code that you'd like to investigate.

For example, you may want to find out more about the setFormatter method that you used in earlier sections of this chapter.

4. Option-double-click the keyword.

While holding down the Option key, double-click setFormatter in the Fusebox.m file. When you do this, a menu appears above the location where you option-double-clicked, listing the various methods in Cocoa named *setFormatter* (see Figure 3-18).

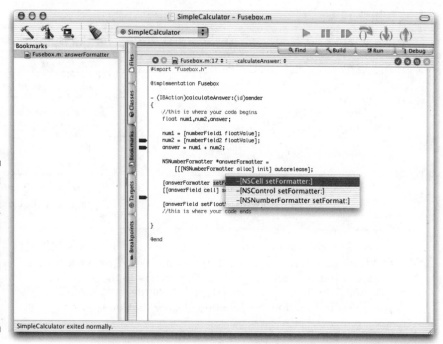

Figure 3-18:
Option-double-click any valid keyword in the code editor to view its documentation.

5. **Choose a keyword from the menu.**

Select the appropriate `setFormatter` method (hint: it's labeled *-[NSCell setFormatter:]* in the menu) to view its documentation. You're using the `setFormatter` method of the `NSCell` because you want to change the format of the cell in the text field.

Building the Final Application

Now that you've set up your project, altered its source code, and browsed the classes in it, you're ready to build the final application. In Chapter 2 you perform this step by choosing Build➪Build and Run. Project Builder then compiles, links, and executes the resulting application.

You don't always have to build and run, although it's probably the most common method of working in Project Builder. You can build your project without running it by choosing Build➪Build. This compiles, links, and creates the target application but doesn't execute it. If you'd prefer to use the Debugger, choose Build➪Build and Debug. Table 3-2 lists the keyboard shortcuts for the various Build commands.

Table 3-2	Keyboard Shortcuts for the Build Menu	
Function(s)	*Keyboard Shortcut*	*What It Does*
Build	Cmd-B	Builds the current project
Build and Run	Cmd-R	Builds and then executes the current project
Build and Debug	Cmd-Y	Builds the current project and starts the debugger
Clean	Cmd-Shift-K	Cleans the current project by removing all object code from it

In addition to the standard menu items and corresponding keyboard shortcuts, Project Builder gives you easy access to the various build features through buttons in the top-left corner of the main project window. Figure 3-19 shows the location and function of these buttons.

Whenever you click one of these build icons, it turns into a stop sign. While the build or debugging proceeds, you can halt the process. Sometimes it takes a while to complete a build. If you forget to do something before building, it's handy to be able to stop the build operation. That way, you can avoid the wait of completing the build and get back to work.

Build active target

Build and debug active executable

Build and run active executable

Clean active target

Figure 3-19:
Click one
of the
buttons in
your
project's
window
for quick
access to
the build
functions of
Project
Builder.

After you complete a successful build, your new application appears in the
Build folder of your project's main folder in Finder. You can then distribute
and run this application on any other computer that uses Mac OS X, which is
the main goal of programming in Cocoa.

Chapter 4

Interface Builder

· ·

In This Chapter

▶ Finding your way around Interface Builder

▶ Using the Design window to construct an interface

▶ Adding controls to an interface

▶ Editing attributes of a control

▶ Editing and creating new menus

▶ Wiring an interface

▶ Implementing code to use an interface

· ·

The second most important component of Cocoa development (Project Builder is the first) is the Interface Builder application, which you use to create interfaces for your Cocoa projects. It gives you the ability to construct beautiful Aqua interfaces with drag-and-drop ease — without a lick of code. More important, the interfaces you create in Interface Builder follow Apple's stringent Human Interface Guidelines, which means that you have a good chance of producing applications that Mac users (they're a finicky bunch) like to look at and ultimately use.

In this chapter, you take a tour of Interface Builder, examining its functionality as you go. To help you acclimate to Interface Builder, you adapt and improve the calculator application that you created in the chapter on Project Builder (Chapter 3). By the end of this chapter, your calculator will have a new menu, additional interface elements, and added functionality.

A Tour of Interface Builder

To begin working with Interface Builder, copy the files from the Chapter 4 directory to your hard drive. You should always make sure that your Cocoa projects and associated files reside on write-enabled media, which is a hard drive for most people.

You can find the project and files for this chapter on the *For Dummies* Web site at www.dummies.com/extras. The files reside in the following directory:

```
/Book Examples/Chapter 4/Start Code/Calculator
```

After you have the code for Chapter 4 copied to your hard drive, do the following to begin working the project in Interface Builder:

1. **Open the file named CalculatorProject.pbproj.**

   This launches Project Builder and opens the project.

2. **Expand the project's Resources folder in Project Builder to reveal the MainMenu.nib file.**

   MainMenu.nib is the file that holds the interface for your calculator project. Figure 4-1 shows the location of MainMenu.nib in Project Builder.

Figure 4-1:
MainMenu.
nib contains
the inter-
face for
your
project.

3. **In Project Builder, double-click MainMenu.nib to open it in Interface Builder.**

   Although Project Builder and Interface Builder are two different applications, they work together to provide you with a fruitful Cocoa experience.

TECHNICAL STUFF

Incidentally, the *nib* in MainMenu.nib is short for NeXT Interface Builder. Why NeXT? NeXT is the name of the company that Steve Jobs headed before his return to Apple. Apple purchased the NeXT operating system, and it became the core of Mac OS X. The nib file is a carry-over from those days. Cocoa geeks call these nib files. Old habits die hard. Besides that, have you ever tried to pronounce ".aib" (for Apple Interface Builder)? Furthermore, the *NS* that appears at the beginning of class names in Cocoa stands for NextStep, another historical tidbit in Cocoa left over from NeXT.

When you first launch Interface Builder, you may see as many as five different windows. Figure 4-2 shows the various windows as they appear in Interface Builder.

Table 4-1 describes why you need each window and how to display one if it isn't currently visible.

Design window   Palettes window

Figure 4-2: Interface Builder has five main windows.

Info window   nib file window

Main editor window

Table 4-1	Main Windows of Interface Builder	
Window	*How to Display it*	*What You Do With It*
nib file window	Double-click the .nib file in Project Builder	Store the components of your interface file
Design window	Double-click the Window icon in the Instances tab of the nib file window	Use it in your application's interface
Info window	Choose Tools⇨Show Info	View and edit attributes of your interface and the classes that the project comprises
Palettes	Choose Tools⇨Palettes⇨ Show Palettes Design	Drag controls from the Palettes window to a window to create an interface
Menu editor	Double-click the MainMenu icon in the Instances tab of the nib file window	Create, delete, or edit menus for your application

Together these five windows form the main tools of Interface Builder. Using these tools in concert, you can build a complete interface for use in your Cocoa applications.

That's not all Interface Builder can do, though. Interface Builder also lets you create and add classes to your project. Later, you can connect classes to the elements of your interface by clicking and dragging. These connections serve as the bridge between your interface and your code in Project Builder. Finally, Interface Builder takes care of the dirty work of writing code for your interface. With one click, it produces the necessary headers and source code for implementing your interface with Project Builder.

The nib file window

The *nib file window* is the heart of your project's interface. This is where you store the components of your project's interface. The nib file window contains four panes:

- **Instances:** The objects in your nib file
- **Classes:** The classes in your nib file
- **Images:** Graphics files that you can use in your interface
- **Sounds:** Audio files that you can use in your interface

The bulk of your time in Interface Builder will be spent in the first two panes (Instances and Classes). You use the Classes pane to create new classes for your nib file. Figure 4-3 shows the Classes pane.

Figure 4-3:
Use the
Classes
pane to
view the
class hier-
archy of
your nib file.

Later, you make new objects based on these classes. Those objects appear in the Instances pane (see Figure 4-4).

Figure 4-4:
The
Instances
pane dis-
plays the
objects in
your nib
file.

The Instances pane can display its contents in Icon mode or Outline mode, as shown in Figures 4-4 and Figure 4-5, respectively. With Outline mode, you can view the hierarchy of items in your interface. Click the Icon/Outline button (labeled in Figure 4-5) to toggle between the two modes.

By default, each new nib file (that Project Builder creates for you as part of a new project) has four items in its Instances pane:

- ✔ File's Owner
- ✔ First Responder
- ✔ MainMenu
- ✔ Window

Figure 4-5:
Click the
Icon/Outline
button to
switch
between
Icon mode
and Outline
mode.

— Icon/Outline button

The MainMenu and Window are what you should concern yourself with for
now. As you can probably guess, the MainMenu is where you edit the menus
for your interface. The Window is a window object that you can use in your
interface.

Design window

The Design window represents a window in your interface and is where you
add controls. Your user then uses these controls to operate your application.
To view a Design window:

1. **In the nib file window, double-click Window.**

   The contents of the Window object are displayed, as shown in Figure 4-6.

2. **With the window opened, click a control to select it.**

   For example, select the Calculate button.

3. **Press the Option key and move your cursor around the window.**

   As you pass over each control, Interface Builder displays guidelines and
   numbers informing you of the distance between the selected control and
   the one with the cursor over it. Figure 4-7 illustrates the distance
   between the button and the answer field.

Figure 4-6:
The Design
window is
where you
lay out the
controls
for your
interface.

Figure 4-7:
Select a
control and
hold the
Option key
to display
guidelines.

4. With the button still selected, press Option and move your cursor into a section of the window where no control resides.

You see guidelines that define the location of the selected button. Figure 4-8 shows the position of the button in the Calculator interface.

Figure 4-8:
Hold Option
and move
the cursor
outside the
selected
element to
see its
coordinates.

You can move the controls in a Design window by dragging them with the mouse. You can also select a control and move it with the arrow keys. As you move a control around a window, Interface Builder displays guides to help you accurately position the control.

Palettes window

To create an interface, you need an assortment of buttons, sliders, and other controls. The Palettes window provides these controls for you to use in your interface. To view the Palettes that are available to you, do these three steps:

1. Choose Tools⇨Palettes⇨Show Palettes.

The Palettes window appears, with a row of eight buttons across the top of it as shown in Figure 4-9.

Cocoa Menus
Cocoa Views
Other Cocoa Views
Cocoa Windows
Cocoa Data Views
Cocoa Container Views
Cocoa Graphics Views

AppleScript

Figure 4-9:
The Palettes
window
contains a
variety of
controls that
you can
use in your
interface.

2. Click any one of these buttons to view a palette of controls related to that button.

For example, click the second button from the left (Cocoa Views) to view a set of controls that includes buttons and text fields. Each button reveals a different set of controls.

3. Close the window.

Click the close button or choose File⇨Close Window to dismiss the window.

Table 4-2 describes the sets of controls available in the Palettes window.

Table 4-2	Buttons in the Palettes Window
Button Name	*Reveals These Types of Controls*
Cocoa Menus	Menu items that you can use with the Menu editor
Cocoa Views	Buttons, text fields, and number and date formatters
Other Cocoa Views	Sliders, popup buttons, progress indicator, image view, and color well

Button Name	Reveals These Types of Controls
Cocoa Windows	Windows, panes, and drawers
Cocoa Data Views	Browser, text view, table view, and outline view
Cocoa Container Views	View, box, and tab view
Cocoa Graphics Views	Movie view, OpenGL view, and QuickDraw view
AppleScript	ASKDataSource

Chapter 9 goes into detail about the controls in the Palettes window. Most chapters throughout this book also deal with some aspect of the Palettes window. That's because it's an important window! The Palettes window is your main toolbox for creating attractive Aqua interfaces. You'll use it often.

Info window

The Info window is another important tool that you'll use frequently when building an interface. The Info window displays important information about whatever item you're working with in Interface Builder. To see how the Info window works, perform these steps:

1. **Choose Tools⇨Show Info.**

   The Info window appears. The purpose of the Info window is to give you the opportunity to view and edit the attributes of the objects in your nib file.

2. **Open a window from your nib file and the Info window displays the attributes for that window (see Figure 4-10).**

   The Info window is a bit of a chameleon, altering itself to match its surroundings.

3. **Click the Calculate button to select it.**

   The Info window immediately changes to display the attributes of that button.

4. **In the Info window, click the popup button that neighbors the Equiv field and choose Return, as shown in Figure 4-11.**

This simple selection has two effects. First, it changes the Calculate button to a blue color in Interface Builder. When you use the button in your application's interface, however, that blue button will pulsate. The purpose is to draw a user's attention to the button, because it triggers the function that the user most likely wants to perform.

Second, your popup selection causes that button to respond to the Return key on your keyboard. Now, instead of forcing users to click the button with a mouse, they can simply press Return to make a calculation. You gained all that functionality with only one click. Cool!

Figure 4-10:
The Info window gives you access to a variety of window attributes.

Figure 4-11:
Choose Return to give users one-key access to calculations.

Menu editor window

The last window to discuss is the Menu editor. The Menu editor window displays a miniature version of your application's menu bar. You can click a menu to display its menu items. It's also easy to change the text or keyboard shortcut for a menu item or add a new one.

To prepare the menu for your application, follow these steps:

1. **In the nib file window, double-click the MainMenu icon.**

   The Menu editor appears.

2. **Click the New Application menu to open it.**

3. **Double-click the About MyFirstProject menu item and rename it to About SimpleCalculator, as shown in Figure 4-12.**

   You can rename the About menu also by single-clicking it and making the change in the Info window.

Figure 4-12:
Change the
text of menu
items using
the Menu
editor.

4. **Change the Hide NewApplication and Quit NewApplication menus to Hide SimpleCalculator and Quit SimpleCalculator, respectively.**

5. **Edit the text of the top Application menu item from MyFirstProject to SimpleCalculator.**

   Figure 4-13 shows this change.

6. **Choose File⇨Save to save the interface changes.**

7. **Press Cmd-R to test the interface.**

   Interface Builder hides your nib files and its other windows and displays your interface as it would appear in a running application.

Figure 4-13:
Change the
name of the
application
menu.

8. **Select menu items, move the calculator window around, and type numbers in the fields of the window.**

   When you click the Calculate button, though, nothing happens. That's because you aren't using the actual application. This is just the interface.

   Although the About SimpleCalculator menu item looks just fine, you may notice that the application menu isn't displaying its name properly. Rather, it displays Interface Builder to let you know that you're using Interface Builder and not your application to preview the interface.

9. **Choose Interface Builder⇨Quit SimpleCalculator to return to Interface Builder.**

   If you check your application by running it in Project Builder, you'll see the changes that you made to the interface in Interface Builder.

10. **Bring Project Builder to the foreground and press Cmd-R to run your application.**

    Look at the example in Figure 4-14 and you'll see that something is not quite right. The application menu is still stuck with the text MyFirstProject.

    What's going on here? It turns out that your application supplies the text for your application menu item using a string in its InfoPlist file.

Figure 4-14:
Despite
changes to
the menu in
Interface
Builder, your
project still
displays the
incorrect
text in the
application
menu.

11. **Change the InfoPlist file as follows:**

    a. **In Project Builder, expand the Resources folder in the vertical Files tab.**

    b. **Select the InfoPlist.strings.**

    The Code editor displays the contents of this file, which you can edit.

    c. **Change the first line of code to read**

    ```
    CFBundleName = "SimpleCalculator";
    ```

12. **In Project Builder, press Cmd-R.**

    The application menu appears as you'd expect. Figure 4-15 shows the results of your InfoPlist change.

13. **Return to Interface Builder by clicking its icon in the Dock.**

Figure 4-15:
Make adjustments to the InfoPlist. strings file in Project Builder to force the application menu to display properly.

The Interface Building Process

Now that you've surveyed the basics of Interface Builder, it's time to put it to use. To build an interface for a new Cocoa application, you'd normally follow this sequence of steps:

1. **Open a nib file in Interface Builder.**

   Double-clicking the MainMenu.nib resource from your project in Project Builder opens the nib file with Interface Builder.

2. **Add controls to a window in the interface.**

   Open a window from the nib file and drag controls onto it from the Palettes window. Use the Info window to adjust attributes of the various controls.

3. **Create and edit menu items.**

   Open the Menu editor by double-clicking MainMenu in the nib file. Double-click an existing menu item to edit its text. You can create new menus in a few different ways, but one of the easiest is to duplicate an existing menu item and adjust it to suit your needs.

4. **Create a controller class.**

   The controller class works as an intermediary that connects an interface to your code.

5. **Connect the interface.**

   Add outlets and actions to the controller class. Then Control-drag from the controller class to a control (such as a text field) in the interface. In the Info window, click Connect to connect the outlet. Control-drag from a control (such as a button) to the controller class. In the Info window, select an action and click Connect to connect the action to the control.

6. **Create files and add them to Project Builder.**

   Choose Classes⇨Create Files to build and add the header (.h) and implementation (.m) files to the project in Project Builder.

You may recognize these steps from Chapter 2, where you begin creating the calculator project. You have to modify the sequence slightly, though, if you want to update the interface. For example, suppose you want to add a popup button to the interface that lets the user choose from a list of mathematical operations. Instead of being limited to addition, a user can choose to add, subtract, multiply, or divide. This would clearly make for a more useful application.

Remember, though, that you already created the files for your project (as in Step 6 of the preceding list) in Chapter 1 (from which this chapter's code stems). If you drag a new popup button into your application's interface and connect it to a new outlet in the controller class (Fusebox), your source and header files in Project Builder will have no way of knowing about the change. Either you have to alter the source code files by hand or merge new files with the ones you already created.

Why can't you simply follow Step 6 in the preceding list and create files for Project Builder using the Classes⇨Create Files menu? The answer is that you can, but you may not like the result. By creating files in this manner, you run the risk of deleting all your existing work, because the process creates *new* files, deleting the previous files. Interface Builder offers a solution to this dilemma, though. When you attempt to create header and implementation files, Interface Builder asks you (see Figure 4-16) if you'd prefer to overwrite existing files (thus deleting your previous work) or merge the new files with the existing ones (thus retaining your previous work).

Figure 4-16:
To retain previous work, merge your new header and implementation files with existing files.

Because of this special consideration, you need to modify Step 6 in the list of Interface Builder tasks:

6. Create files and add them to Project Builder. If files already exist in your Project Builder project, edit them by hand or merge them with the new files.

   If your project doesn't have header (.h) or implementation (.m) files, create them by choosing Classes⇨Create Files. If they already exist in your project in Project Builder, choose Classes⇨Create Files and click Merge when queried in the dialog that appears. If you're making small changes to your interface, sometimes it's just as easy to edit the header and source code files in Project Builder by hand than to go through the merge process.

When you choose to merge files, Interface Builder launches the FileMerge application, which handles the complex task of merging source code and header files. FileMerge is an important tool, and Chapter 5 goes into more detail about its use.

Improving your existing project to include addition, subtraction, multiplication, and division is simple. Follow the same six steps:

1. Open a nib file in Interface Builder.

   If you don't have you calculator's MainMenu.nib opened in Interface Builder, double-click it from your project in Project Builder.

2. **Add controls to a window in the interface.**

   a. **Open the window for your interface by double-clicking Window in the nib file window.**

      Your interface currently displays a plus sign text field between `numField1` and `numField2` to indicate that the calculator performs addition only.

   b. **Click that text field to select it and press Delete to remove it.**

   c. **In the Palettes window, click the third button in the top row of buttons to display the controls in the Other Cocoa Views pane.**

   d. **Drag a popup button from the Palettes window to the window that holds your calculator interface. Then click the popup button to reveal its contents.**

      By default, the popup has three menu items.

   e. **Select the last menu item in the popup button and choose Edit⇨Duplicate to add a new item to the popup button.**

   f. **Edit the text of each menu item by double-clicking the item and changing the text to mathematical symbols for addition, subtraction, multiplication, and division, as shown in Figure 4-17.**

   g. **Resize the popup button to its smallest width and place it between the two number fields. Because the popup won't quite fit between the two fields, resize the window and move the controls around until the popup does fit.**

Figure 4-17:
Change the items in the popup button to mathematical symbols that represent addition, subtraction, multiplication, and division.

3. **Create and edit menu items.**

   In addition to the popup button, it would be handy to give a user menu access to the different mathematical computations. It's a cinch to add keyboard shortcuts to menus, which in turn can give your users keyboard access to the mathematical choices in the popup button. To create a new menu item:

   a. **Open the Menu editor.**

   b. **Select the Window menu and press Cmd-D to duplicate that menu.**

   c. **From the two Window menus that now appear in your Menu editor, double-click the leftmost one and rename it as Calculate. Press Return to accept the new name.**

   d. **Click the new Calculate menu to select it.**

      In the Calculate menu, you'll see three menu items: Minimize, a blank space, and Bring all to front.

   e. **Select the last two menu items and press Delete to remove them from the menu.**

   f. **Select the Minimize menu item and press Cmd-Shift-I to open the Info window. Select Attributes from the popup menu at the top of the Info window. Alter the attributes of the Minimize menu item to match Figure 4-18.**

Figure 4-18:
Users can choose their favorite operation — currently addition only.

g. **In the popup menu at the top of the Info window, select Connections.**

The Info window displays three lists.

h. **In the bottom list, select the sole action: FirstResponder.performMiniaturize and click the Disconnect button.**

This removes the existing action for this menu item.

i. **Select the Addition menu item and press Cmd-D three times to create three duplicates of it.**

j. **Alter these three new menu items to look like Figure 4-19. You may also want to change the Key Equivalent attribute for each item to the appropriate symbol: +, -, *, and /.**

Figure 4-19:
Users can now choose from all four mathematical operations.

4. **Create a controller class.**

Because you're updating an existing project, this one already has a controller class (named Fusebox). Therefore, you can skip this step.

5. **Connect the interface.**

a. **In the Instances tab of the nib file window, double-click the Fusebox object.**

The Info window appears, displaying the outlets and actions for Fusebox.

b. **Add an outlet named operationPopup, which corresponds to the popup button in your project's window.**

c. **Click the Actions tab of the Info window and create four actions: setAdditionMenu, setSubtractionMenu, setMultiplicationMenu, and setDivisionMenu.**

These correlate to the items in the Calculate menu that appears in your project's menu bar. Figure 4-20 shows the actions for the Fusebox class.

Figure 4-20:
Add four
actions to
Fusebox
to cover
the new
Calculate
menu.

d. To connect your interface, Control-drag from the Fusebox **object in the nib file window to the new** popupButton **in the interface. In the Info window, select the** operationPopup **outlet and click Connect.**

e. Open the Menu editor.

f. Select the Addition menu item from the Calculate menu and Control-drag from it to the Fusebox **class. In the Info window, select the** setAdditionMenu **action and click Connect.**

g. For each menu item in the Calculate menu, Control-drag from the menu item to Fusebox **and connect it to the appropriate action.**

When you're finished, the Info window should look like Figure 4-21.

6. Create files and add them to Project Builder. If the files already exist, edit them by hand or merge them with the new files.

Because your project files already exist in Project Builder, you have to tread carefully here. You've added only four new actions and one outlet to your interface, so it won't be difficult to add them by hand to the existing files. You can also perform a merge. Chapter 5 has more details on how to merge files if you prefer that method.

7. Choose File⇨Save to save the nib file.

That means you're finished with Interface Builder for now.

Figure 4-21:
Connect the
individual
menu items
in the Calcu-
late menu
to the four
new actions.

Using an Interface in Project Builder

Now that you have the interface improvements completed, you need to
return to Project Builder to add some code. For starters, you need to define a
few items in Fusebox.h file. Because you added one outlet and four actions to
the interface, you need to do the same in Fusebox.h:

1. **Change Fusebox.h to read as follows:**

```
/* Fusebox */

#import <Cocoa/Cocoa.h>

@interface Fusebox : NSObject
{
    IBOutlet id answerField;
    IBOutlet id numberField1;
    IBOutlet id numberField2;
    IBOutlet id operationPopup;
}
- (IBAction)calculateAnswer:(id)sender;
- (IBAction)setAdditionMenu:(id)sender;
- (IBAction) setDivisionMenu:(id)sender;
- (IBAction)setMultiplicationMenu:(id)sender;
- (IBAction)setSubtractionMenu:(id)sender;
@end
```

2. **Choose File⇨Save to save the header file.**

3. **Select Fusebox.m to edit its code.**

4. **Modify the** `calculateAnswer` **function by adding an integer that will keep track of the currently selected item in the popup button:**

```
int operation;
```

5. **Find out which item the user has selected from the popup button by sending it the** `IndexOfSelectItem` **message.**

   When you do, it returns the index of the currently selected menu item in the popup button, which you then store in the `operation` variable. The first menu item in a popup button has an index of 0 (zero), so all items in the `operationPopup` control are covered by the indices 0 through 3:

```
operation = [operationPopup indexOfSelectedItem];
```

6. **Now that you know which item the user selected from** `operationPopup`, **you can do the math based on that index:**

```
if (operation == 0)
        answer = num1 + num2;
    else if (operation == 1)
        answer = num1 - num2;
    else if (operation == 2)
        answer = num1 * num2;
    else
        answer = num1 / num2;
```

The completed `calculateAnswer` action looks like this.

```
- (IBAction)calculateAnswer:(id)sender
{
    float num1,num2,answer;
    int operation;

    num1 = [numberField1 floatValue];
    num2 = [numberField2 floatValue];

    operation = [operationPopup indexOfSelectedItem];
    if (operation == 0)
        answer = num1 + num2;
    else if (operation == 1)
        answer = num1 - num2;
    else if (operation == 2)
        answer = num1 * num2;
    else
        answer = num1 / num2;

    NSNumberFormatter *answerFormatter =
```

```
            [[[NSNumberFormatter alloc] init] autorelease];

    [answerFormatter setFormat:@"#,###.00;0.00;(#,##0.00)"];
    [[answerField cell] setFormatter:answerFormatter];
  [answerField setFloatValue:answer];
}
```

To account for the Calculate menu that appears in your menu bar, you
need to add four new actions to Fusebox.m as well: setAdditionMenu,
setDivisionMenu, setMultiplicationMenu, and setSubtractionMenu.
The code is the same for each action, with one exception. When a user selects
a particular menu item, the code changes the operationPopup control to
match the operation in that menu item. For example, if a user selects the
Addition menu, the code sets the index of the operationPopup control to 0
(zero). The Subtraction menu item sets the index of the operationPopup
control to 1, and so on. The code looks like this:

```
- (IBAction)setAdditionMenu:(id)sender
{
    [operationPopup selectItemAtIndex:0];
}

- (IBAction) setDivisionMenu:(id)sender
{
    [operationPopup selectItemAtIndex:3];
}

- (IBAction)setMultiplicationMenu:(id)sender
{
    [operationPopup selectItemAtIndex:2];
}

- (IBAction)setSubtractionMenu:(id)sender
{
    [operationPopup selectItemAtIndex:1];
}
```

The completed Fusebox.m source code file combines the calculateAnswer
action and the new menu item actions into one file. To keep your bearings
straight, here's the completed Fusebox.m file:

```
#import "Fusebox.h"

@implementation Fusebox

- (IBAction)calculateAnswer:(id)sender
{
    float num1,num2,answer;
    int operation;
```

```
    //get the numbers from the two number fields
    num1 = [numberField1 floatValue];
    num2 = [numberField2 floatValue];

    //which item in the popup button menu is selected?
    operation = [operationPopup indexOfSelectedItem];
    //do the math
    if (operation == 0)
        answer = num1 + num2;
    else if (operation == 1)
        answer = num1 - num2;
    else if (operation == 2)
        answer = num1 * num2;
    else
        answer = num1 / num2;

    //format the answer,
    //giving it two decimals
    NSNumberFormatter *answerFormatter =
        [[[NSNumberFormatter alloc] init] autorelease];

    [answerFormatter setFormat:@"#,###.00;0.00;(#,##0.00)"];
    [[answerField cell] setFormatter:answerFormatter];

    //display the answer
    [answerField setFloatValue:answer];
}


// Set the popupButton if a user selects a menu item
// from the Calculate menu.
- (IBAction)setAdditionMenu:(id)sender
{
    [operationPopup selectItemAtIndex:0];
}

- (IBAction) setDivisionMenu:(id)sender
{
    [operationPopup selectItemAtIndex:3];
}

- (IBAction)setMultiplicationMenu:(id)sender
{
    [operationPopup selectItemAtIndex:2];
}

- (IBAction)setSubtractionMenu:(id)sender
{
    [operationPopup selectItemAtIndex:1];
}

@end
```

Choose File⇨Save to save the Fusebox.m file. Then choose Build⇨Build and
Run to see your work in action. The result should be an application that performs addition, subtraction, multiplication, and division. You can choose a
mathematical operation by selecting it from the popupButton in the interface,
choosing it from the Calculate menu in the menu bar, or using the keyboard
shortcuts listed in the Calculate menu. Figure 4-22 shows the completed calculator application.

Figure 4-22:
The
completed
calculator
can add,
subtract,
multiply,
and divide.

If you get lost somewhere during the interface-building process or the code
additions, you can get the completed project from
www.dummies.com/extras. The finished project is in the following directory:

```
/Book Examples/Chapter 4/End Code/Calculator
```

Chapter 5

More Utilities for Cocoa Development

In This Chapter

▶ Merging header and source code files

▶ Creating and adding icons to Cocoa applications

▶ Building installers

The bulk of your development tasks will take place in Project Builder and Interface Builder. However, these aren't the only Apple tools for creating Cocoa applications. Nestled in the Applications folder of your Developer folder, you'll find more than a dozen tools and utilities that can help you create great Cocoa software fast.

Some of these tools assist you in the design phase of Cocoa development, and others help you write better code. Others work well after the programming is complete. This chapter points out the highlights in this collection of tools. Along the way, you use each tool to improve your Cocoa projects and applications.

FileMerge

As you read in Chapter 4, the interface building process consists of six specific steps. The last step looked something like this:

> 6. Create files and add them to Project Builder. If files already exist in your Project Builder project, edit them by hand or merge them with the new files.

After you're finished building an interface in Interface Builder, your last step is to create implementation and header files for that interface. Interface Builder creates them for you and adds them to your project in Project Builder. If you try to add these files to a project that already has those files,

Interface Builder asks you whether you'd like to write over the existing files with the new ones or merge the new files with the old. To preserve your existing code, merge the new files with the old.

To facilitate this merging process, Apple was nice enough to provide you with an application titled, appropriately enough, FileMerge. You can find the FileMerge application in the following location on your hard drive:

```
/Developer/Applications/FileMerge
```

You can use FileMerge by itself as an application, but you're more likely to use it in concert with Interface Builder. In fact, Interface Builder automatically launches FileMerge when you need it.

To demonstrate how FileMerge works, copy this chapter's project from the For Dummies Web site (www.dummies.com/extras) to your hard drive. The project for this chapter is at the following location:

```
/Book Examples/Chapter 5/FileMerge Demo/Start Code/Calculator
```

Open the CalculatorProject.pbproj project file, which is in the Calculator folder. To see the FileMerge option in action, you have to alter something in the interface that causes the implementation or header files to change. For example, you may want to add to your calculator interface another button that calculates the average of the two number fields. This change also requires that you add a new action to the Fusebox class. When you add a new action or outlet to your interface, your project needs a change to its header and implementation files. This is the perfect time to use FileMerge.

To begin working with FileMerge, follow these steps:

1. **Open the MainMenu.nib file.**

   To do so, double-click MainMenu.nib, which is in the Resources folder in Project Builder, as shown in Figure 5-1.

2. **In Interface Builder, click the Interfaces tab of the nib file window.**

3. **Double-click Window to view the calculator interface.**

4. **Drag a new button from the Palettes window to the calculator interface.**

5. **Double-click the new button and change its title (the text that appears on the button).**

   To follow along with the example, change the title to Average, as shown in Figure 5-2.

Figure 5-1:
Open the
MainMenu.
nib file by
double-
clicking it in
Project
Builder.

Figure 5-2:
Add an
Average
button to
your
interface.

6. **To make this new button do something, add an action to the** Fusebox
object:

 a. **In the Instances tab of the nib file window, double-click** Fusebox.

 The Info window appears, displaying the outlets and actions for
 the class.

 b. **Click the Action tab and add a new action.**

 c. **Name the action calculateAverage.**

 Figure 5-3 shows the new action.

Figure 5-3:
Add the
calcu-
late-
Average
action to
Fusebox.

7. **Connect the new button to the** calculateAverage **action.**

To do this step, Control-drag from the Average button in the interface to the Fusebox object in the Instances tab of the nib file window. In the Info window, select the calculateAverage action and click Connect. Figure 5-4 shows the connected action and button.

Figure 5-4:
Control-drag
from the
new button
to the
Fusebox
object and
attach an
action.

These steps were sufficient to require changes in the header and implementation files of this project. Because you added an action to the interface, you need to add that action to the Fusebox.h header file in Project Builder:

```
- (IBAction)calculateAnswer:(id)sender;
```

You also need to implement the action in the Fusebox.m file of the project. The empty shell of the action looks like this:

```
- (IBAction)calculateAnswer:(id)sender
{

}
```

Although you can add this code to your project by hand, why not let Interface Builder help you out? Using the FileMerge application, Interface Builder can add the new action to the existing header and implementation file for you. To add the new action to the project, follow these steps:

1. **In the nib file window, click the Classes tab and select** Fusebox, **as shown in Figure 5-5.**

Figure 5-5:
Select the
Fusebox
class in the
nib file
window.

2. **Choose Classes⇨Create Files for Fusebox.**

3. **In the dialog that appears, select the Fusebox.m and Fusebox.h check boxes in the Create files section, as shown in Figure 5-6.**

4. **Click the Choose button.**

   Interface Builder displays an alert telling you that the header and source files already exist. It asks you whether you'd like to overwrite the files or merge them.

Figure 5-6:
Create files
that
account
for the
changes
in the
Fusebox
class and
add them to
your project.

5. Click Merge.

Interface Builder launches the FileMerge application, which is adept at finding the differences between two files. FileMerge displays the differences between the new and original Fusebox.m and Fusebox.h files. Figure 5-7 shows the differences between the new and original Fusebox.h files. The code displayed on the left side is the new header file. The code on the right side is the existing Fusebox.h file. As you can see, you want the code that appears on the left side.

6. In the popup menu at the bottom-right corner of the FileMerge window, choose the Choose left option, as shown in Figure 5-8.

7. Choose File⇨Save Merge to apply the merge function to the Fusebox.h file and close the window.

When you complete the merge function and close the Fusebox.h file, Interface Builder automatically merges the next file checked. In this case, you'll merge the Fusebox.m file next.

8. Note that Fusebox.m has a large number of differences between the new and existing files (see Figure 5-9).

You definitely want to include the new action that appears in the left side of the FileMerge window, but you don't want to eliminate the code that you already created on the right side of the window.

Figure 5-7: The new file has an action that the existing Fusebox.h file doesn't have.

Figure 5-8: Choose the left side of the FileMerge window for Fusebox.h.

9. Select each of the differences between the two files.

Between these two files is a gutter that displays the differences between the two files. Hold the Shift key and select each difference by clicking its number in the gutter. As you select a difference, its outline becomes bold.

Figure 5-9:
The new and existing versions of Fusebox.m have many differences.

10. **In the popup menu at the bottom-right corner of the window, choose the Choose both (left first) option, as shown in Figure 5-10.**

    This merges the two files.

11. **Choose File⇨Save Merge to apply the merge operation to the Fusebox.m file.**

12. **Choose FileMerge⇨Quit to quit FileMerge.**

13. **Click the Project Builder icon in the dock to bring Project Builder to the foreground. In Project Builder, open the Fusebox.h file to view its contents.**

    As you can see, FileMerge added the new `calculateAverage` action to the header file, while preserving the preexisting header code.

    ```
    /* Fusebox */

    #import <Cocoa/Cocoa.h>
    ```

```
@interface Fusebox : NSObject
{
    IBOutlet id answerField;
    IBOutlet id numberField1;
    IBOutlet id numberField2;
    IBOutlet id operationPopup;
}
- (IBAction)calculateAnswer:(id)sender;
- (IBAction)calculateAverage:(id)sender;
- (IBAction)setAdditionMenu:(id)sender;
- (IBAction)setDivideMenu:(id)sender;
- (IBAction)setMultiplicationMenu:(id)sender;
- (IBAction)setSubtractionMenu:(id)sender;
@end
```

14. Navigate to the Fusebox.m file.

Here you discover that FileMerge retained your prior code and added the shell of a `calculateAverage` action.

Figure 5-10:
The Choose both (left first) option merges the code from the two files, using the left side of the window first.

15. **Add the following code to the** `calculateAverage` **function to complete the file:**

```
- (IBAction)calculateAverage:(id)sender
{
    float num1,num2,answer;

    //get the numbers from the two number fields
    num1 = [numberField1 floatValue];
    num2 = [numberField2 floatValue];

    //calculate the average
    answer = (num1 + num2)/2;

    //format the answer,
    //giving it two decimals
    NSNumberFormatter *answerFormatter =
        [[[NSNumberFormatter alloc] init] autorelease];

    [answerFormatter
        setFormat:@"#,###.00;0.00;(#,##0.00)"];
    [[answerField cell] setFormatter:answerFormatter];

    //display the answer
    [answerField setFloatValue:answer];
}
```

You should recognize the bulk of this code from the `calculateAnswer` action. The final step is to test your results.

16. **Choose Build⇨Build and Run to test the** `calculateAverage` **action. Type a value into each of the number fields, and then click the Average button.**

Although this example merged only one new action into the source and header files, you're probably beginning to see that FileMerge can be very handy when the job is much larger. Consider how time consuming it would be to merge a dozen new actions and several new outlets without the FileMerge application.

IconComposer and the icns Browser

After you design, code, and build a Cocoa application, you may want to apply a few finishing touches before you unleash it on the world. One of the first things that users will notice about your application is its icon. When you first build an application with Project Builder, it assigns a generic application icon, as shown in Figure 5-11.

Figure 5-11:
Project
Builder
assigns a
generic icon
to all
applications
that it
builds.

You can assign a different icon to your application by adding an icon (.icns) file to your project. Before you do that, though, you need an icon file in the first place. Apple gives you two utilities to help you work with icon files: IconComposer and icns Browser. These two utilities are in the Applications folder of the Developer folder:

```
/Developer/Applications/IconComposer
/Developer/Applications/icns Browser
```

IconComposer

IconComposer is a tool for constructing .icns files. You can use it to gather all the possible sizes for a particular icon in one .icns file. To begin using IconComposer, launch it by double-clicking its icon in Finder. You'll see an empty icon template like that in Figure 5-12.

Figure 5-12:
Icon-
Composer
presents
you with a
blank icon
template.

An icns file has seven components. The second column of the IconComposer interface displays the color components of the icns file. At the top of that column is a label: Image RGB/Alpha (32 Bit). This means that you can insert icons with 32 bits worth of color. What are *32 bits worth of color*? The number of colors that any one pixel can represent. A 32-bit icon can display one of millions of colors in any pixel, as well as an Alpha mask. A mask lets you change the transparency of any part of an icon.

To create your own icns file, you need an image-editing application such as Adobe Photoshop, Photoshop Elements, or Graphic Converter. Then follow these steps:

1. **In your image-editing application, create a new RGB document with dimensions of 128 x 128.**

   This is the document you'll use to create an icon image.

2. **Using the various graphics tools in the application, create the image that you want to use as your icon.**

3. **If the image doesn't consume the entire 128 x 128 pixels, delete the unused portions.**

4. **Save the result as a TIFF or Photoshop document.**

   You can use TIFF or Photoshop document formats because they support transparency. For example, if you're using Photoshop, you might save the icon as Thumbnail.psd or Thumbnail.tiff, depending on which format you choose. Figure 5-13 shows a sample image for use in an icon. Note the checkerboard pattern that appears in the background. This represents the unused part of the image. It will be transparent when added to an icon in IconComposer.

After you've completed the design and creation of your icon artwork, you can use IconComposer to build an icon file:

1. **After you create the 128 x 128 image, bring IconComposer to the foreground.**

2. **In the blank icns template, double-click the Thumbnail (128 x 128) icon.**

   IconComposer displays an Open dialog box.

3. **Use the Open dialog box to load the Thumbnail.psd file that you created in the preceding set of steps.**

   This draws the icon in the Thumbnail section of the IconComposer template, complete with a see-through background as shown in Figure 5-14.

Figure 5-13:
Don't forget
to remove
the unused
portions
from the
background.

Figure 5-14:
Double-click
the
Thumbnail
icon and
load the
image in its
place.

4. **Drag the Thumbnail icon to the Huge (48 X 48) icon square in the template.**

5. **When IconComposer asks you whether you want it to scale the Thumbnail icon down to the Huge icon size click the Use a scaled version button (see Figure 5-15).**

Figure 5-15:
Icon-
Composer
can auto-
matically
scale icon
sizes
for you.

6. **When IconComposer asks whether you'd like the Huge one bit mask extracted from the Thumbnail icon, click Yes (see Figure 5-16).**

   The result is a new Huge icon and its mask.

7. **Continue dragging the Thumbnail icon onto the Large and Small icon slots until you've filled the entire IconComposer template with icons, as shown in Figure 5-17.**

   With the template filled with icons, you can save the result as an icns file.

8. **Choose File⇨Save to save the file, and then name it.**

   To follow along with the example, name the file newIcon.icns.

9. **To use this file, drag it into your Cocoa project folder. From there, drag it into the Resources folder of your Cocoa project in Project Builder.**

Figure 5-16:
Icon-
Composer
can also
extract
mask data
from icons.

Figure 5-17:
Drag
from the
Thumbnail
icon to the
remaining
icon slots
to fill the
template.

Don't forget to change the CFBundleIconFile entry in the Info.plist entries. To set the CFBundleIconFile entry, do the following:

1. **Click the vertical Targets tab to view the Target settings for the project.**

2. **In the Targets on the left side of Project Builder, select SimpleCalculator.**

   Expand the Targets menu if you don't see the SimpleCalculator target.

3. **In the right portion of Project Builder, select the Expert View of the Info.plist Entries list.**

   You may have to expand the Info.plist Entries list by clicking the triangle to the left of its name.

4. **Change the value of the CFBundleIconFile value to match the name of your icon file.**

   Figure 5-18 illustrates the value that you need to change. Because the Value column is hidden on monitors with a resolution of 1024 x 768 or smaller, you may need to resize or scroll the window to see it.

The next time you build this project, the resulting application will use the newly added icon as its icon. Double-click the application to launch it, and you'll see the new icon in use as the Dock icon too.

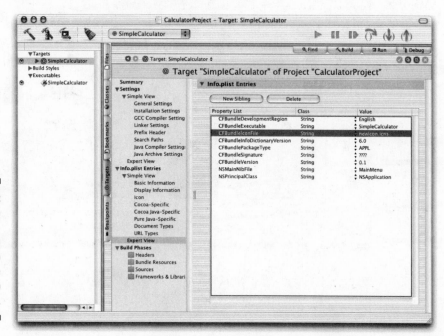

Figure 5-18: Change the CFBundle-IconFile value to affix the new icon to your project.

icns Browser

Unlike the IconComposer application, which lets you create icon files, the icns Browser application is strictly a viewer for icon files. With it, you can view the contents of any icns file, but you can't change those contents. This is handy for finding out why a particular application isn't displaying an icon properly. For example, your application might display a nice looking icon when viewed at 128 x 128, but display nothing at the 32 x 32 size. The icns Browser can help you discover which icon elements are missing so you can correct the situation.

To see how icns Browser works, launch it and choose File➪Open to open the icns file you created with IconComposer. You'll see something that looks like Figure 5-19. Notice that several elements of the icon file are missing.

This icns file doesn't contain all the elements possible in an icns file because you made it for Mac OS X only. The blank elements in this icns file are for maintaining compatibility with earlier versions of the Mac OS. As a Cocoa programmer, you can't target earlier versions of the Mac OS anyway, so forget about that old technology!

Figure 5-19:
Viewing the contents of an icns file.

PackageMaker

After you've built a finished application with Cocoa, you'll no doubt want to distribute it to friends, co-workers, or maybe the world through the Internet. The easiest way to provide your users with an installer for your application is to use the PackageMaker application that Apple provides with the Developer Tools. You can find PackageMaker in the following location on your hard drive:

```
/Developer/Applications/PackageMaker
```

Double-click PackageMaker to launch it. Upon launch, the PackageMaker interface consists of an empty package document. This document stores the settings for your installer. Before you begin adjusting the settings for an installer, you need to perform one preparatory step:

1. **Navigate to Finder and create a folder on your desktop.**

   You can name it whatever you like, but to follow along with the example, call it Parts.

2. **To this folder, add copies of everything that you'd like the installer to install.**

   Presumably, this means the application itself, documentation, and any other supporting files. For the sake of simplicity, add only one item: the SimpleCalculator application.

   If you have many files, consider creating a folder within the Parts folder to hold the files.

3. **Return to PackageMaker.**

A PackageMaker document has five tabs, each with settings that affect the operation of the installer.

✔ Description: The title, version, and description of the installer package

✔ Files: The files you want the package to install

✔ Resources: Additional resources you can add to an installer.

✔ Info: The install location, restart and authorization actions, and installer flags

✔ Version: Version information about the installer itself.

Figure 5-20 shows a blank PackageMaker document.

Figure 5-20:
A new
Package-
Maker
document
consists of
five tabs of
settings.

To make an installer, you need to concern yourself with only a few of these settings. Using just the essentials, you can create an installer in only four steps:

1. **In the Description tab, name the package by entering text in the Title field.**

2. **Click the Files tab to reveal the root directory of the files that you want in this package.**

3. **Click the Choose button to select the folder containing your application.**

   To follow along with the example, select the Parts folder, which contains your SimpleCalculator application.

4. **In the Info tab of your PackageMaker document, click the Choose button and select the Applications folder.**

5. **Create the package.**

   Choose Tools➪Create Package to build a package installer for your application.

After you've built the package, launch it from Finder. You'll see a standard Mac OS X installer for your application, as shown in Figure 5-21.

Figure 5-21:
With
Package-
Maker, you
can build a
customized
installer.

Property List Editor

Each Cocoa application that you create with Project Builder is a bundle. A *bundle* is a folder that looks like an application in Finder. Within that bundle is your application, resources, and some text files in plist format. Files in plist format are XML documents that describe features based on keys and values. For example, you edited the Info.plist file in the "IconComposer" section of this chapter to set an icon for your application. After you build the application, though, there's no way to change this information without rebuilding the application with Project Builder . . . or is there?

Apple includes the Property List Editor application in its suite of Development Tools:

```
/Developer/Applications/Property List Editor
```

With it, you can edit plist files without reading one lick of XML. Choose File⇨ Open and navigate to your SimpleCalculator bundle. In that bundle, you'll find a file named Info.plist. Open that file. You'll see a hierarchical list with Root at the top of the hierarchy. Expand the Root to look like Figure 5-22.

If you'd like to rename your application after it's built, you can change the value of the CFBundleExecutable value that appears in the Property List (to, for example, SimpleCalc). You can even change your application's icon by altering the CFBundleIconFile value (to, for example, anotherIcon.icns) and adding a new icon file to the bundle that matches the new value.

Figure 5-23 shows the Info.plist with edits to the `CFBundleExecutable` and `CFBundleIconFile` values.

After you've finished editing the Info.plist file, choose File➪Save to apply the changes.

Figure 5-22:
Edit your application's Info.plist file using Property List Editor.

Figure 5-23:
Change
`CFBundle-`
`Execu-`
`table` and
`CFBundle-`
`IconFile`
to alter the application's name and icon without rebuilding the bundle.

Part II

Instant Cocoa and the Objective-C Language

The 5th Wave   By Rich Tennant

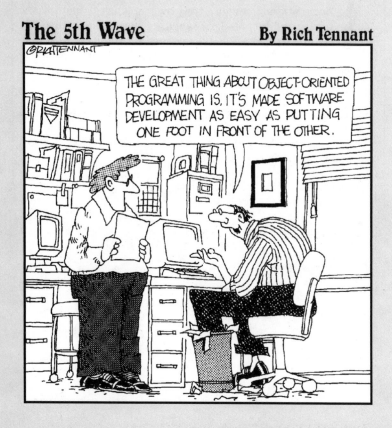

THE GREAT THING ABOUT OBJECT-ORIENTED PROGRAMMING IS, IT'S MADE SOFTWARE DEVELOPMENT AS EASY AS PUTTING ONE FOOT IN FRONT OF THE OTHER.

In this part . . .

Cocoa programmers use their own language, a big brother to the popular C language, called Objective-C. Part II starts by giving you the information you need to decode this cryptic cipher. You see how the Objective-C language operates, how it handles object-oriented programming, and what it shares with its kid sister, C.

Throughout the remainder of Part II, you continue to expand your Cocoa interface knowledge by working with classes, windows, and the huge collection of controls that Cocoa has to offer.

Chapter 6

Cocoa's Flavor of Object-Oriented Programming

In This Chapter

▶ Finding out what's so great about object-oriented programming

▶ Creating classes and objects

▶ Working with outlets and actions

▶ Taking full advantage of object-oriented techniques

*P*erhaps one of the most used terms around computer geeks, *object-oriented programming* has taken the world by storm in the last decade or two. With object-oriented programming, your love life will improve, you'll receive a raise at work, and you'll lose ten pounds overnight. All kidding aside, object-oriented programming was a revolutionary idea for computer programmers when it hit the scene some years back.

Object-oriented programming works by grouping data and functionality into structures called, as you might expect, objects. What this means for you as a Cocoa programmer is that you can write better code faster. It means also that you can reuse that code in different projects, which further expedites your software endeavors.

In this chapter, you explore the exciting (okay, so it's not exactly *exciting*) world of object-oriented programming. First, you consider why you'd even want to use object-oriented programming in the first place. After you're convinced that object-oriented programming is a good thing, the chapter guides you through the basic steps of writing good object-oriented code. The chapter concludes with a look at the benefits of the object-oriented design.

Why Use Object-Oriented Programming?

Object-oriented programming (also known as *OOP*) has drastically altered the way people program computers. Instead of long sequences of hard-to-maintain code, tasks are broken up into functional containers, called *objects*. An object serves as a storage container for data that relates to it.

For example, consider how you might create a program that simulated a zoo. In your zoo, you would presumably have many kinds of animals, each with its own traits, needs, and habitat. If you were to model this in OOP, you'd create an animal object. That object would have a variety of properties describing an animal, such as

- Age
- Weight
- Food requirements
- Habitat requirements

Because this animal object is just a bucket of data, you can use it to describe any animal. When you want to add another animal to your collection, you simply create a new object and fill in its properties, describing that animal.

In addition to storing data, you can also assign functionality to an object. For instance, an animal object might have the following functions:

- Feed the animal
- Set the habitat's temperature
- Vaccinate the animal

By grouping these various functions with the data that they affect, OOP modularizes your code. This makes it easier to maintain and read your code because related items appear together in the source. It's also handy because you can reuse an object as many times as you want. For example, you can add as many animals to your zoo as you want. Alternatively, you can remove animals. It's up to you. With objects, altering one animal object has no effect on another animal object.

Besides all these nerdy reasons for loving OOP, you'll find that this style of programming is often simpler to use. It helps you model things after the real world, which is often what you want to do when programming a computer.

Cocoa Is Classy

To use objects in your applications, you must define them first. OOP calls this definition a *class*. Think of a class as a recipe that describes how to create a particular type of object.

A class, like an object, has properties and functions:

 ✔ The properties of an object are called *instance variables*.
 ✔ The functions of an object are called *methods*.

Unlike objects, however, classes don't store anything. They simply describe how to create an object. This is a subtle but important distinction. After you finish building a class, you can create as many objects as you want with it.

You may be wondering what this instance stuff is about. The word *instance* is a synonym for *object*. The idea is that you are creating an instance based on plans provided by a class. Each instance that you create has a copy of the variables and methods defined in its class. For example, one instance of an animal might weigh 10 kilograms, while another might weigh 100 kilograms. The class serves as the template by which you create as many objects as you need.

In addition to the classes that you create yourself, Cocoa has scores of built-in classes for you to use. If you've read the previous chapters, you've already come across some built-in functions: `NSNumber`, `NSString`, and `NSColor` as well as interface elements such as windows, buttons, and text fields.

Despite being part of the Cocoa framework, built-in classes resemble classes that you create yourself because they have both variables and methods. You use built-in Cocoa classes with your own classes to create object-oriented Cocoa applications.

Designing Your Own Class

To see how classes and objects (make that *instances*) fit into your Cocoa programming, launch Project Builder and create a new Cocoa application project. Open the project's MainMenu.nib file in Interface Builder. The nib file window for MainMenu.nib displays the classes and instances for your project, as shown in Figure 6-1.

Click the Instances tab of the nib file window. Here you find the various classes that make up the Cocoa framework.

Besides the built-in classes, you can also add your own classes to a project. For example, to create an `Animal` class, do the following.

1. **Add a class to the nib file.**

   Click the Classes tab of the nib file window. Scroll all the way to the left edge of the Classes tab and select the `NSObject` class. Then press Return to create a class based on `NSObject`. `NSObject` is a generic class upon which you will base all your Cocoa classes. Name the new class Animal (see Figure 6-2).

2. **Create an instance based on the new class.**

   Select the `Animal` class in the Classes tab of the nib file window. Then choose Classes⇨Instantiate Animal, to create a new instance of the `Animal` class and place it in the Instances tab of your nib file, as shown in Figure 6-3.

Figure 6-2:
Add an
`Animal`
class to
your project.

Figure 6-3:
Create an
instance of
the Animal
class.

3. Create files for the new class.

Double-click the new `Animal` instance to return to the Classes tab. Then
choose Classes⇨Create Files for Animal. All classes in Cocoa have a
header file (.h) and an implementation (.m) file. The header file
describes the elements in the class; the implementation file is where
you add code to make the class functional. When you choose Classes⇨
Create Files for Animal, Interface Builder asks you which files you want
to create. Select both the header and implementation file, as shown in
Figure 6-4.

Figure 6-4:
Create
header and
implementa-
tion files for
the Animal
class.

4. Add instance variables and methods to the class.

In Project Builder, select the new header file and add the following code to it:

```
/* Animal */

#import <Cocoa/Cocoa.h>

@interface Animal : NSObject
{
    int              age;
    int              weight;
    float            idealTemperature;
    int     foodSupply;

}

    - (void)feed;
    - (int)remainingFood;

@end
```

This code defines the instance variables and methods for the Animal class.

The header file starts by including the Cocoa framework:

```
#import <Cocoa/Cocoa.h>
```

The rest of the header file describes the Animal object. A class definition begins with @interface and ceases with the @end keyword. The instance variables of the class appear within braces:

```
{
    int              age;
    int              weight;
    float            idealTemperature;
    int              foodSupply;

}
```

Finally, you declare the methods of the class. In this example, you define two: feed and remainingFood.

```
    - (void)feed;
    - (int)remainingFood;
```

Don't forget the minus sign that precedes the declaration of a method in a class. It indicates that the function belongs to the class.

After you've defined a class, you can implement its methods in the Animal.m file. Navigate to that file in Project Builder and add this code to it:

```
#import "Animal.h"

@implementation Animal

- (void)feed
{
    foodSupply = foodSupply-1;
}

- (int)remainingFood
{
    return foodSupply;
}

@end
```

The implementation file contains the methods (in this case, feed and remainingFood) for your class. For this simple demonstration, feed reduces the foodSupply by one each time. The remainingFood method lets you know how much food is left.

Using an Object

After you're finished defining all the methods and variables for your Animal object, it's time to use it. Return to Interface Builder to add an interface to your project. From the Instances tab, double-click the window to open it. Drag an NSButton and an NSTextField from the Palettes window to the window as shown in Figure 6-5. If you need a refresher on how to create an interface, refer to Chapter 3.

Figure 6-5:
Add a
button and a
text field
to the
interface.

The NSTextField will display the amount of food that remains for the animal, and the NSButton feeds the beast. To use this interface, create a new class. This class will control how the interface works, so it appropriately has the name MyController. It is customary to separate the interface functionality from the data that the interface displays (in this case, the Animal object's data) by using separate classes for each.

Follow these steps to add the MyController class to your project:

1. **Add a class to the nib file.**

   In the Classes tab of the nib file window, select NSObject and press Return to create a new class. Name it MyController.

2. **Add two outlets to the class.**

   Besides the usual variables that you add to a class, you can add instance variables that point to other objects. This special type of instance variable is called an *outlet*. To add an outlet to the MyController class, choose Tools⇨Show Info. Click the Outlet tab and add a new outlet named theTextField (see Figure 6-6). As you may have guessed, this outlet will point to the text field in the interface. Then add another outlet named theAnimal. This outlet will point to the Animal object that you created earlier. Notice how the MyController class acts as an intermediary between the interface (theTextField) and the data (theAnimal). This is an important aspect of Cocoa programming. The next section of this chapter goes into more detail about why this separation of tasks is so useful.

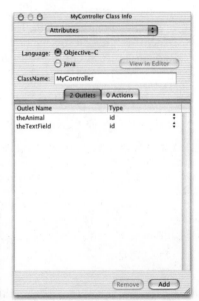

Figure 6-6:
Add two outlets to the class.

3. Add an action to the class.

Just as outlets are special types of instance variables, actions are special kinds of instance methods. They're methods that your interface can trigger. For this example, you need one action: feedAnimal. Like the outlets you created in the preceding step, add the action to the MyController class using the Info window, as shown in Figure 6-7. Note that when you add an action, Interface Builder appends a colon (:) to the action's name. This is normal behavior.

Figure 6-7:
Add an
action to
the class.

4. Create an instance of the MyController class.

Select the MyController class in the nib file window and choose Classes⇨Instantiate MyController to create a new MyController instance. The new instance appears in the Instances tab of the nib file window.

5. Connect the outlets of the MyController instance.

To make your controller object do something, you must connect something to its outlets. You need to connect the NSTextField in your interface to the outlet named theTextField. To do so, Control-drag from the MyController instance to the NSTextField, as illustrated in Figure 6-8. After you've connected the two by Control-dragging, select theTextField in the Info window and click the Connect button. After the theTextField outlet is connected, a small dot is displayed next to its name in the Info window.

Figure 6-8:
Control-drag
from the
MyCon-
troller
instance
to the
NSText-
Field
in the
interface.

Next, Control-drag from the MyController instance to the Animal
instance in the same nib file window. Choose theAnimal in the Info
window and click Connect. Figure 6-9 shows this step. By connecting
these two outlets, your MyController instance knows where to get data
about the animal (theAnimal) and where to display it (theTextField).

Figure 6-9:
Control-drag
from the
MyCon-
troller
instance to
the Animal
instance in
the same
nib file.

6. Connect the action of the MyController **instance.**

Finally, you need to connect the feedAnimal action of the MyController instance to the button in the interface. When a user clicks the button, the feedAnimal action will then fire. To connect the action, Control-drag from the button in the interface to the MyController instance. Choose feedAnimal in the Info window and click Connect. Figure 6-10 shows this connection.

Figure 6-10:
Control-drag from the button in the interface to the MyCon- troller instance.

7. Create files for the new class.

Create files for the MyController class by first selecting the class in the Classes tab of the nib file window. Then, choose Classes⇨Create Files for MyController. Choose to create both the MyController.h and MyController.m files.

To get to the Classes tab of the nib file window quickly, simply double-click the MyController instance.

8. Return to Project Builder to view the files that Interface Builder cre-ated for MyController**.**

In the MyController.h file, you'll see a class definition for MyController like the Animal class from earlier in this chapter:

```
/* MyController */

#import <Cocoa/Cocoa.h>

@interface MyController : NSObject
{
    IBOutlet id theAnimal;
    IBOutlet id theTextField;
}
- (IBAction)feedAnimal:(id)sender;
@end
```

You may recognize a few unusual items in this class: IBOutlet and IBAction. These two data types represent what you might suspect: outlets and actions. Another peculiarity of this code for the Cocoa newcomer is the id in the outlet and action declarations. No, Freud is not involved here. Rather, id represents a pointer to an object — any kind of object. It's a generic pointer that is happy pointing to all types of objects.

Now look at the implementation file for the MyController class. Click the MyController.m file in Project Builder to view its contents. You should see one method (an action, to be precise). The feedAnimal action fires whenever a user clicks the button in this application's interface:

```
#import "MyController.h"

@implementation MyController

- (IBAction)feedAnimal:(id)sender
{
}

@end
```

To make this action do something, you need to add a few lines of code. This action will feed the animal each time and then display the amount of remaining food in the NSTextField. Change the MyController.m file so that it reads like this:

```
#import "MyController.h"

@implementation MyController

- (IBAction)feedAnimal:(id)sender
{
```

```
        [theAnimal feed];
        [theTextField setIntValue:[theAnimal remainingFood]];
}

@end
```

The first new line of code does the feeding. Because you already created the Animal instance and connected an outlet (theAnimal) to it in Interface Builder, all you have to do to feed the animal is call the feed method of the Animal class:

```
[theAnimal feed];
```

The second new line of code displays the amount of food that remains for the animal. To display a numerical value, call the setIntValue method of the NSTextField, passing it an integer. Instead of passing it an actual number, though, we grab an integer value from the theAnimal object by means of its remainingFood method:

```
[theTextField setIntValue:[theAnimal remainingFood]];
```

If you don't quite understand the Objective-C syntax, don't worry. Chapter 7 goes into further detail about how it works. For now, bear with the explanation and come back after Chapter 7 if you want to review. The important part here is that you understand that the feedAnimal action takes care of feeding the animal and displaying the remaining food count.

Go ahead and run the project by pressing Cmd-R. After it compiles and runs, click the button in the interface. You see something that looks like Figure 6-11.

You've encountered an error. We forgot to provide the animal with some food. To give the animal a fighting chance, give him 100 units of food. To assign this value to the Animal instance, navigate to the Animal.m file and add a giveFood method:

```
- (void)giveFood
{
    foodSupply = 100;
}
```

Don't forget to add it to the Animal.h file:

```
- (void)giveFood;
```

Figure 6-11:
Uh-oh! the animal has no food left.

Next, add an `awakeFromNib` method to the `MyController` class. When your application loads its nib file, it sends all objects an `awakeFromNib` message. All you have to do is intercept this message and perform your initializations. In this case, you want to give some food to the animal:

```
- (void)awakeFromNib
{
    [theAnimal giveFood];
    [theTextField setIntValue:[theAnimal remainingFood]];
}
```

When you run the project now, the interface displays the default value of 100 and reduces the `foodSupply` with each click of the button (see Figure 6-12).

Figure 6-12:
Now the animal has food to eat.

How Objects Work Together

Although the example in the preceding section was rudimentary, it described an important element of Cocoa's object-oriented design. In the example, you used three objects to display information about a fictional animal:

✔ `MyController`

✔ `window`

✔ `Animal`

These three instances are important because each fulfills one important role. The MyController instance serves as an intermediary object between the Animal and window instances. The MyController instance retrieves information from the Animal object and tells the window instance to display it.

This trinity of objects has a name in OOP circles: Model-View-Controller (MVC). The main idea behind MVC is that the data (stored in the Animal instance) is a separate entity from the interface (window). By keeping these two things separate, you can reuse the classes in other projects without changing code.

Some programmers love to reuse code because they don't like to work any more than necessary. All programmers can appreciate code reuse, though, because the longer you use code, the more you can consider it bug free. Why throw away all those days, weeks, and years of testing you've performed on a piece of code?

Code reuse means fewer bugs, and fewer bugs mean happier users. Code reuse also means more free time, and more free time means happier programmers (hey, that's you!). By following the MVC methodology, you can increase your chances of producing reusable code.

The example project for this chapter made one assumption of which you should be aware. When you create the Animal class and instantiate it, you create an Animal object. The MyController instance then worked directly with that instance. Normally, you probably wouldn't want to instantiate the Animal class in Interface Builder. That's because you probably want to have more than one animal in your zoo. By creating this one instance, your code was greatly simplified for matters of demonstrating the MVC concept. In Chapter 7, you see how to create objects using code. That way, you can create as many animals as you want.

Another important OOP idea that the example in this chapter illustrates is the idea of accessor methods. Recall that the Animal class stores the amount of food in a variable called foodSupply. Instead of accessing this variable directly, the MyController instance called the remainingFood method of the Animal class. Because this method gives you access to data in the class, it's called an *accessor method*. By using accessor methods, you can further ensure that your classes are reusable.

Use accessor methods whenever possible. You don't crack your friend's head open and read the neurons to know what he or she is thinking. Instead, you access that content by asking your friend to tell you his or her thoughts. The same goes for classes. Don't go poking around in the guts of a class with code. Instead, ask the object to give you access to its data.

Chapter 7

The Basics of Objective-C

In This Chapter

▶ Understanding the grammar of Objective-C

▶ Creating and using your own classes

▶ Naming classes and methods in Objective-C

▶ Using classes provided by the Cocoa framework

*O*bjective-C is the name of the language with which you will program the majority of your Cocoa applications. Although it's not the only language in use, the majority of Cocoa programmers use it for all their Cocoa tasks. Objective-C is an extension to the popular C programming language. If you're a C programmer already, you'll find that Objective-C makes you feel like you're in familiar surroundings, with a few language oddities thrown in. If you aren't well versed in C but know another programming language, you'll probably be able to figure out what's going on anyway.

In this chapter, you examine the basic syntax of Objective-C. After you get the hang of how Objective-C works, you test your skills by creating a project. In the process, you find out how to create instances using code. Next, the chapter runs you through another important topic in Objective-C: class methods. The chapter concludes with a look at the way you should name things in Objective-C. Naming schemes play an important role in Objective-C. As you can see, this chapter is a collection of several small facts. These bits of knowledge form a larger body of information that you'll use every time you program with Cocoa using the Objective-C language.

Objective-C: The Best Language for the Job

Because Objective-C is based on C, you'll find that it's easy to begin writing the former if you're familiar with the latter. All the usual C syntax, C data types, and C pointers are available for you to use in Objective-C. This works out well because you can use your knowledge as well as your existing source code in Cocoa applications.

Objective-C, as you may have guessed, extends C by adding object-oriented features to it. The most basic construct in Objective-C is the capability to execute the methods of an object. To do this, you typically send a message to an object telling it to perform that method. Objective-C uses square brackets to denote that you are sending a message to an object. For a generic object (named `object`), you'd send a message (named `message`) like this:

```
[object message];
```

You should note two things here. First, the syntax of this statement makes it behave much like a command in English. For example, you might say this to a taxi cab driver:

```
Driver, go!
```

In Objective-C, the same command looks like this:

```
[driver go];
```

The second thing you should note about Objective-C is that each line of code ends with a semicolon. Except for the usual places where you might leave one out in C (for example, an `if` statement), Objective-C requires a semicolon at the end of each line of code.

Like traditional C functions, Objective-C lets you pass parameters (also known as *arguments*) to methods. Going back to the taxi analogy, you might want to tell the driver where to go:

```
Driver, go left!
```

In Objective-C, the command might look like this:

```
[driver go:left];
```

For C programmers, the `go` method should seem roughly analogous to a standard C function. If you add another parameter, though, the analogy breaks down. Suppose, for example, that you'd like to pass two parameters (`direction` and `distance`) to the `go` method:

```
[driver go:left distance:10];
```

This syntax may seem a bit weird for C programmers. In Objective-C, the first parameter follows the colon after the name of the method (in this case `go:left`). Each subsequent parameter has a name, followed by a parameter (in this instance, `distance:10`). In contrast, a parallel C function might be

```
go(left,10);
```

In Objective-C, the meaning of the first parameter is usually obvious based on the name of the method. Additional parameters have names to help you identify their purpose.

Like C functions, an Objective-C method can also return a value. If you tell a taxicab driver to go a particular direction and distance, the next you're likely to hear is the price of the fare. You tell the driver to do something. The driver replies with a price. In Objective-C, this works much like it does in C.

```
price = [driver go:left distance:10];
```

Because some methods can return values, Cocoa programmers are fond of nesting them within other methods. Suppose that you based your directions to the cabbie on a map. You know that the driver should go left, but not necessarily how far. In this situation, you might use a map object to find the distance to the desired location, embedding it in the go method.

```
[driver go:left
distance:[map startAt:location1 destination:location2]];
```

Working with Your Own Classes

Because classes form the basis of your Cocoa projects, you'll use them frequently. Most often, you'll create a class to store and manipulate the data for your application. Cocoa geeks call this type of class a *model*. The interface takes care of displaying your data. This is called the *view*. Finally, you'll add a class to mediate between the model and the view. This type of class is a *controller*. To try your hand at working with classes in Objective-C, follow these steps:

1. **Create a Cocoa project.**

   Launch Project Builder and choose File⇨New Project. In the dialog that appears, choose Cocoa Application from the list of choices.

2. **Create a class.**

   You can create classes in Project Builder or Interface Builder. For this class, use Project Builder. Choose File⇨New File. In the window that appears, choose Objective-C Class and click Next. In the next pane that appears, name the implementation file of the new class. Give it the name Driver.m, as shown in Figure 7-1. This is the class you'll use to create a taxi driver object. When you create the Driver class, the header and implementation files — Driver.h and Driver.m — appear in your project.

Figure 7-1:
Create a
class to
represent a
taxi driver.

3. **Create a new controller class.**

   Double-click your MainMenu.nib file in Project Builder to switch to
   Interface Builder. In the Classes tab of the nib file window, select
   NSObject and press Return. Name the new class MyController. This
   class will communicate with your interface.

4. **Create an interface.**

   In Interface Builder, open the default window in your nib file. From the
   Cocoa-Views pane in the Palettes window, add a button (an NSButton),
   a checkbox (also an NSButton), and four NSTextFields to your window.
   You'll use two of the NSTextFields to display the name of your cab
   driver and the fare for your trip. The other two NSTextFields are
   simply labels Fare: and Driver:). Figure 7-2 shows the interface with the
   two empty NSTextFields selected so that you can see them.

Figure 7-2:
The
interface
has two
NSButton
controls
and four
NSText-
Fields.

5. Add outlets to the `MyController` **class.**

For this project, you need to define three outlets as part of the `MyController` class. In the Classes tab of your nib file window, choose the `MyController` class (see Figure 7-3). Choose Tools⇨Show Info to open the Info window, and add three outlets (named `distance-Checkbox`, `driverDisplay`, and `fareDisplay`).

The `driverDisplay` and `fareDisplay` outlets that you add here will give you access to the two `NSTextField` elements in the interface, so you can display the fare and the name of the driver in the interface. The third outlet (`distanceCheckbox`) will permit you to find out whether or not the Distance > 10 miles check box is selected.

Figure 7-3:
Add three outlets to the `MyCon-troller` class.

6. Add an action to the MyController class.

Add one action to `MyController` and name it calculateFare, as shown in Figure 7-4. This is the action that the Calculate Fare button will trigger. When a user clicks this button, the application displays the name of the cabbie and calculates the fare based on one parameter: distance. If the trip is longer than ten miles, the program returns one fare. If the trip is less than ten miles, the program returns a different fare.

Figure 7-4:
Add an
action to
the MyCon-
troller
class.

7. **Create an instance of MyController.**

   In the Classes tab of the nib file window, select the MyController class. Then choose Classes⇨Instantiate MyController. A new MyController instance appears in the Instances tab of the nib file window.

8. **Wire the interface to the MyController instance.**

   You can't do anything with the three outlets and one action until you connect them to the interface. Control-drag from the MyController instance in the nib file window to the NSTextField that neighbors the Fare label. In the Info window, choose fareDisplay and click the Connect button. A small dot appears next to the name of the fareDisplay outlet to indicate that you successfully made a connection.

   Repeat the same process for the other NSTextField and the NSButton that looks like a check box by connecting them to their respective outlets (driverDisplay and fareCheckbox). Figure 7-5 shows the connection between the fareCheckbox outlet and its control in the interface.

9. **Create the files for MyController.**

   In the Classes tab of the nib file window, select the MyController class. Then choose Classes⇨Create Files for MyController. This adds the MyController.h and MyController.m files to your project in Project Builder.

After you've completed your work in Interface Builder, choose File⇨Save to save the nib file. Next, you'll return to Project Builder to add code that makes your project work:

Figure 7-5:
Connect
the outlets
of the
MyCon-
troller
instance
to the
elements
of the
interface.

1. **Return to your project in Project Builder.**

   There you'll find the following four files: Driver.h, Driver.m, MyController.h, and MyController.m.

2. **If the Driver and MyController header and implementation files aren't in the Classes folder already, as shown in Figure 7-6, move them there.**

3. **Click the Driver.h file to view its contents. To this file, add the following code:**

```
#import <Foundation/Foundation.h>

@interface Driver : NSObject {
    NSString *firstName;
}

- (int)go:(int)direction theDistance:(BOOL)distance;
- (NSString *)firstName;
- (void)setFirstName:(NSString *)name;

@end
```

The code begins by including the appropriate header files:

```
#import <Foundation/Foundation.h>
```

The Foundation Kit provides basic functionality for your Cocoa applications. You'll hear more about it later in Chapter 10. Next, the code defines a class named Driver, which inherits functionality from NSObject:

```
@interface Driver : NSObject {
    NSString *firstName;
}
```

Figure 7-6:
Move the
Driver and
MyControl-
ler header
and implem-
entation
files to the
Classes
folder in
Project
Builder.

Almost all classes that you use in Cocoa inherit from NSObject In fact, *all* classes in this book inherit from the NSObject superclass. NSObject is the primary base class for programming in Cocoa. You can think of it as a kind of generic class. It contains methods and variables for creating objects. When you aren't creating a class based on a window, button, or some other existing class, use an NSObject. In this example, you're defining a class (Driver) that has no counterpart in the Cocoa framework. The Driver has one instance variable called firstName that will store the name of the taxi driver.

The rest of the code defines the three methods for the Driver class:

```
- (int)go:(int)direction theDistance:(BOOL)distance;
```

The first method, named go, is what your code will execute when a user wants the driver to take them somewhere. It has two parameters: an integer that represents the direction and a Boolean that represents the distance. For this example, imagine that the cab driver charges one rate for short trips (less than ten miles) and another rate for longer trips. Because this rate scheme includes only two prices, you can use a Boolean variable to determine which rate to charge. A Boolean can have one of two possible values: YES and NO.

The remaining two methods set and get the name of the cab driver. Later, you assign the name of the cab driver using setFirstName when you create an instance from this class:

```
- (void)setFirstName:(NSString *)name;
```

Then when you want to display the name, you ask the `Driver` instance for it using the `firstName` method:

```
- (NSString *)firstName;
```

Finally, `@end` marks the end of the `Driver` class declaration.

Next, click the Driver.m file to reveal its code. To this file, add the following code:

```
@implementation Driver

- (int)go:(int)direction theDistance:(BOOL)distance
{
    if (distance)
        return 10;
    else
        return 5;
}

- (NSString *)firstName;
{
    return firstName;
}

- (void)setFirstName:(NSString *)name
{
if (firstName != name)
    {
        [firstName release];
        [name retain];
        firstName = name;
    }
}

- (void)dealloc
{
    [firstName release];
    [super dealloc];
}

@end
```

This code begins by including the Driver.h file, where the declaration of your `Driver` class resides. Then the code defines the methods for that class. All methods appear in the `@implementation` and `@end` lines. As you know from the header file, this class has three methods. For the sake of simplicity, the go method returns a value of 5 or 10 based on the distance parameter. The `firstName` method returns the value of the `firstName` variable that belongs to the instance. It's perfectly valid to give the same name to a variable and a method of the same class.

Next, the Driver.m file defines the `setFirstName` method. This is where things can get a bit strange. A newcomer to Cocoa might assume that you could assign a value to `firstName` like this:

```
firstName = name;
```

Unfortunately, it's not as simple as that. Because the `name` parameter (that is part of the `setFirstName` method) is a pointer to an `NSString` object, you must be careful to clean house. ("Out with the old and in with the new.") If the value of `name` is different than the value of `firstName`, you must release the `firstName` pointer and retain the `name` pointer. This has to do with memory management in Objective-C.

Because the `firstName` and `setFirstName` methods give you access to the `firstName` variable of the `Driver` class, programmers call these accessor methods. It's best to provide accessor methods when you want to access variables that are internal to a class, rather than have a user poke around in the guts of your class.

The final method in the Driver.m file is `dealloc`, which takes care of releasing the `firstName` pointer. The `dealloc` method begins this process by calling

```
[super dealloc];
```

Now that you've defined a `Driver` class, you may be wondering how you go about using it. Click the MyController.m file in Project Builder and change the code to look like the following listing:

```
#import "MyController.h"
#import "Driver.h"

@implementation MyController

- (IBAction)calculateFare:(id)sender
{

    NSString *name = @"Fred";
    Driver *driver = [Driver alloc];
    int fare;

    [driver setFirstName:name];
  [driverDisplay setStringValue:[driver firstName]];

    fare = [driver go:1 theDistance:[distanceCheckbox
            state]];

    [fareDisplay setIntValue:fare];

    [driver release];
```

```
}

@end
```

First, you declare and assign a value to an `NSString`. Your taxicab company is a small one. It only has one driver, Fred:

```
NSString *name = @"Fred";
```

Working with strings in C can be a nuisance. To get around this problem, Objective-C gives you a convenient method for assigning string literals. Simply place the @ character before the string, as shown in the preceding code snippet. The @ character isn't part of ANSI C, so it may look a tad odd. It signifies the beginning of a string literal.

Then, it's time to use the `alloc` method to create a `Driver` object:

```
Driver *driver = [Driver alloc];

// code here

[driver release];
```

When you create objects using the `alloc` method, it's crucial that you also release them after you're finished using them.

Notice that the object name (`driver`) has a lowercase spelling, but its class (`Driver`) has an uppercase spelling. See the "Naming things in Objective-C" sidebar in this chapter to see why.

After you create a `driver` object, you can begin using its various methods. First, the code assigns a name to the driver object:

```
[driver setFirstName:name];
```

Then you calculate the cab fare using the `go` method:

```
fare = [driver go:1 theDistance:[distanceCheckbox state]];
[fareDisplay setIntValue:fare];
```

In a real-world application, the value of the first parameter might mean something. For this example, you simply pass in a value of 1 to mean left. More importantly, the code passes a second parameter based on the current state of `distanceCheckbox`. The `go` method returns a value for the parameters you pass to it, which you can then display in the interface using the `fareDisplay` outlet.

Press Cmd-R to test your handiwork. If all goes well, you should see something that looks like Figure 7-7.

I kept this example simple so that you could see how the different parts of the project fit together. In case you got lost along the way, however, here's a recap of the steps you performed in creating and using your own class:

1. Created a class (named Driver)

2. Built an interface

3. Added a controller class and connected it to the interface

4. Defined the methods for the Driver class

5. Defined a method for the MyController class

Because the Driver class was just sitting there doing nothing, you had to implement a controller class to use it.

When the user clicks the button in the interface, the calculateFare method of the MyController class creates the driver object, uses its methods, and releases it. Therefore, each time the user clicks the button, the code creates a new object, works with it, and releases it.

Creating Instances without a Fuss

In the preceding section, you created an object using the alloc method of NSObject. You also had to release it when you were finished. Not all objects require this ritual. Some objects release themselves. Consider the earlier example of the NSString:

```
NSString *name = @"Fred";
```

Naming things in Objective-C

Most programming languages have naming conventions, and Objective-C is no exception. Although these so-called rules aren't mandatory, they have the following benefits:

✔ Improve the legibility of your code

✔ Give you hints about code functionality

✔ Make it easier for others to interpret your code

Class names: Class names in Objective-C typically begin with an uppercase letter. Using the class presented earlier in this chapter, Driver is the (capitalized) name of the class. This convention doesn't pertain to only the classes that you create. It applies also to the classes that Apple provides in the Cocoa framework. For example, look at the following built-in class names:

✔ NSString

✔ NSNumber

✔ NSArray

✔ NSImage

Each of these classes begins with a capital letter. Further, they begin with the same two capital letters, *N* and *S*. The classes have this naming system because they're refugees of the NEXT STEP operating system, upon which Apple based Mac OS X. With this little naming convention, you can instantly tell which classes in your code are your own and which ones come from the Cocoa framework.

Project Builder and Interface Builder try to help you remember to capitalize class names. Each time you create a new class with either application, it provides you with a default class name that is capitalized.

Instance names: In contrast to class names, instances begin with a lowercase letter. For example, earlier in this chapter, you created an instance of the Driver class like this:

```
Driver *driver = [Driver
    alloc];
```

The name of the instance is driver. You created an instance of NSString similarly:

```
NSString *name = @"Fred";
```

When you use the lowercase names for your instances, it's easy to discern between instances and classes. This is especially handy when the class and instance names are the same.

File names: Cocoa source code files must follow the prescribed naming scheme. You've already witnessed that Objective-C classes consist of a header file and an implementation file. For example, the Driver class has the following two files.

✔ Driver.m: The implementation file

✔ Driver.h: The interface (or header) file

Although you created and assigned a value to this pointer, you never released it. That's because NSString takes care of that. As a rule of thumb, if you use alloc to create an instance, you have to release that instance when you're finished with it. If you create an object another way, however, you don't have to worry about releasing it.

For example, `NSString` has additional methods for creating instances. Here's a few of them:

- ✔ `+ (id)string`
- ✔ `+ (id)stringWithString: (NSString *)aString`

One thing that you might notice about these methods is that they begin with a plus sign (+). Earlier methods began with a minus sign (-). This is an important difference. Methods preceded by a minus sign are instance methods. You can execute them by sending a message to an instance. For example, you used an instance method named `setFirstName` earlier in this chapter by sending a message to an instance of `Driver`:

```
[driver setFirstName:name];
```

Objective-C calls methods preceded by a plus sign *class methods*. You execute them by sending a message to the class instead of the instance. The `string` and `stringWithString` methods of `NSString` are examples of class methods. To use them, simply pass the message to `NSString`. Don't forget the trailing ":" character at the end of the `stringWithString` method.

```
[NSString stringWithString:]
```

The `stringWithString` method creates and returns a pointer to an `NSString` object using a string that you pass to it. If you'd like to create a copy of the cab driver's name in a new `NSString`, your code would look like this:

```
NSString *newName = [NSString stringWithString:name];
```

Working with Cocoa's Built-in Objects

The majority of the work in this chapter has involved a class that you created: Driver. This is only a small fraction of what you can do in Cocoa. Apple provides a rich set of frameworks with all sorts of great classes that you can use in your own applications. To see the complete list of classes at your disposal, open Project Builder and choose Help➪Cocoa Help. Project Builder displays the table of contents of the Cocoa documentation, as shown in Figure 7-8.

In the Reference Documentation section, find the Objective-C Framework Reference subheading and then the Foundation entry below it. Click Foundation to view its contents. The Foundation Framework contains definitions of numerous classes that you can use in your applications. The classes in Foundation typically have nothing to do with interfaces. Rather, Foundation provides you with a large collection of classes that you'll use for plain-vanilla operations. There are classes for working with numbers, text, dates, and arrays, as well as more sophisticated classes for using files, timers, and processes.

Figure 7-8: Foundation is one of the most important parts of the Cocoa documentation.

When you're searching for a class and the topic has nothing to do with interfaces, check the Foundation documentation first. To use the Foundation Framework in your projects, you must include the Foundation.h header at the beginning of the source file:

```
#import <Foundation/Foundation.h>
```

In addition to the Foundation Framework, Apple provides a rich set of interface-related classes in the Application Kit Framework. Figure 7-9 shows the documentation for the AppKit, as Cocoa veterans call it. You can access it by choosing Help➪Cocoa Help and clicking the Application Kit link below the Objective-C Framework Reference subheading.

To use the Application Kit in your projects, you must include the AppKit.h header at the beginning of the source file:

```
#import <AppKit/AppKit.h>
```

Figure 7-9:
The Application Kit provides you with all the interface classes that you'll need.

Collectively, the Foundation and Application Kit Frameworks form the Cocoa framework. You can use a shortcut to include both the Application Kit and Foundation Frameworks, by simply including the Cocoa.h header file instead:

```
#import <Cocoa/Cocoa.h>
```

Cocoa doesn't use the #include keyword that you may be familiar with from C. Instead, it uses #import. Normally you don't have to worry about these details because Project Builder and Interface Builder usually create the header files for you. If you want to add your own frameworks by hand, however, you need to include the appropriate header and #import line.

Chapter 8

A Window with a View

In This Chapter

▶ Opening, closing, and hiding windows

▶ Positioning windows anywhere on the screen

▶ Tracking open windows

▶ Resizing windows

▶ Changing the appearance of windows

▶ Seeing through a window

▶ Using sheets

*P*erhaps the most important element of any GUI-based application is the window. In fact, it's so important that those guys from Redmond used it to name their operating system. The windows in an application are like pieces of paper that you use to collect ideas, display information, and record input.

Windows in Cocoa are equally important. Mac OS X continues using the fine window traditions that made the Mac OS famous. All the while, Cocoa builds on and improves those ideas from the past with exciting new features. In this chapter, you examine some of the most common window features of Cocoa applications. In the process, you create two projects that demonstrate these features.

Working with Windows

Because windows form the basis for nearly all interfaces, you'll use them often. Some of the most common functions that you'll perform include

✔ Opening and closing windows

✔ Moving windows

✔ Adding windows to the Windows menu

In this section, you discover how to accomplish all these tasks and more.

Opening and closing a window

When you work with windows in your Cocoa projects, you'll typically use Interface Builder to design them. Furthermore, if you leave a window open in Interface Builder when you're designing your interface, that window will is displayed when your application runs. Therefore, it's often unnecessary to issue a command to open a window.

Closing a window is a simple matter:

```
[theWindow close];
```

When you close a window in this fashion, the window is gone. Its contents are gone from memory. It is no more. That means to see the window again, you have to open a new window object.

Hiding and showing a window

If you'd prefer to keep a window around instead of deleting it from memory, you should hide it instead of closing it. Hiding a window is also an easy task to perform. For example, suppose you have an outlet (named theWindow) as part of your controller class. The outlet represents a window in your interface. To hide that window, a hideWindow method might look like this:

```
- (IBAction)hideWindow:(id)sender
{
[theWindow orderOut:sender];
}
```

The orderOut method of the NSWindow class hides a window from view. It still exists in memory; it just isn't visible. To find out whether a window is visible, you can check the return value of the isVisible method:

```
- (IBAction)hideWindow:(id)sender
{
if ([theWindow isVisible])
[theWindow orderOut:sender];
}
```

To make the window appear again, simply use the orderFront method:

```
- (IBAction)showWindow:(id)sender
{
[theWindow orderFront:sender];
}
```

If you'd like a window to appear on the screen and act as the main window, intercepting keystrokes, use the makeKeyAndOrderFront method. Cocoa programmers frequently use this method in the awakeFromNib method to force the main window to the foreground:

```
- (void)awakeFromNib {
    [theWindow makeKeyAndOrderFront:nil];
}
```

Positioning windows

Another important task that you'll need to perform is positioning windows. Before you go bossing windows around, you first need to find out their current position. Use the frame method of NSWindow to discover the origin and size of a window. The method returns an NSRect structure, which contains NSPoint and NSSize describing the window's origin and size, respectively.

After you know a windows origin and size, it's a trivial matter to reposition it. First, set the origin to your liking and call the setFrameOrigin method to apply the new position. This example moves a window ten pixels left of its current position:

```
- (IBAction)moveLeft:(id)sender
{
    NSRect theFrame = [theWindow frame];
    NSPoint theOrigin = theFrame.origin;
    theOrigin.x = theOrigin.x - 10;
    [theWindow setFrameOrigin:theOrigin];
}
```

To position a window in the middle of the screen, use the handy center method. This example centers a window on the screen:

```
- (IBAction)centerWindow:(id)sender
{
    [theWindow center];
}
```

Keeping track of windows

Most Cocoa applications have a Window menu to help users keep track of open windows. Normally, you should use this menu as a list of open document windows. (You probably wouldn't display, say, a toolbar window in the Window menu.) The great thing about the Window menu is that Cocoa takes care of it for you. If your window has the following properties, Cocoa automatically adds it to the Window menu:

✔ Has a title bar

✔ Is resizable

✔ Can become the main window

You can exclude a window from the Window menu by altering any one of these properties. If, on the other hand, you have a window that obeys each of these rules, but you still want it to be left out of the Window menu, use the setExcludedFromWindowsMenu method. The awakeFromNib method is a good place to use this call because the method takes effect when your application launches.

```
- (void)awakeFromNib {
    [theWindow setExcludedFromWindowsMenu:nil];
}
```

Putting windows to work for you

To see how these window features work, do the following:

1. **Launch Project Builder and create a new Cocoa application project.**

   Double-click the Project Builder icon in the Finder to launch it. After it has launched, choose the File➪New Project menu. In the window that appears, select Cocoa Application and click OK.

2. **Create a new window in the MainMenu.nib file.**

   Double-click the MainMenu.nib file in the Resources Group to open the file in Interface Builder. In the MainMenu.nib file window, click the Instances tab. Then, drag a new window from the Cocoa-Windows pane of the Palettes window to the MainMenu.nib file window. To follow along with the example, name this new window MenuWindow. You will use it to control the default window that's already part of the interface.

3. **Open the new MenuWindow and add three buttons to it, as shown in Figure 8-1.**

   For more information on adding buttons, see Chapter 2.

Figure 8-1:
The
MenuWin-
dow has
three
buttons.

4. **Create a controller class.**

   To do so, click the Classes tab of the MainMenu.nib file window. Scroll to the left and select `NSObject`. Press Return to create a new class and name it MyWindowController. Choose Classes⇨Instantiate MyWindowController to create an instance of the new class.

5. **Double-click the new `MyWindowController` instance and add outlets and actions to the instance in the Info window.**

   Add the following outlets: `theMenuWindow`, `theShowButton`, and `theWindow`. Add these actions: `centerWindow`, `moveLeft`, and `showWindow`. For details on adding outlets and actions, see Chapter 2.

   Connect the three new actions to the buttons in `MenuWindow` by control-dragging from each button t the `MyWindowController` instance. Click Connect in the Info window to connect each action.

   Then connect the two window-related outlets to their corresponding windows. Control-drag from the `MyWindowController` instance to each window in the MainMenu.nib file window. Click Connect in the Info window to connect to the appropriate outlet.

   Finally, connect the `theShowButton` outlet to the top button in the `MenuWindow`.

6. **Double-click the `MyWindowController` instance. Choose Classes⇨ Create Files for MyWindowController and add the header and implementation files for the instance.**

7. **Return to Project Builder and add this code to the MyWindowController.m file:**

```
#import "MyWindowController.h"

@implementation MyWindowController

- (IBAction)centerWindow:(id)sender
{
    [theWindow center];
}

- (IBAction)moveLeft:(id)sender
{
    NSRect theFrame = [theWindow frame];
    NSPoint theOrigin = theFrame.origin;
    theOrigin.x = theOrigin.x - 10;
    [theWindow setFrameOrigin:theOrigin];
}

- (IBAction)showWindow:(id)sender
{
```

```
        if ([theWindow isVisible])
            {
                [theWindow orderOut:sender];
                [theShowButton setTitle:@"Show Window"];
            }
        else
            {
                [theWindow orderFront:sender];
                [theShowButton setTitle:@"Hide Window"];
            }
    }

- (void)awakeFromNib {
    [theWindow makeKeyAndOrderFront:nil];
    [theMenuWindow makeKeyAndOrderFront:nil];
}

@end
```

8. **Test the project.**

   To do so, choose Build⇨Build and Run.

Changing the Appearance of Windows

Beauty may be only skin deep, but when it comes to using your application, an attractive interface is mandatory. In this section, you explore some of the possible window settings for nice looking interfaces. These features also enhance the functionality of your applications, so you have some brawn to go with that beauty.

Different windows for different tasks

The standard window of an Aqua interface has a pinstripe background, as shown in Figure 8-2.

This isn't the only kind of appearance that your windows can wear, though. Open a nib file in Interface Builder and display its window by double-clicking it in the MainMenu.nib file window. Then press Cmd-Shift-I to open the Info window. In the Attributes section of the Info window, you'll find a check box for the textured attribute of the window. Click it to radically change the appearance of your window (see Figure 8-3).

Figure 8-2:
A traditional
Cocoa
window
wears
pinstripes.

Figure 8-3:
The rest of
the world
calls this the
*brushed-
metal look,*
but Apple
calls it
textured.

The first time you see the cool metallic look of the textured window, you'll be drawn to make every window of every application with this style. After all, Apple does with many of their applications (such as iTunes and iPhoto).

Before you start clicking the Textured property for every window in sight, keep in mind that the Apple guidelines recommend that you use this window only when hardware is involved. This explains why you see it in all Apple iApps, which use hardware in one way or another. However, it doesn't explain why QuickTime Player uses the textured look, because it *doesn't* interface with hardware. Although textured windows look tempting, try to use them only when necessary. Your users will thank you.

Sizing up your windows

When you want to manually resize a window, use the `frame` method in the same way that you did earlier in this chapter to find out about a window. This gives you access to the window's position and size. Alter the size to your liking and refresh the window using the `setFrame` method. To illustrate, the following method resizes a window to half its current width:

```
- (IBAction)halfAsWide:(id)sender
{
    NSRect theFrame = [theWindow frame];
    theFrame.size.width = theFrame.size.width/2;
    [theWindow setFrame:theFrame display:YES];
}
```

If you'd like to zoom a window without forcing the user to click the zoom button on that window, all you have to do is call the window's `zoom` method. Simple, eh?

```
[theWindow zoom];
```

Setting a window's title

Sometimes you'll want to change the title that appears in the title bar of a window. This is an easy task to perform using the `setTitle` method:

```
[theWindow setTitle:@"My New Window Title"];
```

Of course, you can also set the Title of the window in Interface Builder.

If the window title is the name of a document, use the `setTitleWithRepresentedFilename` method instead of `setTitle`. This method converts from a file path to a window title suitable for viewing:

```
[theWindow setTitleWithRepresentedFilename:theFileName];
```

Windows that you can see through

Adjusting the size and position of a window is rudimentary stuff. So too is changing the title of a window. The next feature, however, will definitely make your users take note. All windows in Cocoa have an opacity setting that allows you to set how see-through a window is. To see this magic in action, use the setAlpha method of NSWindow, passing it a value between 0.0 and 1.0. A value of 1.0 means that a window is fully visible; a value of 0.0 displays a window that's completely transparent. This line of code makes a window 50 percent transparent:

```
[theWindow setAlphaValue:0.5];
```

Figure 8-4 shows the difference between a window with a setAlpha values of 1.0 and 0.5.

Figure 8-4:
Use the setAlpha method to make windows transparent.

Beneath the Sheets

Besides the run-of-the-mill windows that you've used so far, Cocoa offers a special animated window called a *sheet*. It's a window that belongs to another window. Because its functionality is directly connected to another window, it appears from out of the blue at the top of its partner window, as shown in Figure 8-5. You're probably already familiar with sheets because Interface Builder displays one each time you choose the Classes⇨Create Files menu item.

Figure 8-5:
When the functionality of your window is directly tied to another window, display it as a sheet.

A sheet is a special kind of window called a dialog, because it carries on a dialog between your application and the user. Furthermore, a sheet is a particular kind of dialog — a modal dialog. A modal sheet takes over and won't let anything else happen in its parent window until you dismiss it.

Implementing sheets takes some special preparation. To see how they work, launch Project Builder, and create a new Cocoa application. In the project window, double-click MainMenu.nib to open the interface in Interface Builder. Then perform the following steps to add a sheet to your project:

1. **Drag a panel from the Cocoa-Windows panel of the Palettes window (as shown in Figure 8-6) to your MainMenu.nib file window.**

2. **Open the main window (named** Window**) and add a button to it. Open the new panel and add a button to it.**

   The button in the main window will perform an action that displays the sheet. The button in the sheet will close the sheet. Figure 8-7 shows the buttons as they appear in their respective windows.

Figure 8-6:
Add a
panel to
your
nib file.

Figure 8-7:
Add one
button to
the main
window
and one to
the sheet.

3. Create a new controller class.

Click the Classes tab in the MainMenu.nib window. Scroll to the left, select NSObject, and press Return. To follow along with the example, name the new class MySheetController. Create an instance of this class by choosing Classes⇨Instantiate MySheetController.

4. Add outlets and actions.

Add two outlets and two actions to the `MySheetController` class in the Info window. To follow along with the example, name the outlets theBaseWindow and theSheet. Name the actions openSheet and closeSheet.

5. Connect the outlets and actions.

Control-drag from the `MySheetController` instance to the main window and connect it to the `theBaseWindow` outlet. Next, Control-drag from the `MySheetController` instance to the panel in MainMenu.nib and connect it to the `theSheet` outlet.

Then, Control-drag from the button in the main window to the `MySheetController` instance. Connect it to the `openSheet` action. Finally, Control-drag from the button in the sheet panel to the `MySheetController` instance and connect it to the `closeSheet` action.

6. Create the files.

Double-click `MySheetController` in the instances tab of MainMenu.nib. Choose Classes⇨Create Files, and `MySheetController` adds the header and implementation files to your project in Project Builder.

7. Add some code.

Change your MySheetController.m file so that it looks like this (changed lines are shown in boldface):

```
#import "MySheetController.h"

@implementation MySheetController

- (IBAction)closeSheet:(id)sender
{
    [theSheet orderOut:nil];
    [NSApp endSheet:theSheet];
}

- (IBAction)openSheet:(id)sender
{

[NSApp beginSheet:theSheet
    modalForWindow:theBaseWindow
    modalDelegate:self
    didEndSelector:NULL
    contextInfo:nil];
}

@end
```

The `openSheet` method displays the sheet using the `beginSheet` class method of `NSApp`. The `closeSheet` method hides the sheet using the `orderOut` method and disposes of the sheet with `endSheet`.

8. Choose Build⇨Build and Run to see your work in action.

I kept this sheet demonstration simple so that you could see how to display a sheet in your own projects. You can enhance the sheet by adding interface elements to the sheet and wiring them to outlets and actions depending on the desired effect.

Chapter 9

Working with Interface Controls

In This Chapter

▶ Working with button controls

▶ Using slider controls in your project

▶ Animating a progress indicator

▶ Displaying data in a table

T he Mac OS has long been renowned for its graphical user interface. This stems from the fact that people like interacting by using metaphors that relate to the real world. Interface Builder is your tool for creating these metaphors. With it, you build your interface by adding different elements that your users will use to control the application. Because they're controlling the application, Cocoa calls these elements *controls*.

Cocoa has a rich set of interface controls for you to use in your own applications. Using drag-and-drop and a few lines of code, you can add a variety of useful controls to your projects. This chapter guides you through the basics of interface controls in Interface Builder. You'll see how to use each of these controls by adding them to small projects.

By the end of the chapter, you should have enough experience with controls to strike out on your own. The Cocoa framework is a vast one, and nothing prepares you better for programming than practice and experimentation.

Button Controls

Perhaps the most ubiquitous interface element is the button. From the bank's automatic teller machine to the doorbell at your front door, buttons are a nearly universal piece of hardware. Even your mouse and keyboard have button interfaces. Because so many people recognize buttons and know how to use them in the real world, it makes sense that they would be popular in the virtual world as well.

Cocoa puts all sorts of useful and attractive buttons at your disposal. All buttons in Cocoa are of the type NSButton. Most NSButton controls look and act the way you would expect, but some may alter your notion of what constitutes a button.

This section looks at the different types of buttons available to you in Cocoa. To begin working with buttons, launch Project Builder and create a new Cocoa application. Then double-click the MainMenu.nib file to open it in Interface Builder. Open the window found in the nib file window, so that you can start building an interface.

You can find all the NSButton controls in the Cocoa-Views pane of the Palettes window by choosing Tools⇨Palettes⇨Show Palettes. Figure 9-1 shows the Cocoa-Views pane. The NSButton controls appear in the left half of the pane.

Although each of the buttons in Figure 9-1 looks and behaves differently, they are all examples of the NSButton class. This means you could drag a push button to your interface, for example, and later convert it to a square button. You'll see how the buttons differ through the remainder of this section.

Push button

Probably the most recognizable form of NSButton, the push button is a staple of nearly all applications. To add a push button to your interface, simply drag it from the Palette-Views pane of the Palettes window to your window. A typical push button has a centered text label, as shown in Figure 9-2. You can change the text in a button by double-clicking it or by altering the Title entry in the Info window (also shown in Figure 9-2).

Check box

Push button Round button

Figure 9-1:
The Cocoa-Views pane is the home of the NSButton controls in Interface Builder.

Square bevel button

Rounded bevel button

Radio buttons

Figure 9-2:
Push buttons display their functionality using text only.

Besides `Title`, `NSButton` controls have many properties that you can customize. One that you'll use frequently is Equiv (see Figure 9-3). In this little box, you can enter a keystroke that acts as if the user clicked the button with the cursor. Next to the Equiv box in the Info window is a popup menu that lets you select a common keyboard equivalent. The most common keyboard equivalent is Return, which means a user can trigger the push button by pressing Return (or Enter) on the keyboard. You commonly see this sort of functionality on a button labeled OK. When you set it to respond to the Return key, \R appears in the Equiv box and the button automatically takes on a pulsating colorized appearance. The color will be Aqua or Graphite, depending on which appearance setting the user selected in System Preferences. This colorized appearance suggests to users that this button performs the default action for the window in which it appears. For example, when a window has OK and Cancel buttons, often the OK button is the default button. This offers a hint to users that the OK button is probably the button they want to click.

In addition to appearance, an `NSButton` can play a sound when clicked. Just follow these steps to make your button play a sound when it's clicked:

1. **Find a sound to play.**

   Click the Sounds tab in the MainMenu.nib file window. You'll find a number of sounds that you can use. You can also drag your favorite audio files into the nib file window.

2. **Change the Sound setting of the** `NSButton`**.**

   In the interface, click the `NSButton` that you want to alter and open the Info window. In the Sound field, type the name of the sound file that you want to play. Figure 9-4 shows a button that plays the Frog sound.

Figure 9-3:
Set the
Equiv
property to
Return to
make the
button
pulsate.

Figure 9-4:
Type the
name of a
sound file in
the Sound
field.
(Croak.)

3. Test your work.

In Interface Builder, press Cmd-R to test your interface. It should play a
frog sound when you click the button.

Round button

A close relative to the push button is the round button. As its name implies, the *round button* has a circular shape. Two diameters are available for round buttons: 20 and 25 pixels. When you add a new round button to your interface, Interface Builder assigns it a size of 25 pixels. Click the Small setting in the Info window to change the diameter to 20 pixels.

In addition to text, a round button can display icons. To set the icon displayed on a button, perform the following steps:

1. **Add a round button control to your interface.**

   Drag a round button from the Palette-Views pane of the Palettes window to the main window of your interface.

2. **Add an image to your project file to use as the button's icon.**

   Drag your favorite image file from the Finder to your Interface Builder project. When prompted, choose to add the image to your file in Project Builder too. The newly added image appears in the Images tab of the nib file window as well as in your project in Project Builder. Conversely, you could add the image to the project in Project Builder. The addition would simultaneously appear in your nib file. Figure 9-5 shows the location of an image file named arrow in the nib file window.

Figure 9-5:
To use an image file in your interface, drag it to your nib file.

3. Set the button's icon.

Click the Images tab in your nib file window. Drag the arrow image to your round button in the interface. Alternatively, you can set the button's icon manually by entering the name of the image file in the Icon field of the Info window. Figure 9-6 shows the button with the arrow image as its icon. Make sure that any image you use for a button's icon is small enough to fit in the button. Interface Builder will not scale the icon image to fit within the button.

You will find round buttons in use in a variety of roles. Their most common use is as arrow buttons.

Figure 9-6:
Set the icon of a button by entering an image name in the Info window.

Check box

So far, you've looked at buttons that users click to perform an action. Not all buttons have to trigger an action, though. The check box button, for example, is more of a passive control. Rather than firing some action, a check box button indicates a state such as On/Off or Yes/No. Figure 9-7 shows a check box control.

When using check box controls, your code will typically check the state of the control and perform an appropriate operation. To demonstrate, this snippet of code checks the state of a check box control and acts accordingly:

```
if ([prefsCheckbox state])
    // Save Preferences
else
    // Don't Save Preferences
```

Figure 9-7:
A check box button shows the state of a setting.

Square and rounded bevel buttons

Bevel buttons are another style of button available to you. They come in two varieties: square and rounded. Besides the beveled appearance, they differ from standard push buttons and round buttons in that they can display text and icons. Furthermore, they're different in their functionality.

You can use a bevel button like a standard button, which triggers some action when a user clicks it. Beyond this simple button behavior, bevel buttons can also mimic other controls. Like the check box, a bevel button can indicate state by displaying a depressed look. It can also act like a menu by displaying a selection from a list of choices. Figure 9-8 shows the square and rounded bevel buttons in an interface.

Figure 9-8:
Bevel buttons can display text and icons.

Radio Control

The *radio control* is a specialized form of the button that gives a user multiple options. When the user chooses one of these options, the other radio buttons become deselected. Because you typically use more than one radio button at a time, it is customary to use a NSMatrix of radio buttons instead of several individual buttons set to the radio style.

When you drag the radio button control from the Palette-Views window, Interface Builder adds a matrix (or group) of radio buttons to your window. Figure 9-9 shows the NSMatrix that appears in your window when you drag a radio button control from the Palette-Views pane of the Palettes window.

Figure 9-9:
Radio buttons usually appear as part of an NSMatrix.

An NSMatrix is a collection of cells. A radio button resides in each cell in the NSMatrix in Figure 9-9. To edit the text of the particular cell, double-click it. The Title text becomes editable until you click elsewhere in the interface or press Return. You can also change the Title of an NSMatrix element by using the Info window.

To add more radio controls to the NSMatrix, click the NSMatrix in your interface and open the Info window. Change the R field of the Row/Column section, as shown in Figure 9-10. This example shows an NSMatrix with three rows that have edited Titles.

To use this NSMatrix, you need to connect it to an outlet of a controller class.

When connecting an outlet to an NSMatrix, make sure that you Control-drag from the Controller class to the entire matrix, not to an element of the matrix. If one element becomes highlighted when you Control-drag from the controller to the NSMatrix, move the cursor around until a dark outline appears around the entire NSMatrix (see Figure 9-11).

Figure 9-10:
Add rows
to an
NSMatrix
in the Info
window for
that control.

Figure 9-11:
When you
connect an
outlet to an
NSMatrix,
make sure
to attach it
to the entire
control, not
just one of
its elements.

After you have an outlet to the NSMatrix, you can find out which element the user selected by using the selectedRow method of NSMatrix. The selectedRow method returns an integer indicating the index of the currently selected row. Row numbers start from the top, with the first row having an index of 0. To illustrate, here's a sample action that checks the selectedRow of colorRadios. Based on the index, it displays a message in the console telling you which color was chosen:

```
- (IBAction)doSomething:(id)sender
{

    switch ([colorRadios selectedRow])
    {
        case 0:
            NSLog(@"User chose red.");
                break;
        case 1:
            NSLog(@"User chose green.");
            break;
        case 1:
            NSLog(@"User chose blue.");
            break;
    };

}
```

Slider Control

Sliders are the controls you use to represent a range of values. The control gives users an opportunity to select a value in that range by moving (or sliding) the knob of the slider control. The NSSlider is the class behind the slider functions in Cocoa. Unlike the buttons presented earlier in this chapter, the NSSlider controls appear in the Cocoa-Other pane of the Palettes window, as shown in Figure 9-12.

Figure 9-12: The sliders are in the Cocoa-Other pane of the Palettes window.

Sliders come in a variety of styles. They span horizontally or vertically and can display tick marks. Figure 9-13 illustrates the different combinations of styles that sliders can have.

Sliders have two modes of operation: continuous and not continuous. When you check the Continuous property of an NSSlider in the Info window, that slider fires its action any time the user moves it. Conversely, when you uncheck the Continuous property, the slider triggers its action when the user lets up on the mouse button.

Because sliders represent a range of values, they have a minimum and maximum value. They also have a current value, which represents the position of the slider button in the range of minimum and maximum values.

If you want to find out what the current value of the slider is in code, you would do something like this:

```
float x = [theSlider floatValue];
```

You can also set the current position of the slider by using the setFloatValue method:

```
[theSlider setFloatValue:3.0];
```

You aren't restricted to the setFloatValue method. Because NSSlider inherits from NSControl, among other classes, you can use the methods of NSControl to work with the slider. The setFloatValue method is just one method of an NSControl. There are others, which you can view in the built-in documentation (under Help➪Cocoa Help). For example, if you don't care about slider values that contain decimal points, you can use the setIntValue method of the NSControl:

```
[theSlider setIntValue:3];
```

Tab Views

If you like to reduce clutter or if space is at a premium, tab views are for you. The NSTabView is the class in the Application Kit that provides you with tab views for your interface. A *tab view*, as its name implies, is a view consisting of multiple tabs. Figure 9-14 shows a tab view with four tabs. Each tab can hold any number of other controls. As a user clicks a tab, the controls from all other tabs disappear and the controls for the selected tab come into view.

Figure 9-14:
The tab view control helps organize many controls into one confined space.

To use a tab view, simply drag one from the Cocoa-Containers pane of the Palettes window to your interface. To add tabs to the tab view, click once on the tab view and change the number in the Number of Items field in the Info window, as shown in Figure 9-15.

To change the label at the top of each tab, click the tab's text once and change the Label field in the Info window, as show in Figure 9-16.

After you have the number of tabs that you need in your NSTabView, you can add the controls. Just click to select a tab, and then drag the desired controls to that tab. Repeat for the other tabs until you've populated your tab view.

As a Cocoa programmer, you may want to know which tab a user has selected. An NSTabView control can have any number of tabs, which are instances of the NSTabViewItem class. To find out which tab a user has selected, you must first retrieve the NSTabViewItem. Then you pass that result to the indexOfTabViewItem to get the index of the tab. The first tab has an index value of 0 (zero):

```
NSTabViewItem *selectedTab = [myTabView selectedTabViewItem];
int selectedRow = [myTabView selectedTab];
```

Figure 9-15:
Add tabs to
a tab view
using the
Number of
Items field.

Figure 9-16:
Change the
Label field
to alter the
text that
appears at
the top of
each tab.

Making Progress at the Bar

Anyone who has ever used a computer knows that some functions — such as creating a large movie in iMovie or ripping a bunch of MP3 files in iTunes — require a long time to process. As lengthy operations proceed, the thoughtful programmer displays some sort of feedback to let the user know that the computer is working on something. To do this in Cocoa, you use the NSIndicator control.

NSIndicator can display two kinds of progress bars: indeterminate and determinate. You display an indeterminate progress indicator when you don't know how long the process will take, such as when you're searching for files on a hard drive. The indeterminate progress indicator looks like a barber pole.

Use determinate progress indicators when you know how long a process will take to complete, such as when you repeat a task ten times. The window in Figure 9-17 displays one of each type of NSIndicator.

Figure 9-17:
The indeterminate NSIndicator looks like a barber pole. The determinate NSIndicator shows the progress of an operation.

To use the indeterminate NSIndicator control, simply use the startAnimation method. This causes the barber pole to begin moving. The following example calls the startAnimation method using the an outlet named indeterminateProgress:

```
[indeterminateProgress startAnimation:sender];
```

When you've finished processing whatever it is you need to process, you can stop the animation by using the `stopAnimation` method:

```
[indeterminateProgress stopAnimation:sender];
```

When you use a determinate `NSIndicator`, you can set the value of the control using the `setDoubleValue` method. This snippet sets the indicator to the middle position, assuming that the control has a minimum and maximum of 0 to 100, respectively:

```
[determinateProgress setMinValue: 0];
[determinateProgress setMaxValue:100];
[determinateProgress setDoubleValue:50];
```

Table Control

One of the most useful controls that you can add to your applications is the table control. Unfortunately, it's also one of the trickiest to use. With an `NSTableView`, you can display a table or list of data. You'll find the `NSTableView` control in the Cocoa-Data pane of the Palettes window, as shown in Figure 9-18.

Figure 9-18: The `NSTable-View` control can display a table of information.

To begin using an `NSTableView` in a Cocoa project, follow these steps:

1. **Create a new Cocoa application.**

   Launch Project Builder and create a new project by choosing File⇨Project Builder. Name the project simpleTable.

2. **Create the interface.**

   In Project Builder, double-click the MainMenu.nib file to open it in Interface Builder. Drag an `NSTableView` control from the Cocoa-Data pane of the Palettes window to the main window in your interface.

3. Add a controller.

Click the Classes tab in the nib file window. Select NSObject and press Return to create a new class. Name the new class MyDataController. To this new class, add an outlet named tableView, as shown in Figure 9-19. Then, choose Classes⇨Instantiate MyDataController to create an instance of the controller.

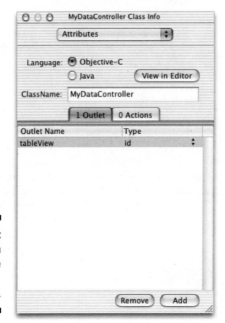

Figure 9-19:
Add an outlet to the Control-ler class.

4. Connect the controller.

Control-drag from the MyDataController class to the center of the NSTableView in your interface, and then click Connect in the Info window.

Be sure to drag to the center of the control. The NSTableView lies within another control called the NSScrollView. As you slowly Control-drag to the center of the control, you will see the focus ring highlight the outer NSScrollView first and then the NSTableView that you want.

5. Connect the data source.

Control-drag from the NSTableView to the MyController class. Select dataSource in the Info window and click Connect. A TableView control must have a data source class that feeds it information. Then connect the `delegate` to `myDataController`. This connection gives you more control over how the `NSTableView` appears in the interface. You'll see it in action in the final part of this section.

6. **Create files for the controller.**

   Click the `MyDataController` class in the Classes tab of the nib file window. Then choose Classes⇨Create Files for MyDataController.

Return to Project Builder and select the MyDataController.h file. Replace the code in MyDataController.h with the following:

```
/* MyDataController */

#import <Cocoa/Cocoa.h>

@interface MyDataController : NSObject
{
    IBOutlet id tableView;
    NSMutableArray *mountedVolumes;
}

- (int)numberOfRowsInTableView:(NSTableView *)tableView;

- (id)tableView:(NSTableView *)tableView
    objectValueForTableColumn:(NSTableColumn *)tableColumn
    row:(int)row;

- (void)tableView:(NSTableView *)tableView
    willDisplayCell:(id)aCell
    forTableColumn:(NSTableColumn *)tableColumn
    row:(int)row;

@end
```

The code begins by declaring the `tableView` outlet and a pointer to an array named `mountedVolumes`. The array will hold the names of all mounted volumes. Then the header declares three methods: `numberOfRowsInTableView`, `objectValueForTableColumn`, and `willDisplayCell`.

The first two methods are mandatory for displaying data in an `NSTableView` control. The `numberOfRowsInTableView` method returns to the row count of the table. The `objectValueForTableColumn` method returns the data for a specific column and row. The idea here is that you don't load a bunch of data into an `NSTableView`. Rather, you load data into some sort of structure (in this case, an array) and let the table ask the `dataSource` class for the data. The `objectValueForTableColumn` method of your class performs this job.

The third method that you're declaring in the header file, named
willDisplayCell, fires each time your table wants to display a row. This
happens because you connected the delegate outlet earlier in this section.
It is not a mandatory method, but it does allow for some nice effects. In this
example, you use this method to colorize the rows of the table.

Next, select the MyDataController.m file and add the following code to it.

```
#import "MyDataController.h"

@implementation MyDataController

- (void)awakeFromNib
{
    int    i;
    NSArray *allVolumes =
[[NSWorkspace sharedWorkspace]
mountedLocalVolumePaths];
    mountedVolumes = [[NSMutableArray alloc] init];

    for (i=0;i<[allVolumes count];i++)
    {
[mountedVolumes addObject:[allVolumes objectAtIndex:i]];
    }
    [tableView reloadData];
}

- (int)numberOfRowsInTableView:(NSTableView *)tableView
{
    return [mountedVolumes count];
}

- (id)tableView:(NSTableView *)tableView
    objectValueForTableColumn:(NSTableColumn *)tableColumn
    row:(int)row
{

    return [mountedVolumes objectAtIndex:row];
}

//colorize rows - requires delegate
- (void)tableView:(NSTableView *)aTableView
willDisplayCell:(id)aCell
forTableColumn:(NSTableColumn *)aTableColumn
            row:(int)rowIndex
{

    [aCell setDrawsBackground:YES];
```

```
    if ( rowIndex % 2 )
        [aCell setBackgroundColor:[NSColor whiteColor]];
    else
        [aCell
setBackgroundColor:
[NSColor colorWithCalibratedRed:0.9
green:0.9 blue:0.9 alpha:1.0]];
}


- (void)dealloc
{
[mountedVolumes release];
 [super dealloc];
}

@end
```

The `awakeFromNib` method starts the source code off by defining and populating the `mountedVolumes` array. It does this using an `NSWorkspace` object to find the names of the mounted volumes. This list can include hard drives, CDs, Zip discs, and other media that "mounts" on your desktop.

Next comes the `numberOfRowsInTableView` method. Because the number of rows in the table matches the number of elements in the array, you return the size of the array.

The next method (`objectValueForTableColumn`) takes care of returning the data to the `NSTableView`. Because the table has only one column, you need not worry about the value of the column. You can simply return the value in that position in the array. The `dealloc` method takes care of releasing the array.

Without adding any other code, this table would display the mounted volumes on your computer. The background of the table would be white with black text. To spruce up the interface a little bit, you can colorize the background of the rows in the table. To do this, you implement the `willDisplayCell` method. The `NSTableView` calls this code each time it needs to display a cell of a table. If the cell is an even-numbered row, the background of the row remains white. Odd-numbered rows get a light gray color using the `colorWithCalibratedRed` method.

Figure 9-20 shows what the result looks like. The names of the volumes will vary depending on which computer you're using.

Figure 9-20:
The completed table lists the mounted volumes on a computer.

Chapter 10

Cocoa Data Types

· ·

In This Chapter

▶ Using the `NSNumber` class

▶ Working with arrays

▶ Understanding Cocoa's Boolean type

▶ Finding out what day it is

· ·

*O*ne of the main tasks that computers do well is manipulate data. Whether you need to calculate the national debt or keep track of the telephone numbers of the players in your poker club, computer programs can ease the task of handling information. Cocoa improves upon the various ways that you work with data in C.

This chapter takes you on a tour of some data types unique to Cocoa. The Foundation Framework defines these data types. You can continue to use the data types that you know from C, but after you see what Cocoa has to offer, you just might stop thinking about those old C types altogether.

Working with Numbers

When you program in Objective-C, you can use all the usual standard C numerical data types for making calculations. If you want to use these values with Cocoa's array objects, however, you're left out in the cold. For this reason, Cocoa offers you the `NSNumber` class. Its main purpose may be to give you a way to add numbers to an `NSArray`. The `NSArray` class is an array class that comes with the Foundation Kit. You'll hear more about it later in this chapter.

To create an `NSNumber` object based on an `int` value of 42, use code like this:

```
NSNumber *n = [NSNumber numberWithInt:42];
```

There are methods for creating NSNumbers based on a variety of numerical types:

- ✔ numberWithDouble
- ✔ numberWithFloat
- ✔ numberWithInt
- ✔ numberWithLong
- ✔ numberWithUnsignedShort

To retrieve values from an NSNumber, use one of the many NSNumber accessor methods. Some of these include

- ✔ doubleValue
- ✔ floatValue
- ✔ intValue
- ✔ longValue
- ✔ unsignedShort

If you want to compare the values of two NSNumber instances, use the isEqualToNumber method. This example shows how to compare two NSStrings named num1 and num2:

```
if ([num1 isEqualToNumber:num2])
    NSLog(@"Numbers are equal");
else
    NSLog(@"Numbers are not equal");
```

Working with Arrays

One of the most common programming tasks that you'll encounter is working with a collection of data. To pull off this task, programmers use *arrays*, which are storage units for a list of data. Cocoa has its own brand of arrays. The NSArray class is at the heart of Cocoa arrays. What makes Cocoa arrays unique is the fact that, unlike traditional arrays, they can store references to instances.

To demonstrate, here's how you would create and populate an array with NSStrings:

```
NSArray *theArray;
   NSString *name1;
   NSString *name2;
   NSString *name3;

   //assign values to the three names
   name1 = @"Maria";
   name2 = @"Mercedes";
   name3 = @"Leopold";

   //create and populate the array
theArray = [NSArray arrayWithObjects:name1, name2, name3,
      nil];
```

Note the `arrayWithObjects` method lets you create an `NSArray` by listing the objects in that array. The last object must always be `nil` to indicate the end of the array.

If you want to find out how many items were in that array, use the `count` method:

```
int i = [theArray count];
```

You can then use the size of the array to retrieve the objects within that array, based on the index. This code snippet displays each item in the array that you just created:

```
NSLog(@"object1=%@",[theArray objectAtIndex:0]);
   NSLog(@"object2=%@",[theArray objectAtIndex:1]);
   NSLog(@"object3=%@",[theArray objectAtIndex:2]);
```

Don't forget that the index is always zero based.

Put it all together and the code looks like this:

```
int i;
   NSArray *theArray;
   NSString *name1;
   NSString *name2;
   NSString *name3;

   //assign values to the three names
   name1 = @"Maria";
   name2 = @"Mercedes";
   name3 = @"Leopold";

   //create and populate the array
```

```
theArray = [NSArray arrayWithObjects:name1, name2, name3,
        nil];

NSLog(@"object1=%@",[theArray objectAtIndex:0]);
NSLog(@"object2=%@",[theArray objectAtIndex:1]);
NSLog(@"object3=%@",[theArray objectAtIndex:2]);

i = [theArray count];
NSLog(@"theArray count = %d",i);
```

The resulting output looks like this:

```
2002-12-18 04:45:54.518 CocoaData2[944] object1=Maria
2002-12-18 04:45:54.520 CocoaData2[944] object2=Mercedes
2002-12-18 04:45:54.520 CocoaData2[944] object3=Leopold
2002-12-18 04:45:54.520 CocoaData2[944] theArray count = 3
```

The NSArray class is handy for storing a group of objects in one place. Its one shortcoming is that you can't alter an NSArray after you've created it. When you can't change something (like an array), Cocoa calls it *immutable*. Conversely, those that you can change are called *mutable arrays*. Thus, Cocoa offers the NSMutableArray. With an NSMutableArray, you can change elements in the array after you create it. This makes it more suitable for maintaining dynamic lists of information. To create an NSArray, you can use its arrayWithCapacity method:

```
NSMutableArray *theArray = [NSMutableArray
        arrayWithCapacity:0];
```

Because you can grow or shrink NSMutableArrays at will, it is safe to create the array with space for zero items.

To add items to an NSMutableArray, use the addObject method:

```
[theArray addObject:name1];
[theArray addObject:name2];
[theArray addObject:name3];
```

To remove an item from the array, use the removeObjectAtIndex. For example, to remove the second name, use code like this:

```
[theArray removeObjectAtIndex:1];
```

Inserting an object is just as easy. Use the insertObject method for that. This example reinserts the second name into the array:

```
[theArray insertObject:name2 atIndex:1];
```

Finally, you may want to replace an element of the array with another object. For this task, use the `replaceObjectAtIndex` method. This snippet replaces the second name in the array with `name3`:

```
[theArray replaceObjectAtIndex:1 withObject:name3];
```

Because `NSMutableArray` inherits from `NSArray`, you can use the methods from earlier in this section to find out the size of the array and to query it for specific elements.

Working with Boolean Data Types

Objective-C has its own Boolean data type: `BOOL`. Instead of the usual `TRUE` and `FALSE` values, Objective-C uses `YES` and `NO`. This code snippet shows some of the ways in which you'd typically use `BOOL` variables:

```
BOOL answerWasFound;

answerWasFound = FindTheAnswer();

if (answerWasFound)
// OR
if (answerWasFound == YES)
```

Besides using `YES` or `NO` for its value, the Objective-C `BOOL` type is important for another reason: It works with other objects in Cocoa. Again, arrays and other types of collection objects expect their elements to be objects themselves. If you wanted to create an `NSArray` of Boolean values in Cocoa, you'd pass the `BOOL` type to the `numberWithBool` class method of `NSNumber`:

```
//create an NSNumber with a BOOL
n = [NSNumber numberWithBool:YES];

//add the NSNumber to an array
[theArray addObject:n];
```

Working with Dates

The `NSCalendarDate` class gives you many options when it comes to working with dates and times. One of the most common tasks you'll perform is finding the current date or time. You can do this in one line of code, using one of the `NSCalendarDate` class methods:

```
NSDate *theDate = [NSCalendarDate date];
```

After you retrieve this date, you can easily convert it into an NSString, suitable for display. Simply use the description method to display the date in standard international format. In this example, you use NSLog to display the date in the console:

```
NSLog(@"theDate = %@",[theDate description]);
```

Figure 10-1 shows output of the description method.

Figure 10-1: Use the description method of NSCalendarDate for a quick look at the date and time.

The description method is okay for quick-and-dirty date displays, but sometimes you want to display the date in a more human-friendly format. The descriptionWithCalendarFormat method can help you build an NSString that holds the date or time. The descriptionWithCalendarFormat method has three parameters. The first one is the only one that you have to worry about for simple date work. That parameter is an NSString that represents the date in the format you desire.

Cocoa gives you lots of flexibility when it comes to formatting your date for display. For example, the following code snippet displays results like those shown in Figure 10-2:

```
NSLog(@"theDate = %@",
  [theDate descriptionWithCalendarFormat:@"%A, %B %d, %Y
          (%I:%M)" timeZone:nil locale:nil]);
```

Figure 10-2:
Use the
descrip-
tionWith-
Calendar-
Format
method to
format the
date.

That odd-looking string that you pass to the descriptionWithCalendar-
Format method dictates which elements of the date you want to display.
Apple calls those strange characters *date conversion specifiers*. Each specifier
is a one-letter code that corresponds to some aspect of the date. In the preceding example, %A represents the name of the day of the week, in this case
Wednesday. Next comes %B, which stands for the name of the month. You can
continue to string together these specifiers until you've built a date in the
format you prefer. Table 10-1 details some of the more common specifiers.
The rest of them are in Project Builder's built-in Cocoa documentation. Click
the Find tab and search for *Setting the Format for Dates* for more information.

Table 10-1	Date Format Specifiers
Code	*What It Represents*
%B	Month name
%m	Month as an integer
%e	Day of the month as an integer
%A	Weekday name
%I	Hours
%M	Minutes
%S	Seconds
%Y	Year

Part III

Putting It All Together: Cocoa Programming in Depth

The 5th Wave By Rich Tennant

Okay—you were right, I was wrong. Cmd—O opens the garage door, and Cmd—Q backs the car out.

In this part . . .

You know how the Developer Tools work, you have a handle on the Objective-C language, and you've even built your own applications. Now it's time to step it up a notch.

Part III elevates your Cocoa skills to new heights. You discover how to add the features found in every cool Cocoa application by creating a variety of programs with a range of functions from text and graphics to audio and video. Every Mac user expects printing capability, so Part III covers that, too.

Chapter 11

Text

In This Chapter

▶ Displaying text

▶ Changing the style of text

▶ Editing text

▶ Saving text to a file

▶ Opening and displaying text files

*E*ver since the first Macintosh computer, Apple has led the pack in design, layout, and typography. Mac OS X continues this tradition by providing some of the best looking text you'll ever see on a computer monitor. Cocoa gives programmers instant access to these wonderful features of OS X.

This chapter shows you how to work with text for a variety of purposes. First, you display some text in a window. Then, you manipulate that text, contorting its sizes and altering its hue. Next, you discover how easy it is to add professional text-editing features to your applications with little or no code. Finally, you save the text from your interface to a file for later recall. Stylized text is a great feature for many types of applications, and Cocoa gives you a wide range of tools for manipulating that text.

Working with Text

Cocoa offers you many controls for working with text in your applications. Which control you use depends on your needs. Some text controls display static text (text that you can't change); others allow full editing (dynamic text). You can display text with any one of the following controls.

✔ `NSTextField`: Displays static or dynamic text. Use this control to display one line of text.

✔ `NSForm`: Like an `NSTextField`, but usually used in a group of `NSForm` controls.

✔ **NSTextView:** The star of the text fields in Cocoa. This baby can work with multiple lines of text. When you think of a word processor, think of `NSTextView`.

This chapter focuses on the `NSTextView` control because it's the most full featured. If you can work with it, you can easily handle the other controls for displaying text.

Build an interface

To get started working with text, you'll need a project and an interface. Perform the following steps to prepare a project for the examples in this chapter.

1. **Create a project in Project Builder.**

2. **Open MainMenu.nib by double-clicking it in the Resources folder.**

3. **In Interface Builder, open the `Window` window from the MainMenu.nib file. To this window, add an `NSTextView`.**

   You can find the `NSTextView` in the Cocoa-Data pane of the Palettes window, as shown in Figure 11-1.

4. **Add two switch-style `NSButtons` to the window.**

   One switch will toggle the display of a ruler in the `NSTextView`. The other switch forces color changes to apply only to a selection. You can find this type of control in the Cocoa-View pane of the Palettes window. Label them as illustrated in Figure 11-2.

5. **Drag two `NSColorWell` controls from the Palettes window to the interface.**

   The `NSColorWell` control resides in the Cocoa-Other pane of the Palettes window. Feel free to label the `NSColorWell` controls using the `NSTextField` control. Figure 11-3 shows the newest additions to the interface. One `NSColorWell` dictates the color of the text in the `NSTextView`. The other will control the background color of that view.

Figure 11-1: The NSText-View control is in the Cocoa-Data pane of the Palettes window.

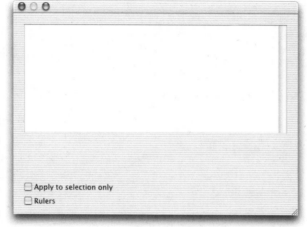

Figure 11-2:
Add two
`NSButtons`
to the
window.

Figure 11-3:
Add two
`NSColor-`
`Well`
controls to
the window.

Add a controller class

As you might expect, the next step is to create a class that will control your interface:

1. **Using Interface Builder, click the Classes tab in the MainMenu.nib file window.**

2. **Scroll all the way to the left of that tab and select** `NSObject`. **Press Return to create a new class.**

3. **Name the class.**

   To follow along with the example, name the class MyTextController. You can see the result in Figure 11-4.

Figure 11-4:
Create a
new class to
act as the
controller.

4. **Add outlets and actions to the class.**

   For starters, define the following outlets for the class by selecting
   `MyTextController` in the Classes tab of the MainMenu.nib file window:

   - `theApplySwitch`
   - `theBackgroundColorWell`
   - `theTextColorWell`
   - `theTextView`

   You may notice that one of the switch-style `NSButtons` is missing. That's
   because it performs its magic through an action. Add the following
   actions to the `MyTextController` class.

   - `setTheBackgroundColor`
   - `setTheTextColor`
   - `toggleTheRuler`

5. **Don't forget to instantiate the class by choosing Classes⇨Instantiate
   MyTextController.**

Wire the interface

To wire the components of your interface to the `Controller` class, perform
the following steps:

1. **Connect the outlets of the appropriate controls to the
   MyTextController object in MainMenu.nib.**

   To do so, simply Control-drag from the `MyTextController` object in the
   Instances tab of MainMenu.nib to the desired control. Connect the two
   by using the Info window. Figure 11-5 shows the `theApplySwitch` outlet
   connected to its switch.

Figure 11-5:
Connect the
outlets
for the
interface.

2. **Next, connect the actions of the** MyTextController **object to the two** ColorWells **and the ruler switch.**

   To connect them, Control-drag from the controls to the MyText Controller object. You can see the toggleTheRuler action connected to its switch in Figure 11-6.

Figure 11-6:
Connect the
actions
for the
interface.

3. **The last step in the interface-building process is to create the implementation and header files.**

   Click the Classes tab in MainMenu.nib and select the MyTextController class. Choose Classes⇨Create Files for MyTextController to add the files to your project in Project Builder.

Add the code

Now that you've assembled the interface for this chapter, it's time to add some code. Before you do, though, perhaps you should know what the project will do. The NSColorWell controls display the standard Color Panel when a user clicks them. Depending on which NSColorWell a user clicks, the Color Panel will alter either the text color or the background color of the NSTextView in the window. Add the code for this functionality in the setTheBackgroundColor and setTheTextColor actions.

```
- (IBAction)setTheBackgroundColor:(id)sender
{
    //set the background color of the NSTextView
    [theTextView setBackgroundColor:[sender color]];
    if ([theApplySwitch state])
        [theTextView setTextColor:[theTextColorWell color]
            range:[theTextView selectedRange]];
    else
        [theTextView setTextColor:[theTextColorWell color]];
}

- (IBAction)setTheTextColor:(id)sender
{
    //set the text color of the NSTextView
    [theTextView setBackgroundColor:[theBackgroundColorWell
            color]];
    if ([theApplySwitch state])
        [theTextView setTextColor:[sender color]
            range:[theTextView selectedRange]];
    else
        [theTextView setTextColor:[sender color]];
}
```

As you can see, setting the background and text colors is as easy as using the setBackgroundColor and setTextColor functions of theTextView. If the state of theApplySwitch is YES, the setTextColor function takes a range as one of its parameters. This allows you to choose which portion of the text you'd like colorized.

You'll want these two ColorWells to display certain text and background colors by default. Use a white background and black text as the default colors and set them in the awakeFromNib function:

```
- (void)awakeFromNib
{
    //set the NSColorWells to preset colors
    [theTextColorWell setColor:[NSColor blackColor]];
    [theBackgroundColorWell setColor:[NSColor whiteColor]];
}
```

The NSTextView control can perform all sorts of other fantastic text manipulation operations besides color. One of these great features is the ruler. With only one line of code, you can incorporate a full-fledged ruler into an NSTextView. In Project Builder, add the following code to the toggleTheRuler action:

```
- (IBAction)toggleTheRuler:(id)sender
{
    [theTextView toggleRuler:sender ];
}
```

Choose Build⇨Build and Run to see your handiwork. Figure 11-7 illustrates the use of a ruler in an NSTextView. Notice that the ruler also permits a user to edit parameters such as alignment and line spacing.

Figure 11-7: With one line of code, you can add a ruler!

Doing Style the Easy Way!

You can continue to add style functions to this project by manipulating the NSTextView directly. This may work great for some projects, but for others, there's a much easier way to stylize text in an `NSTextView`. If you're looking for traditional word-processor styles in your application, Cocoa can deliver!

1. **Return to the MainMenu.nib file in Interface Builder.**

2. **In the Instances tab, double-click MainMenu to open the menu editor.**

3. **Add a Font menu to the menu editor.**

   Drag one from the Cocoa-Menus pane of the Palettes window to the menu editor. As soon as you release the menu, it gains a full Font menu implementation. Notice also that Interface Builder adds a Font Manager object to your Instances tab in the MainMenu.nib file, as shown in Figure 11-8. That's all there is to it!

Figure 11-8:
Add a Font menu to the menu editor for inclusion in your application.

4. **Return to Project Builder to build and run the project.**

You'll quickly discover that all the items in the Font menu work. No code is necessary. No connections are necessary. It doesn't get any simpler than that. Because many types of applications use a Font menu, Apple thought it made sense to include this feature for you. That way, you can add a standardized Font menu to your project without having to worry about how to implement it. Figure 11-9 shows the Font menu in action.

Figure 11-9:
Wow! You
can
implement a
complete
Font menu
without
writing one
line of code.

By now, you should begin to see the power of Cocoa. The high-level classes that Apple includes with Cocoa ensure that your projects maintain a consistent look and feel while providing the full features your users expect from an application.

Manipulating Text

So far, we've been concerned with style over substance. Another important aspect of working with text in NSTextViews is the capability to edit, copy, paste, and alter its text.

Pasteboard manipulations

One common feature that every Mac OS X application has is access to the Pasteboard (sometimes referred to as the Clipboard). Like the Font menu that you implemented earlier, Cocoa takes care of the Edit menu too. Unlike the Font menu, however, you don't have to do anything to implement it. It just works! The Edit menu in OS X offers the typical cut, copy, and paste features that you might expect from an Edit menu. It also implements full-blown spell checking and find functions, as demonstrated in Figure 11-10.

Figure 11-10:
You don't have to do a bit of work to give your application an Edit menu.

Notice, though, that the Edit menu hasn't enabled its Undo and Redo menu items. The fix for this is simple enough:

1. **Double-click the MainMenu.nib file to open it in Interface Builder.**

2. **Open the window for your interface and select** `NSTextView`.

3. **Press Cmd-Shift-I to open the Info window.**

4. **In the Attributes section of the Info window, click the Undo allowed attribute, as shown in Figure 11-11.**

   Now, your users will be able to undo any actions that they perform. You managed to add this useful functionality by clicking one check box.

Manual editing

Sometimes you may want to alter the text in an `NSTextView` without using the Pasteboard. Perhaps the most common editing task that you'll want to perform is to change the text that appears in an `NSTextView`. You can accomplish this task by using the `setString` method of the `NSString` class. First, you create an `NSString` and assign a string to it:

```
NSString* someString = @"Cocoa says Hello!";
```

Figure 11-11:
Click the
Undo
allowed
attribute to
turn on
the Undo
functions
for an
`NSText-`
`View`.

Note the @ character preceding the string. This indicates that it's a Cocoa string, not a traditional C string. After you have `NSString`, it's a simple matter to display it in an `NSTextView`:

```
[theTextView setString:someString];
```

To see how this works, follow these steps:

1. **Open your interface in Interface Builder.**

2. **Add an `NSButton` to the window in your interface.**

3. **Change the button's Title attribute in the Info window to Display NSString.**

4. **Add a new action named `displayAString` to the `MyTextController` instance in the MainMenu.nib file.**

5. **Control-drag from the button to the `MyTextController` instance and connect it to the `displayAString` action in the Info window.**

6. **Return to Project Builder and add the following line to the MyTextController.h file.**

```
- (IBAction)displayAString:(id)sender;
```

7. **Add this method to MyTextController.m:**

```
- (IBAction)displayAString:(id)sender
{
    NSString* someString = @"Cocoa says hello!";
    [theTextView setString:someString];
    [someString release];
}
```

Replacing text is another task that you might like to perform. To replace some portion of the text in an NSTextView, you must first define an NSRange variable. This range describes which part of the string you want to replace. In the preceding example, you used the string "Cocoa says hello!". If you'd like to change the word *hello* to *goodbye*, you'd first find the location of that word in the string. Because the numbering begins at 0, the first letter of *hello* is the eleventh character in the string. Further, the length of *hello* is 5. Thus, to make an NSRange for *hello*, you'd use code like this:

```
NSRange theRange;
theRange = NSMakeRange(11, 5);
```

Then, to replace *hello* with *goodbye*, call the replaceCharactersInRange method of the NSTextView:

```
[theTextView replaceCharactersInRange:theRange
            withString:@"Goodbye" ];
```

Besides editing the text, you'll want to programmatically select portions of the text in an NSTextView. For example, suppose you want to perform a Select All operation. First, create an NSRange representing the entire length of the text. Then call the setSelectedRange method of the NSTextView to select the text:

```
NSRange theRange;
theRange = NSMakeRange(0, [[theTextView string] length]);
[theTextView setSelectedRange];
```

Saving Text for a Rainy Day

Eventually, your users will want to save the text on which they've been working so hard. Cocoa lets you save text in two ways, as

✔ Plain text

✔ Rich text

Plain text is text without any formatting. You see this type of text in HTML and XML documents, SimpleText files (from the Classic Mac OS), and the source code files in your Cocoa projects. When all you care about is the text data in a file and not its formatting, use the plain text format.

Rich text, on the other hand, conveys information about the formatting. You may recognize the rich text format from popular Microsoft applications such as Word. The rich text file format saves formatting data such as fonts, colors, and styles in the file along with the actual text data. If you're building a word processor or a similar type of application in which formatting matters, use the rich text format.

To see how these two file formats work with Cocoa, follow these steps:

1. **Open MainMenu.nib in Interface Builder.**

2. **To the existing window, add two `NSButton` controls. Change their title attributes in the Info window to**

   • Save plain text

   • Save rich text

   Figure 11-12 shows these new buttons.

3. **Add two new actions to the `MyTextController` instance:**

   • `SaveTextFile`

   • `SaveRichTextFile`

Figure 11-12:
Add two
NSButtons
that will
save rich
and plain
text files.

4. **Control-drag from each** NSButton **in the interface to the** MyText Controller **instance in MainMenu.nib. When you let go of the mouse, assign the appropriate action to that button using the Info window.**

5. **Return to Project Builder and add the following lines of code to the MyTextController.h file to declare the two actions:**

```
- (IBAction)openRichTextFile:(id)sender;
- (IBAction)openTextFile:(id)sender;
```

6. **Navigate to the MyTextController.m file and implement the two actions:**

```
- (IBAction)saveTextFile:(id)sender
{
    NSSavePanel *theSavePanel = [NSSavePanel savePanel];
    [theSavePanel setRequiredFileType:@"txt"];
    [theSavePanel setTitle:@"Save as Plain Text"];
    if ([theSavePanel runModal] == NSOKButton)
    {
        [[theTextView string] writeToFile:[theSavePanel
        filename]
            atomically:YES];
    }
}

- (IBAction)saveRichTextFile:(id)sender
{
    NSSavePanel *theSavePanel = [NSSavePanel savePanel];
    [theSavePanel setRequiredFileType:@"rtf"];
    [theSavePanel setTitle:@"Save as Rich Text"];
    if ([theSavePanel runModal] == NSOKButton)
    {
        [[theTextView RTFFromRange:
            NSMakeRange(0, [[theTextView string]
        length])]
        writeToFile:[theSavePanel filename]
        atomically:YES];
    }
}
```

The code for both actions works similarly, with a few exceptions. To begin with, both actions display a SavePanel, so that users can select the name and destination of the file they want to save. The two methods differ on the file type and title that they display in the SavePanel, but otherwise they are identical. To display the panel, each method uses this line of code:

```
if ([theSavePanel runModal] == NSOKButton)
```

The `runModal` method of the `SavePanel` takes care of displaying the modal window. A *modal window* is one in which users are forced into a "mode" of operation. This means they must make a decision (saving a file or halting the operation) before proceeding any further.

When a user clicks a file and clicks the OK button in the `SavePanel`, the `runModal` function of the `SavePanel` returns a value. Instead of worrying about what numerical value it returns, Cocoa provides you with the constant `NSOKButton` indicating that the user clicked the OK button. In this code example, we are checking for the OK button. Conversely, you could check for the Cancel button by using the appropriate constant for that button.

```
if ([theSavePanel runModal] == NSCancelButton)
```

If the users click OK in the `SavePanel`, the code writes the text from the `TextView` to a plain or rich text file. For plain text files, this means using the `writeToFile` method of the `NSString` class:

```
[[theTextView string] writeToFile:[theSavePanel filename]
            atomically:YES];
```

First, you retrieve the text from the text view as an `NSString` using `[theTextView string]` method. Then, save the text file with the `writeToFile` method, passing it two parameters: the name of the file that the user entered in the `SavePanel` and a Boolean value titled `atomically`. If you pass YES as the `atomically` parameter, the `writeToFile` method first writes the data to a temporary file and renames that file after the write operation is finished. If it has a value of NO, `writeToFile` writes the data directly to the file returned by the `filename` method. Set the `atomically` parameter to YES.

The second method in the code listing saves the file to a rich text file. Much of the code in it is identical to the plain text version, with one big exception. Instead of retrieving text from text view with the `string` method of the `NSString` class, you use the `RTFFromRange` method for rich text. This has the effect of retrieving the text with its style information (bold, size, color, and so on) intact:

```
[[theTextView RTFFromRange:
            NSMakeRange(0, [[theTextView string] length])]
  writeToFile:[theSavePanel filename] atomically:YES];
```

The only parameter of the `RTFFromRange` method is an `NSRange` value indicating the portion of text that you want to retrieve from text view. To retrieve all the text, you supply the method with the starting point of the text and the length of text to grab. In this instance, you grab all the text found in the text view, starting from position 0 (zero) and extending the length of the text in the text view:

```
NSMakeRange(0, [[theTextView string] length])
```

After you have `NSString` from `TextView`, `writeToFile` works the same as it does for plain text files, with a minor caveat. When you use the `writeToFile` method, the resulting plain text files have the .txt file extension and rich text files have the .rtf extension.

Retrieving Text

Another important task that you'll likely need to perform regularly is opening text files. To open and read a text file, your code should do the following:

✔ Display an `OpenPanel`, so users can choose which file they want to open

✔ Read the text data from the file

✔ Display that data in an `NSTextView`

To add the capability to open and view plain and rich text files, you'll need to add a few items to the interface:

1. **Open MainMenu.nib in Interface Builder.**

2. **To the existing window, add two additional `NSButton` controls. Change their Title attributes in the Info window to Open plain text and Open rich text.**

   Figure 11-13 shows the new buttons.

3. **Add two new actions to the MyTextController instance:** `OpenTextFile` **and** `OpenRichTextFile`.

4. **Control-drag from each `NSButton` in the interface to the `MyTextController` instance in MainMenu.nib. When you let go of the mouse, assign the appropriate action to that button using the Info window.**

5. **Return to Project Builder and add the following lines of code to the MyTextController.h file to declare these two actions:**

   ```
   - (IBAction)openRichTextFile:(id)sender;
   - (IBAction)openTextFile:(id)sender;
   ```

Figure 11-13:
Add two
NSButtons
to the
interface for
opening
plain and
rich text
files.

6. **Navigate to the MyTextController.m file and implement those two actions:**

```
- (IBAction)openTextFile:(id)sender
{
    NSOpenPanel *theOpenPanel = [NSOpenPanel openPanel];
    if ([theOpenPanel runModal] == NSOKButton)
    {
        NSString *theFileName = [theOpenPanel filename];
        NSString *theFileContents = [NSString
            stringWithContentsOfFile:theFileName];
      [theTextView setString:theFileContents];
        [theFileName release];
        [theFileContents release];
    }
}

- (IBAction)openRichTextFile:(id)sender
{
    NSOpenPanel *theOpenPanel = [NSOpenPanel openPanel];
    if ([theOpenPanel runModal] == NSOKButton)
    {
      NSString *theFileName = [theOpenPanel filename];
        NSData *theRTFData = [NSData
          dataWithContentsOfFile:theFileName];
      [theTextView replaceCharactersInRange:
            NSMakeRange(0, [[theTextView string] length])
          withRTF:theRTFData];
        [theFileName release];
        [theRTFData release];
    }
}
```

In contrast to the examples from earlier in this chapter, in which you saved text files, opening text files requires the use of the NSOpenPanel class. It works in much the same manner as the NSSavePanel. In the two methods for opening text files, you aren't setting the title displayed in the NSOpenPanel (using setTitle) like you did for the NSSavePanel earlier. You certainly could, though.

Like the NSSavePanel, you then display the NSOpenPanel using the runModal method:

```
NSOpenPanel *theOpenPanel = [NSOpenPanel openPanel];
```

If the user selects a text file and clicks OK to open it, runModal returns NSOKButton:

```
if ([theOpenPanel runModal] == NSOKButton)
```

From there, you open the text file, read its contents, and display them in an NSTextView. For plain text files, it's a straightforward process to read in a text file using the stringWithContentsOfFile method of NSString:

```
NSString *theFileName = [theOpenPanel filename];
    NSString *theFileContents = [NSString
            stringWithContentsOfFile:theFileName];
```

Then, to display the text in an NSTextView, you need only one line of code:

```
    [theTextView setString:theFileContents];
```

After you're finished working with the NSString objects, don't forget to dispose of them:

```
[theFileName release];
[theRTFData release];
```

Reading rich text files requires a bit of extra work, but not too much. Instead of using an NSString to read text from a rich text file, you must use an NSData object. Call the dataWithContentsOfFile method of the NSData class to load stylized text from the file into the NSData object:

```
NSData *theRTFData = [NSData
            dataWithContentsOfFile:theFileName];
```

Then to display it in the text view, use the replaceCharactersInRange method:

```
[theTextView replaceCharactersInRange:
          NSMakeRange(0, [[theTextView string] length])
          withRTF:theRTFData];
```

The replaceCharactersInRange method takes two parameters:

- ✔ **NSRange:** The location in the NSTextView where you want to display the text
- ✔ **NSData:** The rich text data that you read from the file

To test your code, choose Build➪Build and Run in Project Builder.

Rich text files play an important role in all sorts of applications. Chapter 17 goes into detail about how you can use rich text content as part of a miniature word processor.

Chapter 12

Graphics

● ●

In This Chapter

▶ Defining colors

▶ Creating a custom view

▶ Drawing rectangles and ovals

▶ Painting irregular shapes

▶ Displaying images

● ●

From the beautiful fonts in a word processor to the "lickable" Aqua interface, the Mac OS has always prided itself on fantastic looking graphics. Mac OS X is no different. With its sophisticated Quartz graphics engine, Mac OS X can produce stunning graphics. Cocoa gives you direct access to these powerful features of Mac OS X.

This chapter covers the basics of getting up and running with graphics in Cocoa. You create a custom View for displaying your graphics and draw on it using a variety of colors, shapes, and images. You even write code to change the opacity of your graphics, giving them the coveted see-through look. So, let's get started creating some digital art!

Cocoa and the Art of Graphics

Before you jump head first into graphics, you should familiarize yourself with a few important Cocoa data structures: NSPoint, NSRect, NSSize, and NSColor. You'll need them to do any type of graphics programming in Cocoa, so they make a good starting point.

Points

Just like in geometry class, Cocoa uses points to designate position on a square grid. To work with points in Cocoa, you use an `NSPoint` structure. `NSPoint` is a structure comprised of two floats (named x and y, respectively). Cocoa graphics defines the bottom-left corner as the origin (0,0). The x value increases as you move to the right. The y value increases as you advance up. This is a different arrangement than most Macintosh and Window programming, where the origin is in the top-left corner.

```
typedef struct _NSPoint {
    float x;
    float y;
} NSPoint;
```

The x and y portion of the structure are the coordinates of the point that you want to represent. To use an `NSPoint` variable, you must first define it:

```
NSPoint thePoint;
```

Then to assign values to the x and y members of an `NSPoint` structure, you use the `NSMakePoint` function. This example creates an `NSPoint` at the location (100,100):

```
thePoint = NSMakePoint(100, 100);
```

Rects and sizes

Closely related to the `NSPoint` structure is the `NSRect` structure. An `NSRect` (*Rect* is short for *rectangle*) is a structure comprised of an `NSPoint` and an `NSSize`:

```
typedef struct _NSRect {
    NSPoint origin;
    NSSize size;
} NSRect;
```

To understand what this means, you also need to know about the `NSSize` structure:

```
typedef struct _NSSize {
    float width;
    float height;
} NSSize;
```

Thus, an NSRect is really a structure of four float values: two for the NSPoint and two for the NSSize. The NSPoint portion describes where the NSRect begins and the NSSize variable describes the dimensions of the NSRect. For Mac programmers who are new to Cocoa, this may take a little getting used to, because the Rect structure used in QuickDraw differs subtlety from the NSRect structure. (A Rect consists of two points.)

To create an NSRect, first declare the NSRect variable:

```
NSRect theRect;
```

Then initialize that variable using the NSMakeRect function. NSMakeRect takes four parameters: x, y, width, and height. For example, this line of code creates an NSRect with an origin at (100,100) and dimensions of 50 x 50:

```
theRect = NSMakeRect(100, 100, 50, 50);
```

Later, if you want to find the origin or size of theRect, use code like this:

```
float theOriginX, theOriginY;
float theSizeW, theSizeH;

theOriginX = theRect.origin.x;
theOriginY = theRect.origin.y;

theSizeW = theRect.size.width;
theSizeH = theRect.size.height;
```

Colors

Cocoa's AppKit includes the NSColor data type to help you work with color in your graphics projects. The easiest way to create and define an NSColor object is to use one of the built-in color preset components. You'll recognize immediately what each one creates, because they have plain-English names. For example, to create an NSColor object that stores the color black, use code like this:

```
//Declare a pointer to an NSColor object
NSColor* theColor;


//create the object
//and assign the color black to it
theColor = [NSColor blackColor];
```

As you may have guessed, this works for many other colors too (blueColor, redColor, and so on). Table 12-1 lists the entire collection of preset components that you can use to create many common colors.

Table 12-1	Preset Color Components
Preset Component	*Color It Produces*
blackColor	Black
blueColor	Bright blue
brownColor	Brown
cyanColor	Light blue
darkGrayColor	Dark gray (for the Canadians, dark grey)
grayColor	Medium gray
greenColor	Bright green
lightGrayColor	Light gray (you were expecting something else?)
magentaColor	Pinkish purple color . . . or is it a purple-ish pink color
orangeColor	Orange
purpleColor	Purple
redColor	Bright red
whiteColor	White
yellowColor	Bright and sunny yellow

Eventually, you'll want some colors that the preset components don't cover. In that case, you have to resort to some of the more sophisticated color methods in the AppKit. The AppKit has three kinds of color spaces that you can use to create colors:

✔ Device dependent (a.k.a. device)
✔ Device independent (a.k.a. calibrated)
✔ Named

When you use *device colors,* you can't be sure that you'll always see the same color across devices. You're probably most familiar with this kind of color, because most home computer monitors and printers display it. Stand any two computer monitors next to each other, and you'll soon discover that they don't produce colors equally. Sure, it's good enough for you to view Web pages, play games, and even create graphics. It also works for many kinds of home printing chores. It's not so good, however, for professional printing, color correction, and similar color tasks.

To get around this color problem, computer and printer manufacturers began creating hardware and software solutions to calibrate their equipment. The idea was that you should be able to see the same kind of output no matter what device you used. The calibration is supposed to account for the peculiarities of your particular device and adjust it to produce accurate colors.

The first two kinds of color spaces in the preceding list correspond to these two types of color: device and calibrated. This chapter uses the device dependent type of color space. The third kind of color space (named) is for even more sophisticated work with color. You can disregard it as well for this book.

The *device dependent* type of color space has three color spaces. A *color space* is just a fancy way of saying "ways of creating color." Normally, you create colors by mixing different amounts of specific base colors. The three mixing schemes that you can use in device dependent color are

- ✔ DeviceRGB: Red, green, blue, and alpha components
- ✔ DeviceCMYK: Cyan, magenta, yellow, black, and alpha components
- ✔ DeviceWhite: White and alpha components

For the rest of this chapter, you have to worry about only DeviceRGB, because it's the best choice for displaying graphics on a monitor. After you get the hang of the DeviceRGB color space, it's easy to use the DeviceCMYK and DeviceWhite color spaces. Therefore, you're not missing anything by forgetting about them for the time being.

Now, it's time to get to the code. Instead of using the colors of the preset components, you can define your own RGB colors using the colorWith DeviceRed function. The function takes four floats as parameters. These four numbers correspond to the three color channels (red, green, and blue) and the alpha channel. Each parameter can have a value between 0.0 and 1.0; 1.0 is full on. The alpha parameter dictates how opaque the color is. A value of 1.0 is completely opaque, and a value of 0.0 is fully transparent.

This numbering scheme contrasts with the colors used in familiar applications such as Web pages and Photoshop documents, where the numbering usually has a range between 0 and 255. To correlate with the Cocoa way of doing things, add 1 to the value of each color component and divide by 256. For example, if you want to convert a Photoshop color with RGB values of (127,63,255) to the RGB values for an NSColor, perform this simple calculation:

```
127 + 1 = 128/256 = 0.5
63 + 1 = 64/256 = 0.25
255 + 1 = 256/256 = 1.0
```

To create an NSColor object in the DeviceRGB color space, use code like this:

```
//Declare a pointer to an NSColor object
NSColor* theColor;

//create the object
//and assign the color black to it
theColor = [NSColor  colorWithDeviceRed:(float)0.0
          green:(float)0.0 blue:(float)0.0
          alpha:(float)1.0];
```

Notice that the red, green, and blue parameters are all set to 0.0. If you wanted to create a red color object, you'd use code like this:

```
//create the object
//and assign the color red to it
theColor = [NSColor  colorWithDeviceRed:(float)1.0
          green:(float)0.0 blue:(float)0.0
          alpha:(float)1.0];
```

The red parameter has a value of 1.0, and the green and blue components have a value of 0.0. By adjusting the alpha value, you can create different shades of the same color. You see more color code later in this chapter, so don't worry if you don't feel entirely comfortable with it yet.

After you create a color object, the only other thing you need to do before working with it is to use the set function. This sets the graphics pen to your desired color:

```
[color set];
```

Yes, it's as easy as that. Again, you'll see more clearly how Cocoa colors work in the code examples in the remainder of this chapter.

Building a Graphics Interface

To begin coding your graphics masterpiece, you need an interface in which to display said graphics:

1. **Launch Project Builder and create a new Cocoa project as shown in Figure 12-1.**

Figure 12-1:
In Project
Builder,
create a
new Cocoa
project by
choosing
File⇨New
Project.

2. **Expand the Resources folder and double-click the MainMenu.nib file to open it with Interface Builder.**

3. **In Interface Builder, click the Classes tab of the nib file window. Scroll the class browser all the way to the left until you see** NSObject.

4. **Click the following in succession:** NSObject, **then** NSResponder, **and then** NSView.

5. **Press Return to create a new** NSView **subclass. Name it MyCanvas, as shown in Figure 12-2.**

Figure 12-2:
Create a subclass of the NSView class and name it MyCanvas.

6. **Click the Instances tab of MainMenu.nib. Open the** `Window` **object in the Instances pane by double-clicking it.**

7. **From the Cocoa Containers pane of the Palettes window, drag a** `CustomView` **object to the** `Window` **object.**

Figure 12-3 illustrates this process.

Figure 12-3:
Add a Custom-View object from the Palettes window to your own window.

8. **Click to select CustomView in the window. Choose Tools➪Show Info. At the top of the Info window, select Custom Class from the popup menu.**

The Info window displays a large collection of class names.

9. **Locate and select the** `MyCanvas` **subclass that you just created, as shown in Figure 12-4.**

Figure 12-4:
Select
MyCanvas
from the
Custom
Class
settings of
the Info
window.

10. **From the popup menu at the top of the Info window, select Size and then set the following values:**

```
★  x = 0
★  y = 0
★  w = 520
★  h = 530
```

Figure 12-5 shows the adjusted `CustomView` values.

Figure 12-5:
Set the x, y,
w, and h
properties
of the
`Custom-`
`View`
object.

11. Select the Window object.

Its attributes appear in the Info window.

If you selected the `CustomView` object and it completely prevents your attempts to click the window behind it, shift-click the `CustomView`. Interface Builder deselects the `CustomView` and in turn selects the window behind it.

12. Change the `Window` size attributes to match those in Figure 12-6.

This interface consists of one window with a `CustomView` (named `MyCanvas`). Your graphics code will draw on this view.

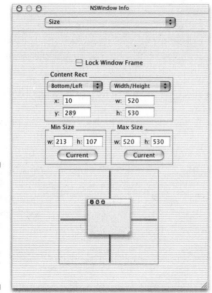

Figure 12-6:
In the Info window, change the size of the `Window` object.

13. Now that you're finished creating the interface, select the `MyCanvas` subclass in the Classes tab of the nib file window.

14. Choose Classes⇨Create Files for MyCanvas to add the header and implementation files to your Project Builder project.

Back in Project Builder, you'll see two new files: MyCanvas.h and MyCanvas.m. MyCanvas.m contains two methods. For most of your drawing needs, you'll focus mainly on the `drawRect` method. This is where you put all your commands to draw to the `MyCanvas` view:

```
- (void)drawRect:(NSRect)rect {
    // Drawing code here.
}
```

The bulk of your drawing code will appear in this method. The `drawRect` function takes care of redrawing your `CustomView`. The other method (`initWithFrame`) that is part of the MyCanvas.m file takes care of setting up the view's frame. You don't need to change anything in this method:

```
- (id)initWithFrame:(NSRect)frameRect
{
  [super initWithFrame:frameRect];
  return self;
}
```

Painting with Lines and Shapes

With your interface readied for displaying graphics, you can now add some code to make it display something. Before you draw something, you have to define what that "something" is. When it comes to defining shapes in Cocoa, paths are the name of the game.

Bezier paths

If you've ever played connect the dots, you're already well on your way to understanding how paths work. A *path* is a collection of points that together form the outline of a shape. For example, a square-shaped path has four points, an octagon-shaped path has eight points, and so on. Cocoa represents paths using a variable of type `NSBezierPath`. Normally, you begin working with paths by declaring a pointer to a `NSBezierPath`:

```
NSBezierPath *thePath;
```

Then you create a path. Your path might form a square, a circle, or some other shape. Because you'll want to create different shapes, Cocoa gives you several methods for creating paths.

One of the most common paths you'll create is the shape of a rectangle. For that, you can use the `bezierPathWithRect` function of the `NSBezierPath` class. It takes a `Rect` (which defines its origin and size) as its sole parameter. Because the `drawRect` function passes in a `Rect` that describes the dimensions of the `MyCanvas` object, you can easily create a rectangular path around `MyCanvas`:

```
- (void)drawRect:(NSRect)rect {
    // Drawing code here.

NSBezierPath *thePath;
thePath = [NSBezierPath bezierPathWithRect:rect];

}
```

Similarly, you can create an oval path the same size as `MyCanvas` by using the `bezierPathWithOvalInRect` function:

```
- (void)drawRect:(NSRect)rect {
    // Drawing code here.

NSBezierPath *thePath;
thePath = [NSBezierPath bezierPathWithOvalInRect:rect];

}
```

Other times, you may not want to limit your `Rect` to the size of `MyCanvas`. In these instances, simply create a `Rect` structure and pass that to the `NSBezier Path` functions. The following example creates a 50 x 50 circular path in the bottom-right corner of the view:

```
Rect theRect;
theRect = NSMakeRect(0, 0, 50, 50);

NSBezierPath *thePath;
thePath = [NSBezierPath bezierPathWithOvalInRect:theRect];
```

Fill a path

After you create a path, it's a simple matter to fill it in with your color of choice. Send the path the fill message and you're finished!

```
[thePath fill];
```

Of course, you'll want to create and set a color first. For example, to fill the entire background of the view with black, your code might look like this:

```
- (void)drawRect:(NSRect)rect {

  //create a path
```

```
NSBezierPath *thePath = [NSBezierPath
        bezierPathWithRect:rect];

//create a black color object
NSColor *theColor = [NSColor blackColor];

//set the color
[theColor set];

//fill the path with the current color (black)
[thePath fill];

}
```

Figure 12-7 shows the results of this code.

Figure 12-7:
Fill the
entire view
for a
background
effect.

You can use the same plan of attack to fill an NSRect that doesn't cover the entire background of the custom view. For example, to draw a white rectangle at the top of the view, use this code:

```
- (void)drawRect:(NSRect)rect {

    //create and define an NSRect
    NSRect theRect = NSMakeRect(70, rect.size.height-235, 120,
            230);

    //define a rectangular path
    thePath = [NSBezierPath bezierPathWithRect:theRect];

    //define a white color object
    theColor = [NSColor whiteColor];

    //set the color
    [theColor set];

    //fill the path with white
    [thePath fill];
}
```

Put the black and white together and you'll see a result like the one shown in Figure 12-8.

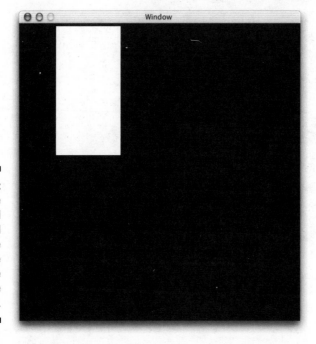

Figure 12-8:
Fill the background in black and fill a white rectangle towards the top of the view.

You aren't limited to filling rectangular paths. Remember that oval-shaped path you created earlier in this chapter? Now is a good time to put it to use. By creating three oval paths and filling them with red, green, and yellow, respectively, you can create a simple traffic light image. Add this code to the end of the `drawRect` function:

```
//*************************************
//      DRAW THE LIGHTS
//*************************************
  //create oval path
  theRect = NSMakeRect(100, rect.size.height-220, 60, 60);
  thePath = [NSBezierPath bezierPathWithOvalInRect:theRect];

  //fill oval in green
  theColor = [NSColor  colorWithDeviceRed:(float)0.0
              green:(float)1.0 blue:(float)0.0
          alpha:(float)1.0];
  [theColor set];
  [thePath fill];

  //create oval path
  theRect = NSMakeRect(100, rect.size.height-150, 60, 60);
  thePath = [NSBezierPath bezierPathWithOvalInRect:theRect];

  //fill oval in yellow
  theColor = [NSColor  colorWithDeviceRed:(float)1.0
              green:(float)1.0 blue:(float)0.0
          alpha:(float)1.0];
  [theColor set];
  [thePath fill];

  //create oval path
  theRect = NSMakeRect(100, rect.size.height-80, 60, 60);
  thePath = [NSBezierPath bezierPathWithOvalInRect:theRect];

  //fill oval in red
  theColor = [NSColor  colorWithDeviceRed:(float)1.0
              green:(float)0.0 blue:(float)0.0
          alpha:(float)1.0];
  [theColor set];
  [thePath fill];
```

The result looks like Figure 12-9.

Window

Figure 12-9:
Add a few
ovals to
create an
image of a
simple
traffic light.

Draw a path

You don't have to fill all paths that you run across. You can also stroke a path. This has the effect of drawing an outline around a path. It's just as simple to stroke a path as it is to fill one:

```
[thePath stroke];
```

You can also use a combination of fill and stroke for different effects. When you do, make sure to perform the stroke functions after the fill function, so that the outline will draw on top of the filled path. For example, suppose that you wanted to draw a black ring around one of the traffic lights. Your code might look like this:

```
//stroke oval in black
theColor = [NSColor blackColor];
[theColor set];
[thePath stroke];
```

This draws a thin outline around the light. If you'd prefer a thicker outline, use the path's setLineWidth function. The default line width is 1, so anything larger produces thicker lines.

```
[thePath setLineWidth: 5];
```

To draw an outline around each of the lights, adjust your drawRect function by adding the boldface code:

```
- (void)drawRect:(NSRect)rect
{

... code omitted ...

//***********************************
//     DRAW THE LIGHTS
//***********************************
    //create oval path
    theRect = NSMakeRect(100, rect.size.height-220, 60, 60);
    thePath = [NSBezierPath bezierPathWithOvalInRect:theRect];

    //fill oval in green
    theColor = [NSColor  colorWithDeviceRed:(float)0.0
                  green:(float)1.0 blue:(float)0.0
              alpha:(float)1.0];
    [theColor set];
    [thePath fill];

    //stroke oval in black
    theColor = [NSColor blackColor];
    [theColor set];
    [thePath setLineWidth: 5];
    [thePath stroke];

    //create oval path
    theRect = NSMakeRect(100, rect.size.height-150, 60, 60);
    thePath = [NSBezierPath bezierPathWithOvalInRect:theRect];

    //fill oval in yellow
    theColor = [NSColor  colorWithDeviceRed:(float)1.0
                  green:(float)1.0 blue:(float)0.0
              alpha:(float)1.0];
    [theColor set];
    [thePath fill];

    //stroke oval in black
    theColor = [NSColor blackColor];
    [theColor set];
    [thePath setLineWidth: 5];
    [thePath stroke];

    //create oval path
    theRect = NSMakeRect(100, rect.size.height-80, 60, 60);
    thePath = [NSBezierPath bezierPathWithOvalInRect:theRect];

    //fill oval in red
    theColor = [NSColor  colorWithDeviceRed:(float)1.0
                   green:(float)0.0 blue:(float)0.0
               alpha:(float)1.0];
```

```
    [theColor set];
    [thePath fill];

    //stroke oval in black
    theColor = [NSColor blackColor];
    [theColor set];
    [thePath setLineWidth: 5];
    [thePath stroke];
}

@end
```

Figure 12-10 shows the result of the code change.

Figure 12-10:
Draw an
outline
around
each of the
lights for an
added
effect.

Fancy-pants paths

So far, you've worked with rectangular and oval paths. Paths need not conform to these two simple shapes, though. A path can be as simple or as complex as you want.

Suppose that you want to display a stop sign next to your traffic light graphic. A stop sign is an eight-sided shape (an octagon). To create a stop-sign-shaped path, simply create eight NSPoint variables and populate them with points that represent the shape of a stop sign. Because it can get tedious tracking the various points in complex paths, Cocoa gives you the ability to define paths relative to the last point in the path. That way, you can define the starting point using the actual coordinates and define the rest of the path relative to that point.

If you want to move that path to another location later, you have to change only one point — the first one. The rest of the path follows the first point without any other code changes. The following code creates the points for a path in the shape of a stop sign. It uses points that are relative to the first point:

```
//*************************************
//  DRAW A STOP SIGN
//*************************************

    // Create the eight points of an octagon (stop sign)
    NSPoint pt1,pt2,pt3,pt4,pt5,pt6,pt7,pt8;

    //Define the points
    pt1 = NSMakePoint(300, rect.size.height-220);
    pt2 = NSMakePoint(100, 0);
    pt3 = NSMakePoint(50, 50);
    pt4 = NSMakePoint(0, 100);
    pt5 = NSMakePoint(-50, 50);
    pt6 = NSMakePoint(-100, 0);
    pt7 = NSMakePoint(-50, -50);
    pt8 = NSMakePoint(0, -100);
```

The first point is relative to the origin of the view. Each of the last seven points has a value that is relative to the point that precedes it in the list. To define relative point positions for a path, use the following guidelines:

- ✔ Positive x value: Path moves to the right
- ✔ Negative x value: Path moves to the left
- ✔ Positive y value: Path moves up
- ✔ Negative y value: Path moves down.

After you define the various points on the path, create the NSBezierPath with the bezierPath class method of the NSBezierPath class.

```
// Create the path
NSBezierPath *stopSign = [NSBezierPath bezierPath];
```

Next, add the points to the path. For the first point, use the moveToPoint function. For subsequent points, use the relativeLineToPoint function, because you should position these points relative to the first point:

```
[stopSign moveToPoint:pt1];
[stopSign relativeLineToPoint:pt2];
[stopSign relativeLineToPoint:pt3];
```

```
[stopSign relativeLineToPoint:pt4];
[stopSign relativeLineToPoint:pt5];
[stopSign relativeLineToPoint:pt6];
[stopSign relativeLineToPoint:pt7];
[stopSign relativeLineToPoint:pt8];
```

Finally, close the path using the `closePath` function:

```
[stopSign closePath];
```

With a path defined, you can apply the usual color, fill, and stroke commands to it. For example, to fill the stop sign in with red and outline it in white, use code like this:

```
// Draw the path
[[NSColor redColor] set];
[stopSign fill];

// Draw the path
[[NSColor whiteColor] set];
[stopSign setLineWidth: 10];
[stopSign stroke];
```

Combined, the code in this section produces result like those shown in Figure 12-11.

Figure 12-11:
Fill and
stroke the
path to see
the stop
sign appear
before your
eyes.

Drawing Text

Besides shapes and paths, Cocoa is quite adept at displaying text in graphics. Before you start drawing text, you need to load that text into an NSString variable. For example, *STOP* is an appropriate string to display on a stop sign:

```
NSString *theString;
theString = @"STOP";
```

You also need to determine the location in the view where you'd like to display the text. Store that position in an NSPoint:

```
NSPoint theTextPos;
theTextPos = NSMakePoint(275, rect.size.height-150);
```

Finally, draw the string with the drawAtPoint function, passing it the NSPoint:

```
[theString drawAtPoint:theTextPos withAttributes:nil];
```

This line of code draws the text at the position determined by the NSPoint. When you run the example, you may be disappointed with the results. The *STOP* string appears in a tiny font and the letters are black, the default text settings. Clearly, you'll want to define how the font looks. To accomplish this, you need to pass something other than nil in the withAttributes parameter of the drawAtPoint function. The withAttributes parameter takes an NSDictionary, so you'll need to declare and create one of those.

An NSMutableDictionary is a container for a collection of items; in this case a collection of text attributes. NSMutableDictionary is a subclass of NSDictionary, so it works in place of an NSDictionary. A *mutable* object is one that you can change sometime after you create it. An *immutable* object is one that you can't change after creating it. Mutable classes (such as NSMutableDictionary) have the word *mutable* in their names. Immutable objects (such as NSDictionary) do not.

```
NSMutableDictionary *theAttributes;

//create the NSDictionary object
theAttributes = [[NSMutableDictionary alloc] init];
```

Next, you add objects to the NSMutableDictionary that represent some text attribute. For example, to set the font to Times with a size of 62, use code like this:

```
[theAttributes setObject:
        [NSFont fontWithName: @"Times" size: 62] forKey:
        NSFontAttributeName];
```

You can set the color of the text in a similar fashion. This code adds a white text color attribute to the NSDictionary:

```
[theAttributes setObject:
    [NSColor whiteColor] forKey:
        NSForegroundColorAttributeName];
```

When you're finished adding text attribute objects to the NSDictionary, simply pass the dictionary object in the withAttributes parameter of the drawAtPoint function:

```
[theString drawAtPoint:theTextPos withAttributes:
        theAttributes];
```

Finally, don't forget to dispose of the NSDictionary:

```
[theAttributes release];
```

The combined code to draw the string on the stop sign looks like this:

```
//************************************
//  DRAW SOME TEXT
//************************************
    //Define a string
    NSString *theString;
    theString = @"STOP";

    //Position the text
    NSPoint theTextPos;
    theTextPos = NSMakePoint(275, rect.size.height-150);


    //Create the NSDictionary object
    NSMutableDictionary *theAttributes;
    theAttributes = [[NSMutableDictionary alloc] init];
```

```
//Add attributes to the NSDictionary
[theAttributes setObject:
    [NSFont fontWithName: @"Times" size: 62]
    forKey: NSFontAttributeName];

[theAttributes setObject:
    [NSColor whiteColor] forKey:
        NSForegroundColorAttributeName];

//Draw the text
[theString drawAtPoint:theTextPos withAttributes:
        theAttributes];

//Dispose of the NSDictionary
[theAttributes release];
```

You can view the results in Figure 12-12.

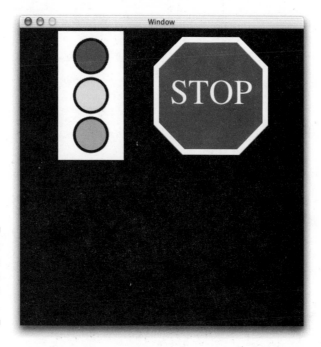

Figure 12-12:
Add text to
the stop
sign to make
it complete.

Displaying an Image

Eventually, you'll grow tired of creating your own graphics and want to display an image file instead. The easiest way to display an image file in your Cocoa app is to add the file directly to the project. For example, if you were to drag an image named face.jpg from Finder to Project Builder, your project might look like Figure 12-13.

Figure 12-13:
Drag an image from Finder to your project for easy access.

To draw this image in a view, you need to add only a few lines of code:

1. **Create an** NSPoint **to hold the coordinates for where you want to display the image.**

   This code creates an NSPoint for the lower-left corner of the view:

   ```
   NSPoint theImagePos;
   theImagePos = NSMakePoint(0, 0);
   ```

2. **Create an** NSImage **object and load the image into it.**

   ```
   NSImage* theImage;
   theImage = [NSImage imageNamed:@"face.jpg"];
   ```

3. **Display the image in the view by calling the** `dissolveToPoint` **function.**

```
[theImage dissolveToPoint: theImagePos fraction:(1.0)];
```

Figure 12-14 demonstrates the `dissolveToPoint` function in action.

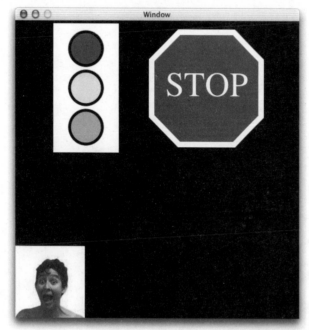

Figure 12-14:
Draw an image in a view by using the `dissolve-ToPoint` function.

The `fraction` parameter of the `dissolveToPoint` function represents the opacity of the image. The smaller the value you use for the fraction, the more transparent it is. A value of 1.0 indicates no transparency; a value of 0.0 denotes complete transparency. Figure 12-15 shows the effect of different opacity settings.

To see how opacity works, add this code to the end of your `drawRect` function:

```
NSPoint theImagePos;
theImagePos = NSMakePoint(0, 0);

NSImage* theImage;
theImage = [NSImage imageNamed:@"face.jpg"];
```

```
int i;
for (i=3; i<7; i++)
{
    [theImage dissolveToPoint: theImagePos
        fraction:(i*0.1)];
    theImagePos.x = theImagePos.x + 130;
}

theImagePos = NSMakePoint(0, 130);
for (i = 7;i<=10;i++)
{
    [theImage dissolveToPoint: theImagePos
        fraction:(i*0.1)];
    theImagePos.x = theImagePos.x + 130;
}
```

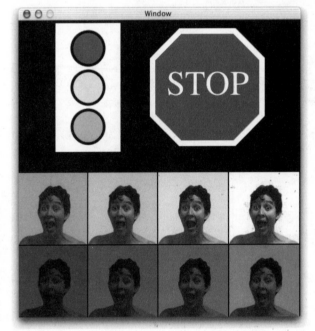

Figure 12-15:
Change the opacity of an image for different effects.

Chapter 13

Managing Your Files

· ·

In This Chapter

▶ Using file paths in Cocoaz

▶ Opening files

▶ Finding out about files

▶ Displaying a Files icon in your interface

▶ Copying, moving, and deleting files and folders

▶ Creating folders

· ·

Almost every device that Apple ships sports some kind of storage device. Whether it's the hard drive in your iPod, a Zip drive on your desktop Macintosh, or a CD burner on your PowerBook, all storage devices share one common trait — they store data. To facilitate this storage, the Mac OS X operating system uses a hierarchical system of files.

Cocoa has a large array of functions that it can perform to make your file manipulation tasks easier. With only a few lines of code, it's a cinch to open, copy, move, and delete any file or folder on your hard drive. This chapter shows you how.

About Files and Folders in Mac OS X

Mac OS X has several types of files. You are undoubtedly familiar with the most basic file type — a document. You use document files every time you save work in your favorite word processor. Later, when you want to view the document, you simple reopen it with your word processor.

Documents aren't the only type of file on your Mac, though. Another important file type is the application. You're probably also very familiar with this type of file, because you use applications to surf the Web, send e-mail, draw pictures, or program with Project Builder. In fact, the whole point of Cocoa programming is to create applications. Carbon applications often come in the form of a single executable file. Cocoa applications, on the other hand, almost never do. Instead, Cocoa applications are a directory (a package) that Finder treats as a single file. The directory contains directories and individual files that contain the executable and supporting files for your application.

To help you keep your documents and applications in order, Mac OS X organizes files in a hierarchical structure of folders. *Folders* are containers of files. A folder can hold documents, applications, or even other folders. Some folders contain your operating system; others are ones that you create and modify yourself.

Computer geeks also refer to folders as *directories*. This chapter uses the terms *folder* and *directory* interchangeably. Not content to keep things simple, geeks also refer to *applications* as *executables*. The two terms are synonyms, so whenever you hear someone say, "place the executable in the directory," you can be sure that they mean "place the application in the folder."

Besides traditional folders, Mac OS X has a special kind of folder called the bundle. Like folders, bundles can hold any number of files and folders. What makes bundles unique is that they can act like applications. If you arrange files and folders within a folder according to Apple's specifications, it constitutes a *bundle*. You can then double-click that bundle to launch the application(s) that reside in it. The idea here is that an application can store its resources (such as pictures, audio, and data) in the same bundle as the application. This keeps the accessory files with the application, while also hiding them from the user. That way, users will be less likely to delete files that are important to the operation of an application.

To confuse naming matters even further, you will also hear the terms *package* and *bundle* used to mean the same thing. Control-click a bundle in Finder and you will find a menu item called Show Package Contents. Choosing it opens the bundle as a folder to reveal its contents.

For years, Macintosh users have happily navigated the files on their hard drives by double-clicking a folder icon to open it. With Mac OS X, newbie Mac users got their first taste of the command line by using the Terminal. There, they discovered the strange and frightening world of paths. *Paths* are a textual method of describing where a file or folder resides on a drive. For example, the Mac OS X Fonts folder resides in the following location:

```
/Library/Fonts
```

Whenever you see the / character, you should think of the word *folder*. You can see in the preceding example that the Fonts folder resides in the Library folder. If your current username is Fred, your home folder is located at this path:

```
/Users/Fred
```

These two examples of paths assume that you're describing a file folder or file on your boot drive. The boot drive contains the operating system that you're using at any one time. If you have other drives connected to your machine, the path of a file or folder located on that machine is preceded by Volumes and the name of the drive. For example, if you have an image file named VacationPhoto.jpg that resides on a drive named Drive2, its path looks like this:

```
/Volumes/Drive2/VacationPhoto.jpg
```

Opening Files and Using Them

To begin working with files, you need a project. The project for this chapter displays important information about any file or folder that a user selects. You'll be familiar with the information, because all of it appears in the Get Info window of Finder.

Building the interface

The interface consists of a button and a whole bunch of NSTextField controls. Users will click the button to select a file or folder. Then the application displays information about that file or folder in the various NSTextField controls. To create the interface for this project, perform these steps:

1. **Create a new Cocoa project in Project Builder, naming it File Demo. After it opens, expand its Resources folder and double-click the MainMenu.nib file to open it in Interface Builder.**

2. **In Interface Builder, open the Window window from the MainMenu.nib file. To this window, add the following seven NSTextField controls from the Palette window.**

   - File Location

   - File Name

   - YES, if a file exists; NO, if it doesn't

- YES, if a file is a folder; NO, if it isn't
- File Creation Date
- File Modification Date
- File Size

Change the Title attribute of each NSTextField to blank (that is, delete all the text in each field). You'll use these controls to display information about a file or folder.

3. **To help you make sense of these seven NSTextFields, add seven more NSTextField controls to the window. Change the Title attribute in the Info window for each of these new NSTextFields to describe what the previous seven will display.**

   Figure 13-1 shows what the interface should look like at this point with all fourteen NSTextField controls. You'll notice a large number of circles indicating the border of each NSTextField. This is to show you the position of each NSTextField, even if it doesn't currently have a Title.

Figure 13-1:
Add 14
NSText
Field
controls to
the window.

4. **Next, add an NSButton control to the window. Using the Info window, change the Title attribute of the button to Select File or Folder, as shown in Figure 13-2.**

Figure 13-2:
Add an
NSButton
that users
will click to
select a file
or folder.

5. **Finally, add an** NSImageView **to the window. Resize it to dimensions of**
   128 x 128 using the Info window.

   This view is where you'll display a file's icon later in this chapter.

Now that you have an interface in place, you need to create a controller class.
Perform the following steps:

1. **In the MainMenu.nib file window, click the Classes tab.**

2. **Create the new class.**

   Scroll to the left edge of the MainMenu.nib file window. Select NSObject
   and press Return. Name the new class MyFileController, as shown in
   Figure 13-3.

Figure 13-3:
Add a
subclass
titled
MyFile
Con-
troller
to the
MainMenu.
nib file.

3. **Add eight outlets to the** `MyFileController` **class.**

   These eight outlets should have descriptive names that tell you the purpose of each. You'll connect seven of them to the `NSTextFields`. The eighth outlet connects to the `NSImageView`. Name them as shown in Figure 13-4.

Figure 13-4:
Add eight outlets to the class.

4. **Add an action to the class.**

   Add an action to the class in the Info window and name it selectTheFile.

5. **Instantiate** `MyFileController`.

   Choose Class⇨Instantiate MyFileController to create an instance of this class.

6. **Connect the interface to the** `MyFileController` **outlets.**

   In the Instances tab of the MainMenu.nib file window, Control-drag from the `MyFileController` instance to each of the `NSTextFields` in your interface's main window. Click Connect in the Info window to connect each control to its corresponding outlet in the instance. Next, Control-drag from the `MyFileController` to the `NSImageView` control. Click Connect in the Info window to connect the control to the `fileIconDisplay` outlet.

7. **Connect the interface to the `MyFileController` action.**

   Control-drag from the `NSButton` in the interface to the MyFileController instance in the MainMenu.nib file window. Click Connect in the Info window to connect the button to the `selectFile` action (see Figure 13-5).

Figure 13-5: Connect the button in your interface to the `select File` action.

8. **Create the files for the `MyFileController` class.**

   In the Classes tab of the MainMenu.nib file window, click the `MyFileController` class. Then choose Classes⇨Create Files for MyController to create the Project Builder files for your class.

Open sesame . . . er, panel

Now, you can finally return to Project Builder to add some code to make this interface functional. Don't forget about the goal of this project — to select a file and report information about it. To display information about a specific file or folder, you need to use Cocoa's `OpenPanel` class. With the `OpenPanel` class, you can display an Open dialog that allows a user to select a file or folder. When you use an `OpenPanel`, you typically follow four basic steps:

1. Create an instance of `OpenPanel`.

2. Alter the attributes of the `OpenPanel` instance.

3. Display the `OpenPanel` for the user and wait for the user to do something with it: select a file and click OK or cancel the operation.

4. Do something with the file that the user selected.

To see how `OpenPanel` works in Cocoa, perform these four steps.

1. **Create an `OpenPanel` instance.**

   You do so in the same way that you create other objects in Cocoa:

   ```
   NSOpenPanel *theOpenPanel = [NSOpenPanel openPanel];
   ```

2. **Alter the attributes of the `OpenPanel` by calling one or more of its methods.**

   For example, to change the Title of the `OpenPanel`, use the `setTitle` method.

   ```
   [theOpenPanel setTitle:@"Choose a File or Folder"];
   ```

   The `setTitle` method of the `OpenPanel` is a method provided by the `NSWindow` superclass. Because the `OpenPanel` is a subclass of `NSWindow`, it can take advantage of the `NSWindow` methods. The `OpenPanel` class also has methods of its own. For example, you'll want to tell the `Open Panel` which files a user may open or select. By default, an `Open Panel` lets users choose any document or application that they want, but they can't choose folders. You can remedy the situation by adding a call to the `setCanChooseDirectories` method of the `OpenPanel`. This method takes one parameter, a Boolean. If you set it to YES, users can select folders in the `OpenPanel`. If you set it to NO (or if you don't use this `setCanChooseDirectories` method at all), users will not be able to choose folders in the `OpenPanel`.

   ```
   [theOpenPanel setCanChooseDirectories:YES];
   ```

3. **Display the `OpenPanel`.**

   You have several options when it comes to displaying `OpenPanel`. The most basic way to display one is to use its `runModal` method, which returns an integer upon completion.

   ```
   int i = [theOpenPanel runModal];
   ```

   The result of this line of code is the modal dialog shown in Figure 13-6.

Choose a File or Folder

From: Fonts

- Comic Sans MS
- Copperplate.dfont
- Courier New
- Didot.dfont
- Futura.dfont
- Georgia
- GillSans.dfont
- HelveticaNeue.dfont
- Herculanum.dfont
- MarkerFelt.dfont
- Optima.dfont
- Papyrus.dfont
- Taipei.dfont

Kind: Data-fork font suitcase
Size: 308 KB
Created: 18 Jul 2002
Modified: 18 Jul 2002

Go to:

Add to Favorites   Cancel   Open

Figure 13-6:
Display an
OpenPanel
using the
runModal
method.

4. **Find out what the user did with the** OpenPanel.

   To find out whether the user clicked OK or Cancel in the OpenPanel,
   you must examine the value that runModal returns. If the user clicked
   OK, the return value is NSOKButton, a constant that Cocoa provides for
   you. If the user cancels the open operation instead, the return value is
   NSCancelButton.

   ```
   int i = [theOpenPanel runModal];
   if (i == NSOKButton)
   {
   NSLog(@"The user clicked OK!");
   }
   ```

Rather than create a new variable just to check the return value, it's customary to wrap the runModal command into the if statement.

```
if ([theOpenPanel runModal] == NSOKButton)
{
NSLog(@"The user clicked OK!");
}
```

Finding a file's path, name, and more

After you discover that a user has clicked OK in the OpenPanel, you should
inquire as to which file or folder the user selected. By using the filename

method of the OpenPanel class, you can get the path to that file or folder in the form of an NSString:

```
NSString *theFilePath = [theOpenPanel filename];
```

To display the path in the interface, call the setStringValue method of the filePathDisplay outlet:

```
[filePathDisplay setStringValue:theFilePath];
```

Besides the path of the file, you can discover all sorts of interesting things about a file using the NSFileManager class. First, create a new NSFileManager object using the defaultManager method:

```
NSFileManager *theManager = [NSFileManager defaultManager];
```

Then call the various NSFileManager methods to find out information about a file. For example, to retrieve the file name from the selected file, use the displayNameAtPath method. Because the method returns an NString, you can nest the call to display it in the interface. In this case, display it using the outlet named fileNameDisplay:

```
[fileNameDisplay setStringValue:
        [theManager displayNameAtPath:theFilePath]];
```

If you'd like to know whether the file exists, use the fileExistsAtPath method of the NSFileManager:

```
if ( [theManager fileExistsAtPath:theFilePath ] )
    [fileExistsDisplay setStringValue:@"YES"];
else
    [fileExistsDisplay setStringValue:@"NO"];
```

If you want to find out whether the selected file is a directory, use the alternate version of the fileExistsAtPath method. The alternate version has two parameters: the file's path and a pointer to a Boolean. After this call completes its execution, the Boolean value holds a value of YES if the file in the first parameter is a directory:

```
if ( [theManager fileExistsAtPath:theFilePath ] )
    [fileExistsDisplay setStringValue:@"YES"];
else
    [fileExistsDisplay setStringValue:@"NO"];
```

You can also find out a fair amount about a file using the fileAttributes AtPath method, but first you need to create an NSDictionary. Use an NSDictionary here instead of an NSMutableDictionary, because there is no need to change the data in that dictionary. You are simply filling in the NSDictionary so you can read its contents. Because you aren't making any changes to the data in that dictionary, you can safely use the NSDictionary class instead of NSMutableDictionary.

```
NSDictionary *theFileAttributes = [theManager
        fileAttributesAtPath:theFilePath
        traverseLink:YES];
```

Note that the fileAttributesAtPath method returns an NSDictionary. An NSDictionary is a data structure that holds a collection of different values. This NSDictionary returns a collection of data about a file or folder, including the following:

- ✔ File size: The size of a file or folder, measured in bytes
- ✔ Creation date: The date the file or folder was created
- ✔ Modification date: The date the file or folder was last modified

To extract this data from the NSDictionary object, use the objectForKey method of the NSManager instance:

```
NSNumber *theFileSize;
NSDate *theModificationDate;
NSDate *theCreationDate;

if (theFileSize = [theFileAttributes
        objectForKey:NSFileSize])        [fileSizeDisplay
        setIntValue:(int)theFileSize];

if (theModificationDate = [theFileAttributes
        objectForKey:NSFileModificationDate])
    [fileModifiedDisplay
        setStringValue:(NSString*)theModificationDate];

if (theCreationDat = [theFileAttributes
        objectForKey:NSFileCreationDate])
    [fileCreatedDisplay
        setStringValue:(NSString*)theCreationDate];
```

Viewing a file's icon

The icon is another great feature of Finder. Without icons, we'd be stuck back in the dark days of DOS. Yikes! Fortunately, it's easy to work with icons in Cocoa. But before you grab an icon from a file, you must create an NSFileWrapper. An NSFileWrapper is an object that stores a file's data in memory. For this example, though, you'll use it to load the file's icon into memory. To create an NSFileWrapper instance, initialize it with the path that you found earlier:

```
NSFileWrapper *theFileWrapper = [ [[NSFileWrapper alloc]
initWithPath:theFilePath] autorelease];
```

Then extract the icon from the file using the icon method of the NSFile
Wrapper. This call returns an NSImage, which you can then display in the
NSImageView of the interface. Because you want to view the icon at dimensions of 128 x 128, stretch the icon to the size of the NSImageView using set
ImageScaling before displaying it. NSScaleToFit is just one of a few scaling
values that you can place in this parameter. To see the others, Option-double-
click the word *NSScaleToFit* to view the online documentation for this call:

```
NSImage *theIcon = [theFileWrapper icon];
[fileIconDisplay setImageScaling:NSScaleToFit];
[fileIconDisplay setImage:theIcon];
```

With your icon code in place, the complete code listing for the selectFile
action is as follows:

```
- (IBAction)selectTheFile:(id)sender
{
    NSOpenPanel *theOpenPanel = [NSOpenPanel openPanel];
    [theOpenPanel setTitle:@"Choose a File or Folder"];
    [theOpenPanel setCanChooseDirectories:YES];

    if ([theOpenPanel runModal] == NSOKButton)
    {
        NSString *theFilePath = [theOpenPanel filename];

        //Display the file's path
        [filePathDisplay setStringValue:theFilePath];

        NSFileManager *theManager = [NSFileManager
            defaultManager];
        [fileNameDisplay setStringValue:[theManager
            displayNameAtPath:theFilePath]];

        //Does the file really exist at this path?
        if ( [theManager fileExistsAtPath:theFilePath ] )
[fileExistsDisplay setStringValue:@"YES"];
        else
            [fileExistsDisplay setStringValue:@"NO"];

        //Is the file a directory?
        BOOL isFolder;
        if ( [theManager fileExistsAtPath:theFilePath
            isDirectory:&isFolder] && isFolder )
            [fileDirDisplay setStringValue:@"YES"];
        else
            [fileDirDisplay setStringValue:@"NO"];
```

```
        //Get file attributes
        NSNumber *theFileSize;
        NSDate *theModificationDate;
        NSDate *theCreationDate;
        NSDictionary *theFileAttributes =
[theManager fileAttributesAtPath:theFilePath
traverseLink:YES];
        if (theFileSize =
[theFileAttributes objectForKey:NSFileSize])
            [fileSizeDisplay setIntValue:(int)theFileSize];
        if (theModificationDate =
[theFileAttributes objectForKey:NSFileModificationDate])
            [fileModifiedDisplay
            setStringValue:(NSString*)theModificationDate];
        if (theCreationDate =
[theFileAttributes objectForKey:NSFileCreationDate])
            [fileCreatedDisplay
            setStringValue:(NSString*)theCreationDate];

        //Retrieve and draw the file's icon
        NSFileWrapper *theFileWrapper = [ [[NSFileWrapper
            alloc]
initWithPath:theFilePath] autorelease];
        NSImage *theIcon = [theFileWrapper icon];
        [fileIconDisplay setImageScaling:NSScaleToFit];
        [fileIconDisplay setImage:theIcon];
    }
}
```

To test your work, choose Build⇨Build and Debug. The result should look like Figure 13-7.

Figure 13-7: With the NSFile Manager and NSFile Wrapper, you can easily display a variety of tidbits about a file.

Reading from and writing to documents

Many types of files are on your hard drive. Each file type has its own format, whether it's text, graphics, fonts, or audio. Cocoa has built-in functions to deal with common file formats. For example, Cocoa is adept at working with text documents of all sorts. Refer to Chapter 11 to get the scoop on working with text files.

Graphics is another place where Cocoa shines. Whether you need to view a PICT file, save a JPEG file, or convert a view to PDF, Cocoa and the underlying QuickTime engine of Mac OS X have you covered. You can find information about working with graphics files in Chapter 12.

Multimedia is yet another highlight of the Mac OS. Chapter 16 discusses the use of audio and video files in your applications. There, you'll find the code you need to view QuickTime movie files as well as play a variety of audio files.

If you're an experienced C or C++ programmer, keep in mind that all standard C file functions are available to you in Cocoa, too.

Working with Files and Folders

Copying and moving files are important functions that you may want to perform in your applications. To add these features to your project, follow these steps:

1. **Open your MainMenu.nib file in Interface Builder again.**

2. **To your main window, add two new NSButtons and change their titles.**

   To follow along with the example, change the Title of one button to Copy File to Desktop. As you may have guessed, when users click this button, they can select a file. The application then duplicates that file, placing it on the desktop.

   Change the Title attribute of the other NSButton to MoveFile to Desktop.

3. **Add a new action to the MyFileController class in the Info window.**

   To follow along with the example, name the action copyTheFile.

4. **Connect the action to the button.**

   To do so, Control-drag from the button to the MyFileController instance in the nib file.

5. **Save your interface and return to Project Builder.**

6. **In Project Builder, add the new actions to the MyFileController.h file, placing them after the** selectTheFile **action.**

The resulting header file looks like this.

```
/* MyFileController */

#import <Cocoa/Cocoa.h>

@interface MyFileController : NSObject
{
    IBOutlet id fileCreatedDisplay;
    IBOutlet id fileDirDisplay;
    IBOutlet id fileExistsDisplay;
    IBOutlet id fileIconDisplay;
    IBOutlet id fileModifiedDisplay;
    IBOutlet id fileNameDisplay;
    IBOutlet id filePathDisplay;
    IBOutlet id fileSizeDisplay;
}
- (IBAction)selectTheFile:(id)sender;
- (IBAction)copyTheFile:(id)sender;
- (IBAction)moveTheFile:(id)sender;
@end
```

Copying files and folders

To copy a file or folder, you need two things:

 ✔ Source path: The path to the file that you want to copy
 ✔ Destination path: Where you want the file copy to reside

You can get the source file from the OpenPanel class covered earlier in this chapter. You could do something similar for the destination using the SavePanel, but this time you know where you want the resulting file to appear: on the desktop. Therefore, you can create your own path that points to a new file on the desktop.

First, you know that the Desktop folder resides in the user's Home directory. You can gain access to it using the NSHomeDirectory function in the Foundation class. Then, simply tack on additional parts of the path using the stringByAppendingPathComponent method (say *that* five times fast!).

```
NSString *theDestination = [ [NSHomeDirectory()
    stringByAppendingPathComponent:@"Desktop"]
    stringByAppendingPathComponent:theFileName ];
```

Finally, copy the file by using the `copyPath` method of the `NSFileManager` class. Pass it the source path, the destination path, and `nil` for the handler:

```
[theManager copyPath:theFilePath
toPath:theDestination handler:nil];
```

The resulting `copyTheFile` action looks like this:

```
- (IBAction)copyTheFile:(id)sender
{
    NSOpenPanel *theOpenPanel = [NSOpenPanel openPanel];
    [theOpenPanel setTitle:@"Choose a File or Folder to
            copy"];
    [theOpenPanel setCanChooseDirectories:YES];

    if ([theOpenPanel runModal] == NSOKButton)
    {
        NSString *theFilePath = [theOpenPanel filename];
        NSFileManager *theManager =
[NSFileManager defaultManager];
        NSString *theFileName =
[theManager displayNameAtPath:theFilePath];

        NSString *theDestination =
[ [NSHomeDirectory()
            stringByAppendingPathComponent:@"Desktop"]
            stringByAppendingPathComponent:theFileName ];

        [theManager copyPath:theFilePath
toPath:theDestination handler:nil];
    }
}
```

Moving files and folders

Moving a file is just as simple as duplicating one. In fact, for this demonstration, the code is identical to the `copyTheFile` action, except for one line. Instead of the `copyPath` method, use the `movePath` method. The code for your `moveTheFile` action looks like this:

```
- (IBAction)moveTheFile:(id)sender
{

    NSOpenPanel *theOpenPanel = [NSOpenPanel openPanel];
    [theOpenPanel setTitle:@"Choose a File or Folder to
            move"];
    [theOpenPanel setCanChooseDirectories:YES];
```

```
    if ([theOpenPanel runModal] == NSOKButton)
    {
        NSString *theFilePath = [theOpenPanel filename];
        NSFileManager *theManager =
[NSFileManager defaultManager];
        NSString *theFileName =
[theManager displayNameAtPath:theFilePath];

        NSString *theDestination =
[ [NSHomeDirectory()
            stringByAppendingPathComponent:@"Desktop"]
            stringByAppendingPathComponent:theFileName ];

        [theManager movePath:theFilePath
toPath:theDestination handler:nil];

    }
}
```

Deleting files and folders

Sometimes you'll want to delete files from a drive. Rather than bore you with another identical code example, I'll simply tell you that the code to delete a file resembles the copyTheFile and moveTheFile except for the last command. Look up the removeFileAtPath method in the NSFileManager documentation. Doing so will give you experience in looking up calls in the documentation and provide you with an ample amount of time to consider why you would want to use this call.

Delete a file and it's gone! Permanently. Make sure that your users know that a deletion will occur and always give them a way out.

Creating folders

To create a folder on your drive, use the createDirectoryAtPath method of the NSFileManager. You need to pass it two parameters. You should recognize the first parameter as the path where you would like to create the folder. The second parameter lets you set various attributes of the folder. You won't use this second parameter very often, so you can simply set it to nil.

To show the createDirectoryAtPath method in action, the following code snippet creates a folder on the desktop titled MyNewFolder:

```
- (IBAction)createAFolder:(id)sender
{
    NSString *theDestination = [ [NSHomeDirectory()
        stringByAppendingPathComponent:@"Desktop"]
        stringByAppendingPathComponent:@"MyNewFolder" ];

    [theManager createDirectoryAtPath:theDestination
        attributes:nil];
}
```

If you use this action, don't forget to define it in the header file:

```
- (IBAction)createAFolder:(id)sender;
```

Then, add an action to `MyFileController` and connect it to a new `NSButton` in Interface Builder. Figure 13-8 shows the completed interface for this chapter.

Figure 13-8:
The completed Files project can display information about a file or folder as well as perform a variety of file tasks.

Sometimes it's easiest to simply add actions and outlets to your project in Project Builder and your nib file in Interface Builder, rather than relying on those applications to talk to each other.

To test your work, return to Project Builder and press Cmd-R.

Chapter 14

Printing with Cocoa

• •

In This Chapter

▶ Understanding the process of printing in Cocoa

▶ Adjusting the page settings

▶ Running a print job

▶ Printing to PDF files

• •

*A*lthough Cocoa's on-screen display of graphics and text is world class, that doesn't mean Apple forgot about printing. Known for decades as one of the innovative adopting forces behind technologies such as Postscript and laser printing, Apple continues in this tradition by adding easy-to-implement printing features to Cocoa. This chapter shows you how to add printing features to your Cocoa applications. Although printing has been a messy topic for programmers in the past, Cocoa makes it simple to implement some sophisticated printing features to your projects. You'll love the consistency that Apple provides you, the Cocoa programmer, and your users will love the professional printing results that your application implements.

How Printing Works in Cocoa

To help you achieve great results that address all your printing needs, Cocoa offers a collection of important classes for printing in Mac OS X. You use these classes together to add printing to your applications:

▶ NSView: Printing to a page is as simple as drawing text and graphics in an NSView. The demonstration in this chapter builds on the graphics example presented in the Graphics chapter (Chapter 12).

▶ NSPageLayout: This class is responsible for displaying the Page Setup panel. Typical applications display this panel when a user chooses File⇨Page Setup. You users will invoke the Page Setup panel to choose the orientation of the printed page. They can also set the paper size in the Page Setup panel. When the user has finished adjusting the printing properties of the NSPageLayout object, the NSPageLayoutObject saves the results in an NSPrintInfo object.

✔ NSPrintInfo: NSPrintInfo is a storage class that holds the settings and options for printing. NSPrintInfo stores the settings from the Page Setup panel as well as the page count, margins, and other items that appear in the NSPrintPanel.

✔ NSPrintPanel: When you choose File⇨Print from most applications, you see an example of the NSPrintPanel. The NSPrintPanel is responsible for managing the settings of a print job. Like the NSPagePanel, NSPrintPanel stores its settings in an NSPrintInfo object.

✔ NSPrintOperation: This class takes care of creating the printed page. It displays the Print panel and carries out the print job.

To help you envision how the printing process works in Cocoa, here's a list of the basic steps involved:

1. **Your application draws some text or graphics in a view.**

   This drawing can occur in any view, whether it's a view in a graphics application, a word processor, or even the background of a window. Cocoa can print from them all.

2. **The user chooses File⇨Page Setup.**

   Your application displays the Page panel, where the user selects the paper size and orientation of the page. Figure 14-1 shows the Page panel. When finished, the user dismisses the panel and your application stores the settings in a PrintInfo object.

3. **The user chooses File⇨Print**

   Your application displays the Print panel, where the user tweaks the settings for the print job. Figure 14-2 shows a typical Print panel. When the user finishes preparing the print job, he or she may dismiss the panel by clicking Cancel or start the print job by clicking OK.

Figure 14-1:
Use the
Page panel
to adjust
settings for
the pages
in your
print job.

Figure 14-2:
Use the
Print panel
to adjust
settings for
the print job.

4. **Print the view.**

   Your application sets up the print operation using the Page panel and
   Print panel settings that you stored in the `PrintInfo` object. Then you
   print the view. The view's `drawRect` takes care of drawing the graphics
   or text, just as it does on the screen.

Tweaking the Page Settings

The first step of your printing journey begins with the Page panel, where
your users select the paper size and page orientation. If you have access to
multiple printers, you'll also choose a Format For option to get the dimensions
of a printable area. The dimensions help you avoid cropping around the edges.

To begin working with printing, copy the Start source code for this chapter to
your hard drive. (To download the code, go to `www.dummies.com/extras`.)
It's essentially a project based on the completed project from Chapter 12.
Because you can print using any view, you can use the graphics view from
Chapter 12 as your printable canvas.

Open the Project Builder project for this chapter. Double-click the Main-
Menu.nib file to open the interface for this project in Interface Builder. After
the nib file is opened, follow these steps to add a print controller to the
project:

1. **Create a new class.**

   Click the Classes tab in the nib file window. In the leftmost list of
   classes, click `NSObject`. Press Return to create a new class. Name it
   `MyPrintController`. Figure 14-3 shows the new class.

Figure 14-3:
The
MyPrint-
Control-
ler class
will take of
all printing
tasks.

2. **Add an outlet and two actions to the** `MyPrintController`.

In the Info window, add an outlet named `myCanvasView` to the `MyPrintController` class. Then add two actions to the controller. Name them `printOnePage` and `showPagePanel`. The `showPagePanel` action will take care of displaying the Page panel and storing its settings. The `printOnePage` action will handle the tasks of displaying the Print panel and print executing the print job.

3. **Create an instance of** `MyPrintController`.

In the Classes tab of the nib file window, select the `MyPrintController` class, and then choose `Classes`⇨Instantiate MyPrintController.

4. **Connect the MyPrintController instance to the interface.**

Control-drag from the `MyPrintController` instance to the view in the main window of your interface. Select the `myCanvasView` outlet in the Info window and click Connect. Figure 14-4 shows the connected `myCanvasView` outlet.

Next, connect the two actions to the menu for this project as follows. Control-drag from the Page Setup menu item to the `MyPrintController` instance. Select the `showPagePanel` action in the Info window and click Connect. Do the same for the Print menu item and the `printOnePage` action in the Info window.

5. **Create the files for** `MyPrintController`.

In the Classes tab of the nib file window, select `MyPrintController`. Choose Classes⇨Create Files for MyPrintController to add the header and implementation files to your project in Project Builder.

Return to Project Builder and click the MyPrintController.h file to view its contents. Change your MyPrintController.h file to read as follows:

```
/* MyPrintController */

#import <Cocoa/Cocoa.h>

@interface MyPrintController : NSObject
```

Figure 14-4:
Connect the
one outlet
and two
actions
of the
MyPrint-
Control-
ler
instance.

```
{
    IBOutlet id myCanvasView;
    NSPrintInfo *thePrintInfo;
}
- (IBAction)printOnePage:(id)sender;
- (IBAction)showPagePanel:(id)sender;
@end
```

The only real change here is the line

```
NSPrintInfo *thePrintInfo;
```

This sets up a pointer to an NSPrintInfo object so that you can store settings that the user makes in the Page and Print panels.

Next, click the MyPrintController.m file and change its code to read

```
#import "MyPrintController.h"

@implementation MyPrintController

- (IBAction)showPagePanel:(id)sender {

    int i;
    thePrintInfo = [NSPrintInfo sharedPrintInfo];
```

```
        NSPageLayout *pageLayout = [NSPageLayout pageLayout];
        i = [pageLayout runModalWithPrintInfo:(NSPrintInfo
            *)thePrintInfo];

   }

@end
```

The showPagePanel method first populates the thePrintInfo variable
with the NSPrintInfo value, which is shared by all applications. Then
the code creates an NSPageLayout instance and displays it using the
runModalWithPrintInfo method. By passing thePrintInfo to the
runModalWithPrintInfo method, the Page panel will retain its settings
in thePrintInfo when the user dismisses it. So far, this code is functional
but not terribly interesting. You can run it and choose File⇨Page Setup to
view and play around with the settings in the Page panel.

Setting Up the Print Job and Printing the View

To add printing, all you have to do is implement the printOnePage method
that you created in the last section of this chapter. Click the
MyPrintController.m file in Project Builder and change its code to read

```
#import "MyPrintController.h"

@implementation MyPrintController

- (IBAction)showPagePanel:(id)sender {

    int i;
    thePrintInfo = [NSPrintInfo sharedPrintInfo];
    NSPageLayout *pageLayout = [NSPageLayout pageLayout];
    i = [pageLayout
runModalWithPrintInfo:(NSPrintInfo *)thePrintInfo];

}

- (IBAction)printOnePage:(id)sender
{

thePrintInfo = [NSPrintInfo sharedPrintInfo];
NSPrintOperation *thePrintOperation;

thePrintOperation =
```

```
[NSPrintOperation printOperationWithView: myCanvasView
          printInfo:thePrintInfo];

[thePrintOperation setShowPanels:YES];
[thePrintOperation runOperation];

}

@end
```

The `printOnePage` method takes care of running the Print panel and executing the print job. First it creates an `NSPrintOperation` instance using the class method named `printOperationWithView`. You pass this method a view to print and an `NSPrintInfo` instance, and it returns an instance of `NSPrintOperation`. Then if you want to display the Print panel (this step is optional, but typical of most applications), call the `setShowPanels`, passing it a Boolean value of `YES`. Finally, to run the print job, use the `runOperation` method of the `NSPrintOperation`. Cocoa takes care of everything else for you, including dismissing the Print panel and printing the view.

Printing to Places Other Than a Printer

So far, you've implemented some pretty boring stuff. Printing is nice, but it's become a standard requirement on all applications and operating systems. When it comes to printing, Cocoa really shines in its capability to print directly to PDF files. Instead of printing your view to a standard printer, you can ask Cocoa to save it to a PDF-formatted file instead. PDF is a standard format for publishing and printing documents. In the past, you had to rely on third-party solutions when it came to creating PDF content on the fly. With Cocoa, it's as easy as adding a few lines of code to your project.

Before you begin adding PDF features to your project, you may be surprised to know that you already have one form of PDF printing. When users choose File➪Print, they adjust settings for the print job using the Print panel. At the bottom of this panel is a button labeled Save as PDF. By clicking that button, users can print directly to a PDF file.

You can save to PDF in this manner only on Mac OS X 10.2 (Jaguar) and later. Earlier OS X installations require you to use the Output Options pane of the Print sheet if you want to print to PDF. From there, you must select Save to File and then select PDF to create the file.

There's a more elegant solution if you don't like the fact that users have to open the Print panel to print to PDF:

1. **Open the MainMenu.nib file in the project for this chapter.**

2. **Add a new push button to the existing interface.**

   Figure 14-5 shows what the interface should look like.

Figure 14-5:
Add a new button that users will click to print to a PDF file.

3. **Add a new action to the** `MyPrintController` **class.**

   Click `MyPrintController` in the Classes tab of the nib file window and add a new action named `printToPDF` in the Info window, as shown in Figure 14-6.

4. **Connect the new action to the interface.**

   Control-drag from the new button in your interface to the `MyPrintController` instance in the nib file window. Select `printToPDF` in the Info window and click Connect.

Return to Project Builder and add the new `printToPDF` action to the MyPrintController.h file:

```
/* MyPrintController */

#import <Cocoa/Cocoa.h>

@interface MyPrintController : NSObject
{
    IBOutlet id myCanvasView;
    NSPrintInfo *thePrintInfo;
}
- (IBAction)printOnePage:(id)sender;
- (IBAction)showPagePanel:(id)sender;
- (IBAction)printToPDF:(id)sender;
@end
```

Figure 14-6:
Add a new action titled `printTo-PDF` to the `MyPrint-Controller` class.

Then implement the `printToPDF` method in the MyPrintController.m file:

```
- (IBAction)printToPDF:(id)sender
{
    NSRect theRect;
    NSData *theData;

    theRect = [myCanvasView bounds];
    theData = [myCanvasView dataWithPDFInsideRect: theRect];
    [theData
        writeToFile: [@"~/Desktop/MyView.pdf"
stringByExpandingTildeInPath]
        atomically: YES];
}
```

Just to keep matters simple, this method creates a PDF file on the desktop. The code starts by getting the bounds of the `NSRect` that surrounds the view. Then, using those bounds, `dataWithPDFInsideRect` provides us with raw PDF data for use in a file. From there, it's just one more line of code to save the data to a file using the `writeToFile` method. You can view the resulting PDF with popular PDF viewers such as Apple's Preview application and Adobe's Acrobat viewer.

Although this method doesn't exactly use printing classes, don't forget that you can print from your project with the Print panel. For this reason, PDF is part of the printing chapter.

Chapter 15

Cocoa on the Internet

*T*he last decade of personal computing has witnessed explosive growth in networking technologies. Consequently, the vast majority of personal computer owners use the Internet, many on a daily basis. Among the various means of communication available to a user on the Internet, the World Wide Web and e-mail stand out as the two main tools that everyone uses.

In this chapter, you explore the wild and wooly world of the Internet and see how it applies to Cocoa programs. The chapter starts by showing you how to load Web pages, download files, and render HTML in your own projects. Later, you add e-mail features to your application as well. By the end of this chapter, you'll have a fully functional project that performs some important Internet functions. Although it's not necessarily the kind of application you'll want to use for your next best-selling killer app, it will serve as a handy reference for future projects.

Interacting with the Web

Just a few short years ago, no one had ever heard of the Internet or the World Wide Web. Now, even your dog has a domain name, an e-mail address, and an online storefront. Computer users have eaten up all that the Internet has to offer and in the process have become discerning consumers. They expect instant connectivity to any Web site in the world. Luckily, Cocoa has you covered. Perhaps the two most popular tasks on the Web are viewing Web pages and downloading files. With only a few lines of code, Cocoa gives you the ability to offer these important Internet functions in your own applications.

Loading a Web page in a browser

Loading a URL into a Web browser is one of the most common Internet-related tasks that you'll want to perform. It comes in handy for directing users to online documentation, to a download page where they can get the latest version of your application, or even to your Web-based store to purchase software.

Because viewing Web pages is a task that you perform so frequently, Cocoa provides a class to handle the dirty work for you: NSWorkspace. The NSWorkspace class gives you easy access to miscellaneous utilities. Every application has one, and only one, NSWorkspace object. By calling the openURL method of the NSWorkspace instance, you can load and view a URL using the default Web browser.

To use your application's NSWorkSpace instance, and, more important, its openURL method, use code like this:

```
[[NSWorkspace sharedWorkspace] openURL:theURL]
```

This code snippet works by calling the sharedWorkspace class method of NSWorkspace. From there, it's a simple matter of calling the openURL method and passing it a valid URL in the form of an NSURL. You can define an NSURL using a hard-coded URL:

```
NSURL *theURL = [NSURL URLWithString:@"http://www.wiley.com"];
```

If you'd like users to supply the URL in an NSTextField (with an outlet named theURLField) in your app's interface, you might do something like this instead:

```
NSURL *theURL = [NSURL URLWithString:[theURLField
        stringValue]];
```

Because openURL returns a Boolean value, you can determine whether the command executed successfully. For example, if you were to create an action named loadWebPage, the code might look like this:

```
- (IBAction)loadWebPage:(id)sender
{
    NSURL *theURL = [NSURL URLWithString:[theURLField
            stringValue]];

    if ( [[NSWorkspace sharedWorkspace] openURL:theURL] )
        NSLog(@"URL Loaded");
}
```

If the openURL method performs as it should, the code displays a URL Loaded message on the screen.

Downloading files

Another important feature that you may want to add to your Cocoa applications is the capability to download files from the Internet without using a browser. You can use download functionality for a variety of situations:

- Offer instant one-click access to the latest version of your application on the Web

- Download and display HTML help files from your Web site

- Retrieve a file from the Web that lists the current version of your application

Cocoa makes it a cinch to offer all these features and more. With only two lines of code, you can download a file from the Web to your hard drive. This example loads the main Web site from the *For Dummies* home page:

```
NSURL *theURL = [NSURL
        URLWithString:@"http://www.dummies.com"];
NSData *pageData = [theURL resourceDataUsingCache:YES];
```

Like the browser code from earlier in this chapter, you first define an NSURL. In this example, the URL is hard-coded to www.dummies.com. Although this may suffice for some purposes, other times you'll want to be more flexible in your approach to creating a URL. Because the URLWithString parameter is an NSString, you can use any of the usual NSString functions with it, including retrieving the URL from the interface.

Don't forget that an NSURL doesn't necessarily have to point to a file somewhere on the Web. It can also point to a file on your local hard drive. For example, you can use the initFileURLWithPath method of NSURL to build a URL to a local file, based on its path. Check the built-in Cocoa documentation in Project Builder to see the complete list of NSURL methods.

After you create and define an NSURL, call its resourceDataUsingCache method to begin downloading the file into memory. In the preceding code snippet, pageData points to data in memory. From there, it's a simple matter to transfer that data from memory to a file on your hard drive. For example, if you want to save a simple HTML document to your desktop, just call the writeToFile method of the NSData class. However, note that if you pass a relative path (for example, ~/Desktop/download.html) to the writeToFile method, you must expand it into a full URL with the stringByExpandingTildeInPath method:

```
if ([pageData writeToFile:[@"~/Desktop/download.html"
        stringByExpandingTildeInPath]
        atomically:YES])
{
NSLog(@"download successful");
}
```

One shortcoming of this "download and save to disk" approach is that it functions in a synchronous manner. Your application won't do anything else until the file has finished downloading. This may suffice for small downloads, but larger downloads become troublesome. The solution is to use the `load-ResourceDataNotifyingClient` method instead of `resourceDataUsing-Cache`:

```
[theURL loadResourceDataNotifyingClient:self usingCache:YES];
```

This method enables you to perform other functions while downloading the file. If you implement the `URLResourceDidFinishLoading` method, Cocoa notifies you when the download finishes, giving you the chance to access the data. For example, to save the download to an HTML file on the desktop, implement the `URLResourceDidFinishLoading` method like this:

```
- (void)URLResourceDidFinishLoading:(NSURL *)sender
{
NSData *pageData = [sender resourceDataUsingCache:YES];
if ([pageData writeToFile:[@"~/Desktop/download.html"
stringByExpandingTildeInPath] atomically:YES])
    {
        NSLog(@"download successful");
    }
    else
    {
        NSLog(@"download failed");
    }
}
```

Just because you're downloading and saving an HTML file in this example doesn't mean that you're limited to HTML downloads. You can download any kind of file that you want. To download a JPG image, for instance, simply change the URL and name of the destination file to indicate that it's a JPG file:

```
NSURL *theURL = [NSURL
URLWithString:@" http://purplee.net/images/cocoa_cover.jpg"];
...
if ([pageData writeToFile:[@"~/Desktop/download.jpg"
        stringByExpandingTildeInPath]
                            atomically:YES])
...
```

Displaying HTML

After you download an HTML file, it might be advantageous to display it in your interface. Using an `NSTextView`, it's straightforward to render simple HTML documents. This means that images aren't displayed — only the frames and text in the HTML source.

First create an NSAttributedString. This string will hold the rendered HTML. Then pass the pageData pointer from the preceding section to the initWithHTML method of the string. Finally, display the HTML in an NSTextView using the setAttributedString:

```
NSAttributedString *attrString = [NSAttributedString alloc];
[attrString initWithHTML:pageData documentAttributes:nil];
[[theHTMLView textStorage] setAttributedString:attrString];
[attrString release];
```

Putting it all together

To put all these HTML skills to use, create a new Cocoa application project in Project Builder. Next, open the MainMenu.nib file in Interface Builder by double-clicking the MainMenu.nib file. Then perform the following steps to create the interface:

1. **Add two NSButton controls, an NSTextField, and an NSTextView to the main window of your interface.**

   Change the Title attributes of the two buttons to Load URL with Client and Load URL Manually, respectively. Adjust the sizes of the window, the NSTextField, and the NSTextView to look like Figure 15-1. Feel free to label the interface too. You'll use the NSTextField as the source of the URL to download. The NSTextView is where you'll display the rendered HTML.

2. **Create a new class named MyInternetController.**

   In the Classes tab of the MainMenu.nib file window, click the NSObject and press Return to create a new class: MyInternetController. Choose Classes⇨Instantiate MyInternetController to create an instance of the new class.

Figure 15-1:
The Internet demo interface has two buttons, an NSText-Field, and an NSText-View.

3. **Add two outlets and two actions to the** `MyInternetController` **class.**

   In the Instances tab of the MainMenu.nib file window, double-click the `MyInternetController` instance. In the Info window, add two outlets named theHTMLView and theURLField. Then add two actions named loadWebPage and loadWebPageManually, as shown in Figure 15-2.

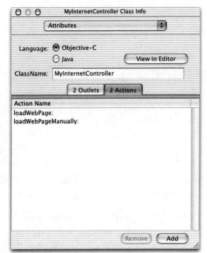

Figure 15-2:
Add two outlets and two actions to the My-Internet-Control-ler class.

4. **Connect the outlets and actions to the interface.**

   Control-drag from the Load URL with Client button in the window to the `MyInternetController` instance in the MainMenu.nib window and connect the button to the `loadWebPage` action. Then Control-drag from the Load URL Manually button to the `MyInternetController` instance and connect that button to the `loadWebPageManually` action. Next, Control-drag from the `MyInternetController` instance to the `NSText-Field` control. Select the `theURLField` outlet in the Info window and click Connect. Finally, Control-drag from the `MyInternetController` instance to the `NSTextView` control. Select the `theHTMLView` outlet in the Info window and click Connect.

5. **Create the files for the class.**

   Double-click the `MyInternetController` instance and then choose Classes⇨Create Files for MyInternetController to add the header and implementation files for this class to your project in Project Builder.

Return to Project Builder and change the MyInternetController.m file to read as follows:

```
#import "MyInternetController.h"

@implementation MyInternetController

- (IBAction)loadWebPage:(id)sender
{
NSURL *theURL = [NSURL URLWithString:[theURLField
          stringValue]];

   if ( [[NSWorkspace sharedWorkspace] openURL:theURL] )
       NSLog(@"URL Loaded");
}

- (IBAction)loadWebPageManually:(id)sender
{
NSURL *theURL = [NSURL URLWithString:[theURLField
          stringValue]];
[theURL loadResourceDataNotifyingClient:self usingCache:YES];
}

- (void)URLResourceDidFinishLoading:(NSURL *)sender
{
NSData *pageData = [sender resourceDataUsingCache:YES];
   if ([pageData writeToFile:[@"~/Desktop/download.html"
stringByExpandingTildeInPath] atomically:YES])
       {
           NSLog(@"download successful");
           NSAttributedString *attrString =
           [NSAttributedString alloc];
           [attrString initWithHTML:pageData
           documentAttributes:nil];
           [[theHTMLView textStorage]
           setAttributedString:attrString];
           [attrString release];
       }
       else
       {
           NSLog(@"download failed");
       }
}
```

Choose Build➪Build and Run to test your work. The result looks like Figure 15-3.

Figure 15-3:
The finished
product
downloads
an HTML file
and renders
it in the
window.

Sending E-mail from a Cocoa Application

Downloading Web pages is just one of Cocoa's many networking skills. Cocoa
is equally adept at e-mail. With a few simple lines of code, you can create an
e-mail message in your favorite e-mail client. With a few more lines of code,
you can take care of sending the e-mail too. E-mail features in an application
are handy for several uses:

- ✔ Provide a contact e-mail in an About Box
- ✔ Give users the opportunity to automatically send you bug reports
- ✔ Format an e-mail message in an existing client
- ✔ Spam tools, but you wouldn't dare do that, would you? Would you?

In this section, you add e-mail features to the demo project that you created
earlier in this chapter.

Sending e-mail from your favorite client

When you click an e-mail link on the Internet, your Web browser instructs
your e-mail client to open a new message, often with the To and Subject fields
completed for you. It's simple to add this kind of functionality to a Cocoa
application. In fact, if you followed along earlier when loading a URL in a
browser, you're well on your way to creating an e-mail message.

The main difference between creating an e-mail message and loading a URL in a browser is the format of the URL. Whereas a typical URL in a browser looks like this:

```
http://www.dummies.com
```

an e-mail URL looks like this.

```
mailto:yourFriend@email.com
```

Otherwise, you handle the two URLs identically. To create an e-mail addressed to your friend, simply pass the e-mail URL for that friend to the `openURL` method of the `NSWorkspace` class. For example, to send your friend an e-mail, use code like this:

```
NSURL *theURL =
[NSURL URLWithString:@"mailto:yourFriend@email.com"];
if ( [[NSWorkspace sharedWorkspace] openURL:theURL] )
        NSLog(@"Email Loaded");
```

If you know HTML, you've probably already guessed that it's possible to add other attributes to the e-mail address. If you want to attach a subject to an e-mail, simply tack it to the end of the e-mail URL preceded by `?subject=`, as follows:

```
mailto:yourFriend@email.com?subject=Important Message
```

You can also CC and BCC your other friends using a simple e-mail URL. The following e-mail URL sends an e-mail to yourFriend@email.com with a Subject heading of *Important Message*. The same message will also go to your other friend (otherFriend@email.com):

```
mailto:yourFriend@email.com?subject=Important Message
?cc=otherFriend@email.com
```

Keep on tacking the new parameters to the end of the e-mail URL address to suit your needs. Just remember to always precede each parameter with a question mark. Pass this URL to the `openURL` method of the `NSWorkspace` to launch your e-mail client and create a new e-mail according to your specifications, as shown in Figure 15-4.

 E-mail clients use the question mark character as a separator, so you can't use it as-is in a URL. Instead, you must use an *escape sequence* if you want to include a ? in your subject. For example, to send an e-mail with the subject *Ready?*, modify the `mailto` URL as follows:

```
mailto:yourFriend@email.com?subject=Ready%3F
```

Figure 15-4:
Creating an
e-mail is as
easy as
loading
a Web page
in your
browser.

Sending e-mail from your own apps

Giving your users a way to contact you by e-mail is a useful feature, but sometimes it may not fit your needs. This may be true for a variety of reasons, including the following:

- ✔ You're creating an e-mail application.
- ✔ You can't guarantee that your user will have an e-mail client installed.
- ✔ You don't want to reply by using an additional e-mail client.

Cocoa offers you the opportunity to send e-mail from your own applications. Before you start sending e-mails en masse, though, you need to perform a preparatory step. E-mail functions aren't part of the frameworks that typically accompany the average Cocoa project. Instead, Apple stores the e-mail functions in the Message framework. To use e-mail in your project, you must first add the Message framework to your project.

1. **Add the Message framework to your project.**

   To add the framework, choose Project➪Add Frameworks.

2. **Choose the Message.framework file.**

   In the dialog that appears, select Message.framework, which you can find in the System directory.

   `/System/Library/Frameworks`

3. Move the Message framework to the Frameworks folder.

After you add the framework, drag it to the Frameworks folder in your project, as shown in Figure 15-5.

With the Message.framework in place, its' time to send some e-mail. You'll be amazed at just how easy it is to send an e-mail with Cocoa:

1. Create a handful of `NSStrings` **that represent different parts of an e-mail message:**

```
NSString *theEmailDest = @"yourFriend@email.com";
NSString *theSubject = @"Important Message";
NSString *theBody = @"Hello there!";
```

2. Call the `deliverMessage` **method of the** `NSMailDelivery` **class.**

Because `deliverMessage` is a class method, you don't have to create an `NSMailDelivery` object before using it. The `deliverMessage` method has parameters for the message, the subject of the e-mail, and the recipient. Furthermore, it returns a Boolean value, telling you whether or not the delivery occurred.

```
    if ( [NSMailDelivery
deliverMessage:theBody subject:theSubject
      to:theEmailDest] )
      NSLog(@"Email Sent");
    else
      NSLog(@"Email Not Sent");
```

That's all there is to it! For this to work, however, users must set the correct e-mail server information in the Internet panel of System Preferences (see Figure 15-6).

Adding e-mail functions to the project

To see all these great e-mail functions in action, return to the project that you created earlier in this chapter. Open the MainMenu.nib file in Interface Builder and perform the following steps:

1. **Add two new buttons to the interface.**

   Label them Send Email with Client and Send Email Manually, respectively.

2. **Add an** NSTextField **to the interface.**

   Add a text label next to the NSTextField to let users know that this field is where they should enter a destination e-mail address. You can see the resulting interface in Figure 15-7.

3. **Add an outlet and two actions to the** MyInternetController **class.**

   Double-click the MyInternetController class in the Instances tab of the MainMenu.nib file window. Then in the Info window, add an outlet named theEmailField, so you can retrieve the e-mail addresses that users enter. Then add two new actions to the class named sendEmailManually and sendEmailWithClient. Figure 15-8 shows the Info window displaying all four actions of the MyInternetController class.

Figure 15-7:
Add two
NSButtons
and an
NSText-
Field
to the
interface.

Figure 15-8:
Add two
actions and
one outlet
to the My-
Internet-
Control-
ler class
for the
e-mail
functions.

4. **Connect the interface to the** `MyInternetController` **class.**

   Control-drag from the Send Email with Client button to the `MyInternet-Controller` instance in the Instances tab of the MainMenu.nib file window. In the Info window, connect the button to the `sendEmail-WithClient` action. Then, Control-drag from the Send Email Manually button to the `MyInternetController` instance. In the Info window, connect the button to the `sendEmailManually` action. Finally, connect the `theEmailField` outlet of the `MyInternetController` class to the interface by Control-dragging from the `MyInternetController` instance in the MainMenu.nib file window to the `NSTextField` in the main window of your interface. Click Connect in the Info window to make the connection.

5. Update the project files.

Because you already created the files for your class earlier in this chapter, you want to be careful not to destroy them.

Double-click `MyInternetController` in the Instances tab of the Main-Menu.nib file window. Choose Classes⇨Create Files for MyInternet-Controller. In the window that appears, make sure to uncheck the MyInternetController.m, as shown in Figure 15-9. This has the effect of creating only a new header file. You will change the implementation file (MyInternetController.h) by hand.

Figure 15-9:
Select
MyInternet-
Controller.h
only, when
adding the
new actions
and outlets
to Project
Builder.

Return to Project Builder and update the code in MyInternetController.m. The revised code looks like the following. Note the additional `#import <Message/NSMailDelivery.h>` statement at the beginning of the code; this statement permits use of the Message framework:

```
#import "MyInternetController.h"
#import <Message/NSMailDelivery.h>

@implementation MyInternetController

- (IBAction)loadWebPage:(id)sender
{
    NSURL *theURL = [NSURL URLWithString:[theURLField
            stringValue]];

    if ( [[NSWorkspace sharedWorkspace] openURL:theURL] )
```

```
        NSLog(@"URL Loaded");
}

- (IBAction)loadWebPageManually:(id)sender
{
    NSURL *theURL = [NSURL URLWithString:[theURLField
          stringValue]];
    [theURL loadResourceDataNotifyingClient:self
          usingCache:YES];
}

- (void)URLResourceDidFinishLoading:(NSURL *)sender
{
    NSData *pageData = [sender resourceDataUsingCache:YES];
      if ([pageData writeToFile:[@"~/Desktop/download.html"
stringByExpandingTildeInPath] atomically:YES])
        {
            NSLog(@"download successful");
            NSAttributedString *attrString =
            [NSAttributedString alloc];
            [attrString initWithHTML:pageData
            documentAttributes:nil];
            [[theHTMLView textStorage]
            setAttributedString:attrString];
            [attrString release];
    }
        else
        {
            NSLog(@"download failed");
    }
}


- (IBAction)sendEmailWithClient:(id)sender
{

  NSString *theURLString = @"mailto:";
  theURLString =
[theURLString stringByAppendingString:[theEmailField
          stringValue]];

  NSURL *theURL = [NSURL URLWithString:theURLString];

  if ( [[NSWorkspace sharedWorkspace] openURL:theURL] )
      NSLog(@"Email Loaded");

}

- (IBAction)sendEmailManually:(id)sender
{
    NSString *theEmailDest = [theEmailField stringValue];
    NSString *theSubject = @"Important Message";
```

```
    NSString *theBody = @"Hello there!";

    if ( [NSMailDelivery deliverMessage:theBody
            subject:theSubject to:theEmailDest] )
        NSLog(@"Email Sent");
    else
        NSLog(@"Email Not Sent");
}

@end
```

To see the results of your hard work, choose Build⇨Build and Run. If your project sends the e-mail successfully, you'll see the *Email Sent* message.

Chapter 16

Multimedia

. . . .

In This Chapter

▶ Playing system sounds

▶ Playing audio files

▶ Building an audio player project

▶ Playing movies with Cocoa

▶ Loading and using dozens of other media formats

. . . .

Working with text and creating files are useful functions for your applications, but they aren't always the most exciting functions. Multimedia, on the other hand, *is* exciting. Cocoa continues the long Macintosh tradition of providing high-quality multimedia features for you to use in your projects.

In this chapter, you discover how easy it is to add sophisticated multimedia features to your applications. First, you explore audio by creating a simple application that plays audio files from a number of sources. Then you delve into the real fun — movies! By building a movie player application, you'll see how easy it is to add dynamic QuickTime content to your Cocoa projects. By changing only one line of code, you'll also see how to (dis)play many other kinds of media beyond QuickTime movies.

Listening to Audio

The Macintosh has long been a popular machine with audio aficionados. Cocoa continues in this tradition, offering a complete set of tools for producing audio with your own apps. Some of the possibilities that Cocoa offers are

✔ Playing sounds that reside in your application's bundle

✔ Playing sounds that reside in the Mac OS X System folder

✔ Playing sounds from anywhere on your hard drive

Besides playing audio files that reside in a variety of locations, Cocoa can play many different audio file formats. In the past, you had to know about the various file formats to use them. Cocoa takes away this necessity and lets you play common audio file formats such as AIFF, MP3, and WAVE without knowing anything about them:

Playing system sounds

The QuickTime engine stands at the heart of Cocoa's multimedia toolbox. QuickTime takes away the guesswork of dealing with a variety of media formats. Because QuickTime takes care of knowing the details of each format, you can treat each type of audio file as if it were the same as any other format. To gain access to the power of QuickTime audio, use the NSSound class in Cocoa.

To play audio with the NSSound class, you'll typically follow a simple three-step process:

1. Create an object based on the NSSound class.

2. Load an audio file into the NSSound object.

3. Play the audio.

You usually combine the first two steps into one line of code. The easiest way to load an audio file is by using its name. For example, drag and drop an AIFF file (named someSound.aiff) into your Cocoa project. Then load it into an NSSound pointer using the soundNamed class method:

```
NSSound *theSound = [NSSound soundNamed:@"someSound"];
```

Note that you can omit the .aiff file extension.

Besides loading an audio file that you drag into your project, you can load any sound located in one of the Mac OS X Sounds directories:

```
/Library/Sounds
~/Library/Sounds
```

For example, suppose that you'd like to play the famous Sosumi alert, which Apple ships with Mac OS X. The code is identical, besides a name change:

```
NSSound *theSound = [NSSound soundNamed:@"Sosumi"];
```

After you've loaded a sound, it's a trivial matter to play it:

```
[theSound play];
```

Loading and playing sound files

For some applications, playing sounds that reside in your project is not enough. Suppose that you want your application to play any sound that a user selects. To accomplish this task, follow these steps:

1. **Create an array and fill it with all the sound file types that Cocoa can use:**

   ```
   NSArray *theFileTypes = [NSSound
           soundUnfilteredFileTypes];
   ```

   If you're curious about which types of sounds Cocoa can load and play, you can display them in the console by looping through the elements in the `theFileTypes` array and passing them to `NSLog`:

   ```
   int i;
   for (i=0;i<[theFileTypes count];i++)
       NSLog([theFileTypes objectAtIndex:i]);
   ```

   Figure 16-1 shows the available list of sound file types that a user can open.

Figure 16-1: Cocoa can load and play many types of sound files.

2. **Display an** `OpenPanel`, **restricting the user's choices in that panel to the file types in your array. Restrict the user also to only one file selection in the** `OpenPanel`**:**

   ```
   NSOpenPanel *theOpenPanel = [NSOpenPanel openPanel];
   [theOpenPanel setAllowsMultipleSelection:NO];
   result = [theOpenPanel runModalForTypes:theFileTypes];
   ```

3. **Use the** `initWithContentsOfFile` **method to load the sound (repre-sented by** `theFileName`**) that the user selected in the** `OpenPanel`**.**

Because you restricted the user to opening only one audio file, its path resides in the first element of the array that `OpenPanel` returns:

```
theFiles = [theOpenPanel filenames];
theFileName = [theFiles objectAtIndex:0];
NSSound *theSound = [[NSSound alloc]
        initWithContentsOfFile:theFileName
        byReference:YES];
```

4. **Play the sound as usual:**

```
[theSound play];
```

Building a simple audio player

To see some audio playback code in action, follow these steps:

1. **Create a new Cocoa project in Project Builder. After the project opens, double-click the MainMenu.nib file to edit the interface in Interface Builder.**

2. **In Interface Builder, add three** `NSButton` **controls to the main window of your interface. Resize the window and change the Title attributes of the three buttons so that they look like the ones in Figure 16-2.**

3. **In the Attributes section of the Info window, uncheck Close and Resize for the window.**

Figure 16-3 shows the position of the two attributes.

Figure 16-2:
Add three
buttons to
your Audio
Player
interface.

4. **Create a class named MyAudioController.**

Click the Classes tab in the MainMenu.nib file and scroll to the leftmost point in that window. Click `NSObject` and press Return to create a new class. Name it MyAudioController, as shown in Figure 16-4.

5. **Add three outlets to the** `MyAudioController` **class using the Info window.**

Name the outlets playAppSound, playSoundFile, and playSystemSound.

Figure 16-3:
Uncheck
the Close
and Resize
attributes of
the audio
player
window.

Figure 16-4:
Create a
new object
based on
NSObject.

6. **Create an instance of the class in MainMenu.nib.**

   To do so, choose Classes⊅Instantiate MyAudioController.

7. **Create the header and implementation files in Project Builder.**

   To do so, double-click the new instance and choose Classes⊅Create Files for MyAudioController. Instead of connecting the outlets and actions in Interface Builder this time, you'll do it later in Project Builder.

8. **Return to Project Builder and drag an AIFF file from Finder to your project.**

   Make sure that the AIFF file has the name someSound.aiff.

Navigate to the MyAudioController.m file and add the following code:

```
#import "MyAudioController.h"

@implementation MyAudioController

- (IBAction)playAppSound:(id)sender
{
    //play a sound file that is part of the project
    NSSound *theSound = [NSSound soundNamed:@"someSound"];
    [theSound play];
}


- (IBAction)playSoundFile:(id)sender
{
    int result;
    NSArray *theFiles;
    NSString *theFileName;

    //fill an array with all
    //of the file types that Cocoa can use
    NSArray *theFileTypes = [NSSound
            soundUnfilteredFileTypes];

    //display the sound file types in the console
    int i;
    for (i=0;i<[theFileTypes count];i++)
        NSLog([theFileTypes objectAtIndex:i]);

    //create and display an open panel
    NSOpenPanel *theOpenPanel = [NSOpenPanel openPanel];
    //permit users to open only one file at a time
    [theOpenPanel setAllowsMultipleSelection:NO];
    result = [theOpenPanel runModalForTypes:theFileTypes];

    if (result == NSOKButton) {
        //which files did the user select - only one in this
            case
        theFiles = [theOpenPanel filenames];
        //get the path to the chosen file
        theFileName = [theFiles objectAtIndex:0];
        //create, load, and play the audio file
        NSSound *theSoundFile = [[NSSound alloc]
            initWithContentsOfFile:theFileName
            byReference:YES];
        [theSoundFile play];
    }
}

- (IBAction)playSystemSound:(id)sender
{
    //play a sound file that accompanies the operating system
```

```
      NSSound *theSound = [NSSound soundNamed:@"Sosumi"];
      [theSound play];
}
 @end
```

You should recognize most of the code in this listing. The `playAppSound` and `playSystemSound` methods have identical code. They load a sound from the project's bundle or from one of the system folders that contains sounds. The `playSoundFile` method, on the other hand, permits users to open any sound files that they want for immediate playback.

If you want to stop the playback of an audio file, simply call the `stop` method of the `NSSound` class:

```
[theSound stop];
```

You have to make a few minor changes to your code if you want to add this functionality to a new button. Because a stop function would presumably reside in a new method of the `MyAudioController` class, your first change would be to declare the `NSSound` instance as a member of the class, not as a variable in the `playSoundFile` method, as in the previous code listing. Therefore, to implement a stop feature, your altered MyAudioController.h file would look like this.

```
/* MyAudioController */

#import <Cocoa/Cocoa.h>

@interface MyAudioController : NSObject
{
    NSSound *theSound;
}
- (IBAction)playAppSound:(id)sender;
- (IBAction)playSoundFile:(id)sender;
- (IBAction)playSystemSound:(id)sender;
- (IBAction)stopSoundFile:(id)sender;

 @end
```

Note also that you defined a new action in the process: `stopSoundFile`. Return to your MyAudioController.m file and change the second-to-last line of code in the `playSoundFile` method:

```
theSoundFile = [[NSSound alloc]
          initWithContentsOfFile:theFileName
          byReference:YES];
```

Then implement the `stopSoundFile` method in MyAudioController.m This method will stop any audio playback that `playSoundFile` started. Of course, you don't want to stop playback unless there is any audio already playing. To find out whether the sound file is currently playing, use the `isPlaying` method of the `NSSound` class. The completed `stopSoundFile` method looks like this.

```
- (IBAction)stopSoundFile:(id)sender
{
    if ([theSoundFile isPlaying])
        [theSoundFile stop];
}
```

Incidentally, you aren't required to create actions in Interface Builder. Actions are just as valid if you declare and define them in Project Builder. You still have to connect actions to their desired interface elements in Interface Builder, though, so we'll do that now:

1. **Return to Interface Builder by double-clicking the MainMenu.nib file in the Resources folder of your project in Project Builder.**

2. **In the MainMenu.nib file window of Interface Builder, double-click the** `MyAudioController` **instance.**

   This displays the Classes tab and selects the `MyAudioController` class.

3. **Choose Classes⇨Read MyAudioController.h.**

   When you choose this menu item, Interface Builder checks the header files for any changes. Because you added a new action named `stopSoundFile` in Project Builder, Interface Builder updates the MainMenu.nib file, adding the new action as shown in Figure 16-5.

Figure 16-5:
If you add actions or outlets in Project Builder, Interface Builder can find them in the header files and update the .nib file accordingly.

4. **Add a new button to the main window of your interface. Label it Stop Sound File.**

   Figure 16-6 shows the result.

Figure 16-6:
Add a new button to the interface for halting playback of a sound file.

Audio Demo

Play Application Sound

Play System Sound

Play Sound File

Stop Sound File

5. **Connect the new button to the** `stopSoundFile` **action.**

   Control-drag from the new button to the `MyAudioController` instance in the Instances tab of the MainMenu.nib file window. Click Connect in the Info window to connect the action to the button.

6. **Choose File⇨Save to save the MainMenu.nib file.**

7. **Return to Project Builder and choose Build⇨Build and Run to test your work.**

   When testing, initiate playback of an audio file that has a long duration using the Play Sound File button. As the file plays, click the Stop Sound File button to cease playback.

Watching Movies with Cocoa

Unless you've been living under a rock, you know that Mac OS X is a whiz at playing other kinds of multimedia content as well. QuickTime is a cross-platform multimedia engine that enables users to view, edit, and create all sorts of multimedia content. Chief among the various multimedia formats is the QuickTime movie. With Cocoa, it's easy to add movie playback functions to your applications.

To work with QuickTime content in your projects, Cocoa provides you with two important classes:

✔ `NSMovie`: The movie that you want to view

✔ `NSMovieView`: The player you use to view an `NSMovie`

NSMovie

NSMovie is a wrapper class for QuickTime movies. With it, you can load movies into memory from files or even the Pasteboard. For the demo in this section, you use the initWithURL method of the NSMovie class to load a movie from a file.

Earlier in this chapter, you loaded a sound file using an OpenPanel. Then you used the result from that OpenPanel to open the file using a traditional UNIX path. Mac OS X also lets you designate files according to a URL scheme. Therefore, instead of retrieving the filenames (that is, the paths of the files) from the OpenPanel as you did before:

```
NSArray *theFiles = [theOpenPanel filenames];
```

you should retrieve the URLs of the selected files using the URLs method:

```
NSArray *theSelectedMovie = [theOpenPanel URLs];
```

It's important to get the URL of a movie file because you need it to use the initWithURL method of NSMovie. The initWithURL method loads a movie from a file into an NSMovie instance:

```
NSMovie *theMovie = [[NSMovie alloc] initWithURL:movieURL
        byReference:NO];
```

NSMovieView

After you load a movie into memory, you probably want to display it. For that, you need the NSMovieView class. You can find it in the Cocoa-GraphicsViews panel of the Palettes window in Interface Builder (see Figure 16-7).

Figure 16-7:
Find the
NSMovie-
View by
searching
for the giant
QuickTime
icon.

NSMovieView has several attributes that you can set by hand in Interface Builder or programmatically with code. Figure 16-8 shows the attributes that you can set in Interface Builder.

Figure 16-8:
The
NSMovie-
View
attributes in
Interface
Builder.

The Loop mode attribute controls movie looping during playback. Its default state is Normal. This causes the movie to play until it reaches the end, which causes the playback to stop. You can also set it to Looping, which repeats the movie when the playback head reaches the end of the movie. The Looping Back and Forth setting plays the movie in a forward direction until it reaches the end of the movie, then it plays the movie in reverse until it returns to the beginning of the movie, and then it repeats the process.

The Show Controller attribute toggles the display of the built-in QuickTime controller, which appears at the bottom of the NSMovieView control when you load a movie into it. You'll be familiar with the QuickTime controller if you've ever viewed a QuickTime movie in a Web browser or the QuickTime Player application. The controller lets users control the playback of QuickTime content using a set of familiar buttons. Besides starting and stopping playback, you can rewind and fast forward through portions of the movie as well as adjust the volume during playback. Figure 16-9 shows a typical QuickTime movie controller.

Figure 16-9:
The standard QuickTime controller offers simple playback interface elements.

The Is Editable attribute of `NSMovieView` relates to the Show Controller and Plays Selection Only attributes. By default, Is Editable has a Boolean value of NO (that is, it's unchecked in the Info window). This causes the QuickTime controller to appear as shown in Figure 16-9. When you set Is Editable to YES by clicking the check box in the Info window of Interface Builder and then load a movie in code, you see a controller that looks like Figure 16-10.

Figure 16-10:
The Is Editable attribute toggles between playback and editing interface elements.

Hourglass playhead versus round playhead

The Is Editable attribute causes an `NSMovieView` to display a slightly different QuickTime controller. You can use this type of controller for different purposes, such as to select some portion of the movie. As you can see in Figure 16-11, Shift-clicking permits you to select some or all the movie in the `NSMovieView`. If you select some portion of the movie and set the Play Selection attribute to YES, `NSMovieView` plays only that selection.

Figure 16-11:
Shift-click
the
controller to
select some
section of a
movie in an
NSMovie-
View.

Plays Every Frame is the remaining attribute of the NSMovieView class that you can determine in Interface Builder. When you set this attribute to YES by clicking the check box in the Info window, QuickTime plays each frame of the movie. This yields the smoothest looking results, because it doesn't skip any frames. The downside is that it is computationally intensive. If you're not sure you need it, leave it unchecked. QuickTime plays movies nicely without setting this attribute.

After you've set the desired NSMovieView attributes in Interface Builder, you need to add some code to Project builder to play a movie with it. Presumably, you've already loaded a movie into memory using the NSMovie class. To display that movie in an NSMovieView, add the following code:

```
[movieScreen setMovie:theMovie];
```

This loads the movie into the NSMovieView for playback. Not all movies have similar dimensions, though, so you'll probably want to perform another step to resize the NSMovieView to match its movie. The resizeWithMagnification method will do this for you. You can resize movies to any size you want, including 1.0 (full size with no magnification):

```
[movieScreen resizeWithMagnification:1.0];
```

You can set many other aspects of playback using code. Besides the attributes that you found in Interface Builder, you can set the volume of the movie during playback:

```
[movieScreen setVolume:1.0];
```

Alternatively, if you'd prefer, you can mute the sound:

```
[movieScreen setMuted:YES];
```

The remaining NSMovieView methods give you the opportunity to program-matically alter playback, make a selection, or work with the Pasteboard.

Building a simple movie player

The easiest way to see how movie playback in Cocoa works is to build a player. Follow these steps:

1. **Launch Project Builder and create a new Cocoa application project. Double-click the MainMenu.nib file in Project Builder to open it with Interface Builder.**

2. **From the MainMenu.nib file window, open the main window for your interface. To it, add an NSMovieView control from the Cocoa-GraphicsViews pane of the Palettes window.**

   Be sure to move the NSMovieView into the upper-left corner of the window and resize the window to eliminate extra blank space. Just for fun, you can also click the Textured Window attribute in the Info window to create an iMovie-like window, as shown in Figure 16-12.

Figure 16-12:
Add an NSMovie-View to your window and set the Textured Window attribute to YES.

3. **Click the NSMovieView control and alter its Size attributes to look like Figure 16-13.**

   Make sure to set the springs so that the NSMovieView resizes when users resize the window.

If Interface Builder restricts your window size to something smaller than you'd like, click the Max button in the Info window. The reason it won't resize larger is that you've set a maximum size that you are now trying to exceed. Clicking the Max button sets the maximum size to a new value.

Figure 16-13:
Click the springs in the Info window to make the NSMovie-View resize with the window.

4. **Create a controller class for this interface.**

In the MainMenu.nib window, click the Classes tab. Scroll all the way to the left edge of the Classes tab and click NSObject. Press Return to create a new class and name it MyMovieController. Figure 16-14 shows the new class.

Figure 16-14:
Create a controller class for the project.

5. **To your new controller class, add two outlets and one action in the Info window.**

   Name the outlets movieScreen and theWindow. Name the action openMovie.

6. **Create an instance of the class by choosing Class⇨Instantiate MyMovieController.**

7. **Connect the** MyMovieController **instance to the interface.**

   Control-drag from the new MyMovieController instance to the NSMovieView that you added to the window earlier. Then select the movieScreen outlet in the Info window and click Connect. Connect the MyMovieController instance to the theWindow outlet by Control-dragging from the instance to the window in MainMenu.nib. Select theWindow in the Info window and click Connect.

   Finally, connect the action to the File⇨Open menu in the Menu Editor. From the Menu Editor, Control-drag from the Open menu item to MyMovieController in the Instances tab of the MainMenu.nib file window. Select the openMovie action in the Info window and click Connect.

8. **Now that you've designed the interface, double-click the** MyMovieController **instance in the MainMenu.nib file window and choose Classes⇨Create Files for MyMovieController.**

9. **Return to Project Builder to begin adding code to the new files that Interface builder created.**

In Project Builder, add the following code to the MyMovieController.m implementation file:

```
- (IBAction)openMovie:(id)sender
{
    NSArray *theFileTypes = [NSArray arrayWithObjects:@"mov",
        nil];
    NSOpenPanel *theOpenPanel = [NSOpenPanel openPanel];
    [theOpenPanel setAllowsMultipleSelection:NO];
    int result = [theOpenPanel
        runModalForTypes:theFileTypes];

  if (result == NSOKButton)
  {
        NSArray *theSelectedMovie = [theOpenPanel URLs];
        NSURL *theMovieURL = [theSelectedMovie
            objectAtIndex:0];

        NSMovie *theMovie = [[NSMovie alloc]
            initWithURL:theMovieURL byReference:NO];

        NSRect origFrame = [theWindow frame];
        NSPoint topLeft = origFrame.origin;
```

```
        topLeft.y = topLeft.y + origFrame.size.height;

        [movieScreen setMovie:theMovie];

        NSSize size = [movieScreen sizeForMagnification:1.0];
        size.width = size.width+40;
        size.height = size.height+40;
        [theWindow setContentSize:size];

        [theWindow setFrameTopLeftPoint:topLeft];
        [theWindow display];
    }
}
```

The code starts out by defining an array of file types that a user can open. In this case, you're restricting users to only QuickTime movies:

```
NSArray *theFileTypes = [NSArray arrayWithObjects:@"mov", nil];
```

Then the code presents a standard OpenPanel with which users can select a movie file to open. After they choose a file, get the URL for it and load it into an NSMovie:

```
NSArray *theSelectedMovie = [theOpenPanel URLs];
NSURL *theMovieURL = [theSelectedMovie objectAtIndex:0];
NSMovie *theMovie = [[NSMovie alloc] initWithURL:theMovieURL
        byReference:NO];
```

Next, you want to keep track of the window's size and position for use later:

```
NSRect origFrame = [theWindow frame];
NSPoint topLeft = origFrame.origin;
topLeft.y = topLeft.y + origFrame.size.height;
```

With the prep work out of the way, it's safe to assign the movie to the NSMovieView:

```
[movieScreen setMovie:theMovie];
```

Because we don't know what dimensions this newly loaded movie has, it's best to resize it. You could use the resizeWithMagnification method as described earlier, but this won't account for the resizing of the window that may need to take place.

To get around this problem, you can simply set the size of the window that holds the NSMovieView control. As the window resizes, the NSMovieView also resizes because you turned on the springs in the Info window for the control. To figure out how large to make the window, retrieve the size of the magnified NSMovieView:

```
NSSize size = [movieScreen sizeForMagnification:1.0];
```

Then add 20 pixels to each side of the NSMovieView to account for the border that surrounds it in the window:

```
size.width = size.width+40;
size.height = size.height+40;
```

Finally, resize the window to the new size:

```
[theWindow setContentSize:size];
```

Because Cocoa uses a coordinate system that assigns the origin to the bottom-left corner of a window or an NSMovieView, you may see some behaviors that you don't like. As the window resizes, it has a tendency to jump to some other position on the screen. To maintain the top-left corner position of the window (as you'd expect), use the original window location from earlier in the code to reposition the window:

```
[theWindow setFrameTopLeftPoint:topLeft];
```

Because the current movie may be a radically different size than the one the user loaded previously, it's a good idea to refresh the window. This forces the window to redraw itself and eliminates any leftover artifacts that the previous movie may leave behind during all this resizing and repositioning:

```
[theWindow display];
```

Choose Build➪Build and Run to test the project.

When a movie is not a movie

Playing movies is useful, but QuickTime can do much more. Everyone knows that a traditional movie is a sequence of movie pictures coupled with sounds, but fewer people know that in QuickTime this is only one kind of movie. QuickTime treats all media as a movie.

For example, if you open your favorite audio files as QuickTime movies, QuickTime dutifully plays the audio file. It's also smart enough to alter the NSMovieView according to the type of media you loaded. Figure 16-15 shows the result of loading an audio file as an NSMovie.

Figure 16-15:
QuickTime
can play
much more
than movies.

Some of the possible media file types that you can load into an NSMovie follow:

- ✔ Audio: AIFF, MP3, MP4, WAVE
- ✔ Video: QuickTime .mov, AVI, MPG
- ✔ Graphics: JPEG, TIFF, PICT, BMP
- ✔ 3D: QTVR
- ✔ Animation: Flash

To give a user the option of loading other types of media, simply add them to the theFileTypes array in the code from earlier in this chapter. For example, if you'd like to offer the option of loading a QuickTime movie or a TIFF file, change the code as follows:

```
NSArray *theFileTypes = [NSArray
        arrayWithObjects:@"mov",@"tiff", nil];
```

Cocoa (and subsequently QuickTime) treats both file types equally: as an NSMovie. This means you can load and play (or load and display if it's an image) many kinds of media without special code. This is one of the most powerful features of QuickTime, so use it often! Figure 16-16 shows the NSMovieView with an image loaded into the NSMovie.

Figure 16-16:
QuickTime
will even
display
images.

Although QuickTime movies and graphics have a spatial quality, audio files don't. This means you probably want to forego the additional resizing code when loading an audio file into an NSMovie. If you leave the resize code, it's likely that your movie window will become so small that you won't be able to see the controller when loading an audio file.

Part IV
Advanced Cocoa Topics

The 5th Wave   By Rich Tennant

Well heck, Justin--that's darn impressive! What else can that little programmable robot of yours do? How about sewing up and dressing that incision?

In this part . . .

Cocoa affords you the ability to easily program simple projects, but can it handle other tasks? You bet! Part IV takes you beyond simple Cocoa programming and into the realm of super geeks. You discover how to write applications that use multiple windows as well as how to harness the power of the Mac OS X command line. Part IV concludes with a discussion of how to take advantage of AppleScript in your Cocoa applications.

Chapter 17

Document-Based Applications

● ●

In This Chapter

▶ Building a document-based project

▶ Getting features free

▶ Implementing Save and Open

● ●

*T*hroughout this book, you create simple one-window applications to see how various aspects of Cocoa work. This is okay for testing your skills as you become familiar with Cocoa. But after you're comfortable working with Cocoa, you'll want to venture out on your own and create an honest-to-goodness application. Creating demo projects is one thing, but creating full-fledged applications is quite another.

When you create an application, you have to worry about much more than managing a single window. Many applications use a document-based approach whereby a user creates a document and adds some kind of content to it. If you've ever used a word processor or drawing program, you're probably familiar with this kind of application. In document-based applications, a user might also save a document, open it later, or print it. All these features require a lot of work when you implement them on your own. Fortunately, Project Builder helps by providing a full-featured, document-based project for you to use as a starting point for your own doc-based application.

This chapter guides you through the steps required to build a document-based application. Along the way, you'll implement many different features without having to do much work.

Creating the Project

To begin working with document-based applications, create a new project in Project Builder as follows:

1. **Choose File⇨New Project and select Cocoa Document-based Application from the list shown in Figure 17-1.**

Figure 17-1:
Choose
Cocoa
Document-
based
Application
in the New
Project
Assistant
window.

2. **Click the Next button and save the new project in a location where you can find it later.**

When your new project opens, you'll notice one big difference from projects throughout the rest of this book. The project already contains an instance called MyDocument. You can see it in Figure 17-2.

Figure 17-2:
A document-
based
project
comes
equipped
with a My -
Document
instance.

Click the MyDocument.h file to view its contents:

```
#import <Cocoa/Cocoa.h>

@interface MyDocument : NSDocument
{
}
@end
```

The header file simply defines the MyDocument class as a subclass of the NSDocument class. Like other classes in this book, this is where you'll add outlets and actions later.

Next, click the MyDocument.m file to view its contents:

```
#import "MyDocument.h"

@implementation MyDocument

- (id)init
{
    [super init];
    if (self) {

        // Add your subclass-specific initialization here.
        // If an error occurs here, send a [self dealloc]
            message and return nil.

    }
    return self;
}

- (NSString *)windowNibName
{
    // Override returning the nib file name of the document
    // If you need to use a subclass of NSWindowController or
            if your document supports multiple
            NSWindowControllers, you should remove this method
            and override -makeWindowControllers instead.
    return @"MyDocument";
}

- (void)windowControllerDidLoadNib:(NSWindowController *)
            aController
{
    [super windowControllerDidLoadNib:aController];
    // Add any code here that needs to be executed after the
            windowController has loaded the document's window.
}

- (NSData *)dataRepresentationOfType:(NSString *)aType
{
```

```
        // Insert code here to write your document from the given
                data. You can also choose to override -
                fileWrapperRepresentationOfType: or -
                writeToFile:ofType: instead.
        return nil;
}

- (BOOL)loadDataRepresentation:(NSData *)data
        ofType:(NSString *)aType
{
        // Insert code here to read your document from the given
                data. You can also choose to override -
                loadFileWrapperRepresentation:ofType: or -
                readFromFile:ofType: instead.
        return YES;
}

@end
```

The MyDocument.m file has five methods where you add code to make your application functional. Cocoa is even nice enough to give you full comments on how to use each method. Just for kicks, press Cmd-R to build and run the project. You'll be pleased to know that it already performs many tasks. When it launches, you'll see a single document window, as shown in Figure 17-3.

Figure 17-3:
The new document-based project already does something: It makes documents.

Choose File⇨New to create a new document. The application creates a new document and adds it to the Window menu. You can continue creating new windows as long as you want.

Note that the application has many other features such as a full suite of menus and an About box. At this point, however, you can't save the document because you haven't implemented that functionality yet.

Building the Interface

You need to make a decision about what kind of document-based application you want to create. It could be a word processor, a graphics application, or a checkbook program. In this chapter, you create a simple text editor.

Follow these steps:

1. **Return to Project Builder and double-click the MyDocument.nib file to open it in Interface Builder.**

   You should see a generic document like the one that was shown in Figure 17-3.

2. **Create the interface for this project.**

   Delete the text label that stands at the center of your document window. Then add an NSTextView control from the Cocoa-Data palette to the document window in MyDocument.nib. Resize the NSTextView to your liking. Figure 17-4 shows the new interface.

Figure 17-4:
The text editor interface.

3. Add an outlet to the `MyDocument` **class.**

Click the Classes tab in the nib file window and select the `MyDocument` class as shown in Figure 17-5. Control-click the `MyDocument` class and select the Add Outlet to MyDocument from the contextual menu that appears. In the Info window, name the outlet myTextView. You'll use this outlet to get and set the text in the `NSTextview` of a document.

4. Connect the `myTextView` **outlet to the NSTextView in the interface.**

Click the Instances tab of the nib file window and Control-drag from the File Owner's icon to the `NSTextView` in your document window. Click Connect in the Info window to connect the `myTextView` outlet.

5. Choose File➪Save to save the nib file and then return to Project Builder.

6. Find and click your application in the Targets window. Then expand the Info.plist Entries hierarchy to reveal the Document Types item.

To find your application, click the vertical Targets tab. On the left side of the Targets window, under the Targets (not the Executables) disclosure triangle, you'll see your application.

7. Change the document type of the project to handle rich text files, as shown in Figure 17-6.

Click the default DocumentType entry. In the Extensions box, type **rtf** (without quotation marks). Then, in the OS Types box, type **"RTF"** (that's a quotation mark, RTF, a space, and another quotation mark) in the OS Types field. Finally, click the Change button to apply these fields to the default document type in the list above the fields. This associates the rich text file type with the MyDocument class.

Figure 17-6:
Set an RTF
file type for
your project.

Adding the Code

Now that you've set up the interface and classes in Interface Builder and
added the RTF file type in Project Builder, you can add code to your project.
The MyDocument.h and MyDocument.m files that you created with Interface
Builder appear in your project. You need to add code to these two files to
make the application work.

In Project Builder, add an outlet and an NSData pointer to your MyDocument.h
interface file by entering the code that follows. The NSData object will hold
the contents of your rich text file.

```
#import <Cocoa/Cocoa.h>

@interface MyDocument : NSDocument
{
    IBOutlet id myTextView;
    NSData *fileContents;
}
@end
```

Then, navigate to your MyDocument.m implementation file and change its code to read as follows:

```
#import "MyDocument.h"

@implementation MyDocument

- (NSString *)windowNibName
{
    return @"MyDocument";
}


//save the file
- (NSData *)dataRepresentationOfType:(NSString *)aType
{
    [fileContents release];
    fileContents = [[myTextView
            RTFFromRange:NSMakeRange(0,[[myTextView string]
            length])] retain];
    return fileContents;
}


//open the file
- (BOOL)loadDataRepresentation:(NSData *)data
        ofType:(NSString *)aType
{
    fileContents = [data retain];
    return YES;
}



- (void)windowControllerDidLoadNib:(NSWindowController *)
        aController
{
    [super windowControllerDidLoadNib:aController];
    [myTextView
            replaceCharactersInRange:NSMakeRange(0,[[myTextVie
        w string] length])
                    withRTF:fileContents];

}


- (void)dealloc
{
    [fileContents release];
    [super dealloc];
}

@end
```

The big changes in this file are in `dataRepresentationOfType`, `loadDataRepresentation`, and `windowControllerDidLoadNib`. The `dataRepresentationOfType` method takes care of saving the file. Notice how it doesn't really do anything with files. Instead, it returns the data that the application should save to the file. The application takes care of the rest!

The `loadDataRepresentation` and `windowControllerDidLoadNib` methods handle the task of opening a rich text file. The `loadDataRepresentation` method receives the incoming data from the file and lets the application know whether or not it was successful. Then the `windowControllerDidLoadNib` method takes care of displaying the text in the `NSData` instance named `fileContents`.

To test your work, press Cmd-R. You should be able to open and save rich text files. When you open a file, your application displays its contents in a new window. Notice too, that the application's other menus work too. You can close a window by pressing Cmd-W or even use spell-checker on a document.

The beauty of using a Cocoa Document project is that Cocoa takes care of a lot of the work for you. You don't have to do much work to implement a large assortment of features. Besides making it easy on you, Cocoa makes it easier on your users. By using the default behaviors that Cocoa document-based apps provide you, your users will be familiar with their operation.

Chapter 18

Cocoa and the Command Line

● ●

In This Chapter

▶ Using command-line utilities in Cocoa

▶ Populating arguments for a command

▶ Executing a command

● ●

For years, Mac users have stayed safely (and presumably happily) on the sidelines when it came to text-based computing. After all, the Macintosh was supposed to be an alternative to traditional text-based operating systems such as DOS. In an ironic twist, Mac OS X reintroduced Mac users to computing through text-based commands. Being a UNIX variant, Mac OS X has all the usual UNIX tools, including command-line utilities.

Although the command line is a popular addition to Mac OS X, some people don't appreciate the geekier side of computing. Those folks liked their old Mac GUI operating system and don't see any reason for changing. To help them out, Cocoa programmers have been creating GUI applications that utilize the great command-line utilities beneath the hood of Mac OS X.

Cocoa makes it easy to call command-line utilities in your projects. This chapter leads you through the steps necessary to create a Cocoa application that wraps a command-line utility.

Wrapping Command-line Utilities

To issue text commands to your Mac, you typically use a terminal application, such as the Terminal.app program that accompanies Mac OS X. With this tool, you enter various text commands at a prompt and press Return to execute them.

These commands cover many different aspects of working with your computer. In Mac OS X, you'll find commands for working with files, editing text, diagnosing problems with your system, and more. Not all commands are boring utilities for geeks. Some commands are actually fun. In this chapter, you focus on the banner command.

The banner command creates giant-sized text banners. Each letter in the message of the banner consists of many smaller characters. The banner command typically takes one argument: the text of the message that you want to show in the banner. For example, if you type this in a terminal:

```
banner "hi"
```

the banner command returns the textual display shown in Figure 18-1.

The one big drawback of using command-line utilities is that they require the use of a terminal. The Terminal application that comes with Mac OS X (located at /Applications/Utilities/Terminal.app) consists of a window where you can enter and execute text-based commands. Mac users like GUI applications, though. Enter Cocoa.

Cocoa provides a class named NSTask that enables you to issue command-line commands from your GUI applications. Create an instance of NSTask in the usual manner:

```
NSTask *banner;
banner=[[NSTask alloc] init];
```

Figure 18-1:
Run banner "hi" to view a large banner with that message.

Then, you need to let the NSTask know which command you want to perform. You do this by telling it where to find the command. The banner command resides in the /usr/bin directory. Use the setLaunchPath method to set the location of the command:

```
[banner setLaunchPath:@"/usr/bin/banner"];
```

Next, define the arguments that you want to pass to the command using the setArguments method of NSTask. In this example, add "hi" to an NSArray, which you in turn pass to setArguments:

```
[banner setArguments:
[NSArray arrayWithObject:@"hi",nil]];
```

Finally, execute the command by sending the launch message:

```
[banner launch];
```

For commands that don't return anything, that's about all you need to do. The banner command, however, returns a large string that forms a picture. To capture the text that the command returns, you need to set the destination for its output, in this case an NSPipe named output:

```
NSPipe *output=[[NSPipe alloc] init];
[banner setStandardOutput:output];
[banner launch];
```

After you issue the launch message, you need to convert the output contents to a string that you can display in an interface. Use this fancy bit of code for that task:

```
NSString *theResult;
theResult=[[NSString alloc]
initWithData:[[output fileHandleForReading] availableData]
encoding:NSASCIIStringEncoding];
```

Creating the Project and Building the Interface

Now that you have a basic feel for how the NSTask class works, you can build an application that uses it. Launch Project Builder and create a Cocoa project by choosing File⇨New Project⇨Cocoa Application. When the new project opens, double-click the MainMenu.nib file to open it in Interface Builder. To create the interface, follow these steps:

1. **Add an** NSTextView **to the window.**

   Add an NSTextView control to your interface by dragging one from the Cocoa-Views palette to the main window. Double-click the NSTextView and change its font to Monaco using the Font⇨Show Fonts menu. With the NSTextView selected, choose Size from the popup menu at the top of the Info window and alter its springs to match Figure 18-2.

Figure 18-2:
Alter the
Size settings
of the
NSText-
View.

2. **Add an** NSButton **to the window.**

   Drag an NSButton to the main window of your interface and change its Title to Create. Then alter the springs in the Size section of the NSButton Info window, as shown in Figure 18-3.

3. **Add an** NSTextField **to the window.**

   Drag an NSTextField to the main window of your interface. Then alter its springs in the Size section of the NSTextField Info window as shown in Figure 18-4.

Figure 18-3:
Alter the
Size settings
of the
NSButton.

Figure 18-4:
Alter the
Size settings
of the
NSText-
Field.

4. **Rearrange the controls to your liking.**

The completed interface for the example in this chapter appears in Figure 18-5.

Figure 18-5:
The completed banner project interface.

5. **Create a controller class.**

Click the Classes tab in the nib file window and select the NSObject. Press Return to create a new class, and name it MyController.

6. **Add two outlets and an action to the class in the Info window.**

Name the outlets outputField and bannerField. Name the action createBanner.

7. **Create a new instance of the MyController class.**

To do so, choose Classes⇨Instantiate MyController.

8. **Connect the two outlets by Control-dragging from the MyController instance to the elements in the interface.**

Control-drag from the MyController instance to the NSTextView and connect it to the outputField outlet. Next, Control-drag from the MyController instance to the NSTextField and connect it to the bannerField outlet.

9. **Connect the NSButton to the action.**

Control-drag from the NSButton to the MyController instance and connect it to the createBanner action, as shown in Figure 18-6.

Figure 18-6:
Connect the
NSButton
to the
create
Banner
action.

10. **Before you leave Interface Builder, select the MyController class in the Classes tab of the nib file window. Choose Classes⇨Create Files for MyController to add the implementation and interface files to the project in Project Builder.**

Adding the Code

Now it's time to put it all together. Select the MyController.h file and make sure it looks like this:

```
/* MyController */

#import <Cocoa/Cocoa.h>

@interface MyController : NSObject
```

```
{
    IBOutlet id bannerField;
    IBOutlet id outputField;
}
- (IBAction)createBanner:(id)sender;
@end
```

Then navigate to the MyController.m file. Using the code from earlier in this chapter combined with the outlets and action you added to the nib file, alter your MyController.m file to read as follows:

```
#import "MyController.h"

@implementation MyController

- (IBAction)createBanner:(id)sender
{
    NSTask *banner;
    NSPipe *output=[[NSPipe alloc] init];
    NSString *theResult;

    banner=[[NSTask alloc] init];
    [banner setLaunchPath:@"/usr/bin/banner"];
    [banner setArguments:[NSArray
            arrayWithObject:[bannerField stringValue]]];

    [banner setStandardOutput:output];
    [banner launch];

    theResult=[[NSString alloc]
        initWithData:[[output fileHandleForReading]
            availableData]
        encoding:NSASCIIStringEncoding];

    [outputField setString:theResult];

    [output release];
    [banner release];
}

@end
```

To test the project, press Cmd-R. When the built application launches, enter some text in the NSTextField and click the Create button. If all goes well and you entered *hi* as the banner text, you should see results like those shown in Figure 18-7.

Figure 18-7:
The finished
application
displays
banners!

Chapter 19

Cocoa and AppleScript

· ·

In This Chapter

▶ Mixing Cocoa and AppleScript for fun and profit

▶ Speaking text from a Cocoa project

▶ Launching applications with AppleScript

▶ Recording voices to AIFF files

· ·

*F*or years, the Macintosh operating system has had a secret weapon: AppleScript. With AppleScript, Mac users have been able to control their applications using an English-like scripting language. Cocoa enables you to take advantage of the power of AppleScript in your own applications. With a simple script and a few lines of Objective-C code, you can harness the enormous possibilities that AppleScript affords you.

In this chapter, you create a project that demonstrates how to use AppleScript in a Cocoa application. Along the way, you discover the different methods you can use to add AppleScript to your projects. You also find out how to boss around a few different applications. More important, your project will gain great new features without much effort.

What's So Great about AppleScript Anyway?

AppleScript makes a great addition to a Cocoa developer's toolbox of tricks. AppleScript is a system-wide scripting language that permits you to control many different applications. Because you can control multiple applications at once, many programmers use AppleScript to automate their work flow.

AppleScript is great for a variety of reasons:

✔ AppleScript gives you control of different applications.

✔ You can find a large number of freely available scripts on the Internet.

✔ AppleScript gives you access to sophisticated features that would be impossible or impractical to implement on your own.

AppleScript's real power stems from that last entry. When you're writing Cocoa applications for personal use, sometimes all you want is a quick-and-dirty hack to fulfill your needs. In these cases, you probably don't mind how the interface works or what additional applications the Cocoa project requires. All you care about is the functionality of your application.

AppleScript gives your Cocoa project instant access to the powerful features that reside in many different applications. If your graphics application supports AppleScript, your Cocoa project can utilize it to perform graphics tasks. QuickTime Player has extensive AppleScript support, so you can use that for all sorts of interesting multimedia applications. The list goes on. The point here is that AppleScript can help you achieve your goals more smoothly and accomplish things faster.

AppleScript doesn't just benefit Cocoa. The reverse also holds true. Although AppleScript provides you with lots of great interapplication features, it's not a particularly visual method of programming. Using Cocoa, you can easily add graphical front ends to your favorite AppleScripts, making them behave more like their big brothers, the GUI applications.

Creating the Project and Building the Interface

To begin working with AppleScript in a Cocoa application, follow these steps:

1. **Create a new Cocoa application project.**

   To do so, launch Project Builder and choose File⇨New Project.

2. **Double-click the MainMenu.nib file to open it in Interface Builder.**

3. **Create an interface.**

   The interface for this project consists of one window with three NSButton controls and one NSTextField. The three buttons will perform the following functions:

   • Say "Hello"

   • Launch the iMovie application

   • Speak the text from the NSTextField to an AIFF file

   Drag the three buttons to the main window in your interface to match the completed interface in Figure 19-1.

You aren't limited to using AppleScript files as the source of your AppleScript source code. You can also define AppleScript code directly in your Cocoa code. This works well for short scripts, when you don't feel like going to the hassle of creating and adding an AppleScript file to your project. To see how this works, add the following code for the btnAction2 method:

```
- (IBAction)btnAction2:(id)sender
{

    NSString *theCode=
[NSString stringWithFormat: @"tell application \"iMovie\" to
        launch"];

    NSAppleScript *theScript=[[NSAppleScript alloc]
        initWithSource:theCode];
    [theScript executeAndReturnError:nil];
    [theScript release];

}
```

The btnAction2 method begins by creating an NSString that holds a complete AppleScript. In AppleScript, the script looks like this:

```
tell application "iMovie" to launch
```

As you probably guessed, this short script launches the iMovie application. Next, the code creates an NSAppleScript object and populates it with the NSString (theCode) that you just created.

Finally, execute the AppleScript by sending the executeAndReturnError method. Again, you can test your work so far by pressing Cmd-R and clicking the iMovie button in the application's interface.

The final step for this project is to add the code for the btnAction3 method. This method grabs the text from the NSTextField in the application's interface and speaks it. Instead of speaking it aloud, though, it saves the resulting audio to an AIFF file.

Before you implement the btnAction3 method, consider a raw AppleScript code snippet from Apple:

```
set the target_file to choose file name
with prompt "Name and location for the sound file:"
default name "voice.aiff"
say this_string using default_voice saving to target_file
```

The first line of the script displays a Save dialog box with a specific prompt and default file name. The user then names the target file and clicks Save, after which the result goes into the `target_file` variable. Next, the script speaks a string (named `this_string`) using a voice (stored in the `default_voice` variable) and saves the result in the file that the user chose (`target_file`).

Because this script is only two lines long, you can insert it into your Cocoa code, but first you must prep it. The first thing you need to do is add escape characters to the script to avoid problems with the quotation marks. Because a quotation mark signals the beginning or end of an `NSString` declaration, you must add backslash (\) directly before each quotation mark that's part of the script. While you're at it, you can also customize the prompt to your liking. Furthermore, because this script consists of two lines of code, you need to tack a newline character (\n) to the end of the first line of code. The modified script looks like this:

```
set the target_file to choose file name
with prompt \"Save as AIFF:\"
default name \"voice.aiff\"\n
say this_string using default_voice saving to target_file
```

Of course, you also need to replace `this_string` and `default_voice` with something concrete. Mac OS X has many different voices from which to choose. for this example, use the `"Fred"` voice.

Because you have an outlet to the `NSTextField` in the interface, you can grab its contents to use in place of `this_string`. Because this script will be one long `NSString`, you can replace `this_string` with %@ and add the outlet to the end of the `NSString`. The further modified script looks like this:

```
@"set the target_file to choose file name with
prompt \"Save as AIFF:\"
default name \"voice.aiff\"\n
say \"%@\" using \"Fred\" saving to target_file",[speechField
        stringValue]
```

Now that you've converted your script into a suitable `NSString`, you can add it to the code. The completed `btnAction3` method follows:

```
- (IBAction)btnAction3:(id)sender
{

    NSString *theCode=[NSString
        stringWithFormat: @"set the target_file to choose
            file name with prompt \"Save as AIFF:\" default
            name \"voice.aiff\"\n say \"%@\" using \"Fred\"
            saving to target_file",[speechField stringValue]];

    NSAppleScript *theScript=[[NSAppleScript alloc]
        initWithSource:theCode];
```

```
        [theScript executeAndReturnError:nil];
        [theScript release];

}
```

The completed MyController.m file declares all three actions, each of which drives one of three AppleScripts:

```
#import "MyController.h"

@implementation MyController

- (IBAction)btnAction1:(id)sender
{
    NSURL *theURL=[NSURL fileURLWithPath:
 [[[NSBundle mainBundle] resourcePath]
 stringByAppendingPathComponent:@"Scripts/speakText.scpt"] ];

    NSAppleScript *theScript;
    theScript=[[NSAppleScript alloc]
            initWithContentsOfURL:theURL error:nil];

    NSString *theResult=[[NSString alloc] initWithString:
            [[theScript executeAndReturnError:nil]
            stringValue]];

    [theScript release];
    [theResult release];
}

- (IBAction)btnAction2:(id)sender
{

    NSString *theCode=[NSString stringWithFormat: @"tell
            application \"iMovie\" to launch"];

    NSAppleScript *theScript=[[NSAppleScript alloc]
            initWithSource:theCode];
    [theScript executeAndReturnError:nil];
    [theScript release];

}

- (IBAction)btnAction3:(id)sender
{

    NSString *theCode=[NSString
        stringWithFormat: @"set the target_file to choose
            file name with prompt \"Save as AIFF:\" default
            name \"voice.aiff\"\n say \"%@\" using \"Fred\"
            saving to target_file",[speechField stringValue]];

NSLog(theCode);
```

```
    NSAppleScript *theScript=[[NSAppleScript alloc]
        initWithSource:theCode];
    [theScript executeAndReturnError:nil];
    [theScript release];

}


@end
```

Part V
The Part of Tens

The 5th Wave   By Rich Tennant

Oh come on—
how fatal
can it be?

FATAL
ERROR

In this part . . .

To help make your experience more fulfilling, Part V gives you important tips that speed up your Cocoa development as well as Web locations for Cocoa code, demos, and assistance.

Chapter 20

Ten Tips to Make Cocoa Programming Easier

· ·

In This Chapter

▶ Use keyboard shortcuts

▶ Use Class Browser

▶ Read the documentation

▶ Adjust the window count

▶ Use drag and drop

▶ Use `init` and `awakeFromNib`

▶ Don't forget the methods of the superclass

▶ Position items with Cocoa coordinates

▶ Use guidelines in Interface Builder

▶ Reuse code

· ·

As you familiarize yourself with Objective-C and Cocoa, you're bound to run across various tips and tricks that you'll want to remember. This chapter attempts to reduce the amount of time you have to wait until you discover some of those tips and tricks.

Use Keyboard Shortcuts

One of the easiest ways to speed up your Cocoa programming is to take advantage of the multitude of keyboard shortcuts available to you in Project Builder and Interface Builder. Table 20-1 lists some of the common keyboard shortcuts that Project Builder and Interface Builder share.

Table 20-1	Keyboard Shortcuts Shared by Project Builder and Interface Builder
Shortcut	*What It Does*
Cmd-S	Saves a file
Cmd-O	Opens a file
Cmd-M	Minimizes a window to the Dock
Cmd-?	Displays help for Project Builder or Interface Builder
Cmd-N	Creates a new file in Project Builder or a new nib file in Interface Builder
Cmd-Q	Quits the application
Cmd-R	Runs a project or an interface

Besides the run-of-the-mill keyboard shortcuts, you can help your Cocoa programming along by using the keyboard shortcuts of the pros. Table 20-2 lists some keyboard shortcuts that will give a decided advantage.

Table 20-2	Keyboard Shortcuts Used by the Pros
Shortcut	*What It Does*
Option-double-click *keyword*	In Project Builder, looks up the keyword's definition in the Cocoa documentation
Cmd-Z	Goes back in time whenever you make a mistake. Project Builder and Interface Builder offer multiple Undos.
Cmd-Shift-F	Finds all instances of your search term in the Cocoa documentation.
Control-click	Control-click (or right-click if you have a multibutton mouse) anywhere in Project Builder or Interface Builder to reveal a large menu of context-sensitive functions.

Read the Documentation

It seems too much of a cliché to say it, but your best bet for accelerating your Cocoa programming is to read the manual. Some documentation explains how the Developer Tools work; other documentation details the various classes and methods of Cocoa. You can view the built-in documentation by choosing Help⇨Cocoa Help. You can also read the documentation by visiting Apple's Developer Web site:

```
developer.apple.com/techpubs/macosx/macosx.html
```

Use Class Browser

In addition to using the standard documentation that's part of Project Builder, you can browse the various classes in Cocoa using Class Browser. Click the vertical Classes tab in Project Builder to display Class Browser. The Browser displays all the classes in Cocoa in a structured fashion. This gives you instant access to the definitions of the accessor functions of Cocoa classes.

Adjust the Window Count

Setting up your work environment to best suit your needs is another quick way to improve your Cocoa programming experience. Project Builder can operate with a different numbers of windows, and it's up to you to set the number of windows with which you feel most comfortable.

Throughout this book, I use the single-window setting in the Task Templates section of the Preferences window. Some people don't appreciate having all the various components of Project Builder in one window and like to stretch out a bit. For them, Project builder offers a few other settings that force various Project Builder functions to appear in different windows.

Choose Project Builder⇨Preferences and click the Task Templates button in the Toolbar to adjust the window count setting.

Use Drag and Drop

Drag and drop has long been an attractive feature of the Macintosh operating system. Project Builder and Interface Builder continue in this tradition, offering many different drag-and-drop features.

You can add files to Project Builder from Finder by dragging them into your project window. These files include source code files, frameworks, image files, HTML documents, rich text documents, and .icns icon files.

When you create classes in Project Builder, you can let your nib file know about them by dragging the header files for those classes from Project Builder to the Interface Builder nib file window. In Interface Builder, drag and drop is, perhaps, the most important interface operation. You use drag and drop to create the entire interface.

Initialize and Awaken!

When your application loads its nib file, Cocoa creates the objects in that file and calls the `init` method. Next, your application sets the outlets for your interface and calls the `awakeFromNib` method. Because the application sets the outlets after the `init` method, you can't use any methods that rely on outlets. Because `awakeFromNib` loads after the outlets are set, you can use code that replies on outlets.

As a basic rule, try to add initialization code to the `init` method of your object. If it doesn't work properly or yields a compiler error, move that initialization code to the `awakeFromNib` method for that object.

Don't Forget the Superclass

One of the great features of object-oriented programming is the fact that it has a hierarchical structure. This has a wonderful benefit called *inheritance*. Because every class in Cocoa (with the exception of `NSObject`) is a subclass of some other class (or classes) above it in the class hierarchy, every class has more methods than those listed for its particular type. This can be confusing at first for some beginners.

Consider this example. The `NSTextField` and `NSTextView` controls in Cocoa seem like they should work in a similar fashion because they both display text. By taking a quick look at the documentation, however, you find that they are very different controls. The `NSTextView` control doesn't have a method for setting its text. In the documentation for `NSTextView`, you'll notice that it is a subclass of `NSText`. `NSText`, on the other hand, does have a method for setting the text of the view: `setString`. You may be tempted to use the `setString` method with an `NSTextField` control. It's a good guess but an incorrect one.

Like the `NSTextView`, the `NSTextField` control has no direct method for setting its text. Because it's a subclass of the `NSControl` class, you can use the `setStringValue` method from that class. The lesson here is that if you expect a control to have some kind of method and it doesn't, check one of the superclasses of that class to see whether one of them has the function you need.

Position Items with Cocoa Coordinates

Programmers who are migrating to Cocoa from other languages may be surprised to discover that Cocoa bases all its measurements on a different coordinate system. Whereas most computer languages define the upper-left corner of a view as the origin, Cocoa designates the bottom-left corner as the origin. You may remember this arrangement as Quadrant I from your high school trigonometry class.

If you're familiar with PDF and PostScript, you can skip this tip. You're already living in an upside-down world. PDF and PostScript use the same coordinate system that Mac OS X uses — and this is no accident. NeXT based its image model on Display Postscript. Mac OS X continued with this tradition by basing its image model on PDF, which is essentially PostScript in a document model.

Use Guidelines in Interface Builder

When it comes to building interfaces, Apple insists that you follow many guidelines to ensure the best Aqua experience. Frankly, there are too many guidelines to keep them all straight. To help you out, Interface Builder offers a great feature in the form of Guidelines. As you drag controls around your interface, Interface Builder displays lines in the interface to help you align controls and place them according to the Aqua Human Interface guidelines.

Pay attention to these interface suggestions! They make it a snap to follow the stringent interface guidelines in Mac OS X and help you create software that follows standard norms. This results in software that's easier to use by more people. If you follow your own guidelines, you're bound to hear complaints. Macintosh users expect a certain user experience. If you stray from it, your users won't be happy.

Reuse Your Code

The guiding principle of object-oriented programming is code-reuse, and Cocoa is no different. In fact, many programmers claim that Cocoa code is some of the *most* reusable code around, because Cocoa programmers separate form from function through the Model-View-Controller paradigm.

To reuse a nib file, simply drag it into your project in Project Builder. To reuse a class, drag its implementation (.m) and header (.h) files into your project in Project Builder. It's as simple as that!

Chapter 21

Ten Great Web Sites for Cocoa Developers

. . . .

In This Chapter

▶ *MacTech* magazine

▶ CocoaDev

▶ CocoaDev Central

▶ MacTelligence

▶ Cocoa Mailing List Archive

▶ Vermont Recipes

▶ Scotland Software

▶ iDevGames

▶ HyperJeff Network

▶ Stepwise

. . . .

The Internet is a virtual treasure chest for Cocoa developers. On the Web, you'll find scores of sites offering Cocoa source code, demo projects, tutorials, instruction, and even personal assistance. This chapter touches on ten important Web sites that will improve your Cocoa experience by offering help and insight into how to program most effectively in Cocoa. You'll find links to professional Cocoa development companies as well as individual Web sites.

MacTech Magazine

www.mactech.com

MacTech magazine is the premiere Macintosh programming print journal for the English-speaking part of the world. The publication covers a wide range of Macintosh-related topics, including plenty of wholesome Cocoa goodness. You'll see articles and tutorials in *MacTech* from Cocoa professionals such as

Andrew Stone (of Stone Software fame) and Dan Wood (the creator of the popular Watson Internet application). I'm a regular contributor as well. Although leaning towards the advanced programmer, *MacTech* sometimes has articles for beginners.

CocoaDev

www.cocoadev.com

CocoaDev is a site devoted entirely to Cocoa programming and is one of the first places you should look for common questions and code snippets. CocoaDev maintains important lists of Cocoa links, Cocoa book reviews, and tutorials. One of their best features is the CocoaSampleCode section, where different programmers submit code snippets for all kinds of everyday Cocoa tasks.

CocoaDev Central

www.cocoadevcentral.com

Another Cocoa-centric site, the similarly named CocoaDev Central offers many useful code samples and demo projects to satisfy your lust for Cocoa. Focusing primarily on Cocoa tutorials, CocoaDev Central has some longtime Cocoa programmers on their staff who really know their stuff.

MacTelligence

www.mactelligence.com/info/CocoaLinks.tpl

MacTelligence is not strictly a Cocoa site, but they do have a nice collection of Cocoa links. You'll find a variety of links here, from simple beginner projects to advanced frameworks.

Cocoa Mailing List Archive

cocoa.mamasam.com

One of the great things about the Internet is that you can use it to pose questions to experts from all over the world. The Cocoa Mailing List Archive is a collection of short question-and-answer threads related to Cocoa programming. Read questions that people have posted and see the answers that others give. If you're ever stuck, this is a great resource for solving your problem. Plus, it's always cool to know that a programmer in Japan helped another programmer in Ohio, who in turn offered assistance to a developer in Germany. The Web is a crazy place!

Vermont Recipes

www.vermontrecipes.com

Bill Cheeseman is a veteran Cocoa (and NEXTStep) programmer — and it shows. He presents clear and descriptive cookbook-style tutorials for Cocoa programmers. Considered classics among the Cocoa community, the Vermont Recipes are some of the first Cocoa tutorials that appeared on the Web. Bill has also compiled those recipes into a new book titled *Cocoa Recipes for Mac OS X: The Vermont Recipes* (published by Peachpit Press).

Scotland Software

www.scotlandsoftware.com/products/source/

Based in Scotland (well, duh!), Scotland Software is a company that specializes in Macintosh software. Although not primarily a Cocoa site, Scotland Software does post some useful Cocoa projects for you to download. They cover handy topics such as graphics, networking, and icons. This site is a little pearl in the giant Cocoa ocean, so don't miss it.

iDevGames

www.idevgames.com

iDevGames is a Web site devoted to Macintosh game programming. They have regular content about the Mac game development community, including book reviews, industry interviews, commentary, tutorials, and source code. Although iDevGames doesn't focus only on Cocoa programming, they regularly post Cocoa projects and source code. Even if you aren't programming games, the source code samples usually offer glimpses into other kinds of functionality besides gaming.

HyperJeff Network

osx.hyperjeff.net/Apps/CocoaSource.html

Hosted by Jeff, the HyperJeff Network strives to post original, high-quality content. The site covers many topics that interest Jeff, including Macs, physics, and mathematics. His Cocoa section has a nice list of Cocoa applications that include free source code. Want to see what kinds of applications other Cocoa programmers are making? Check with Jeff!

Stepwise

www.stepwise.com

After you get the hang of Cocoa, you'll probably spend a fair amount of time at the Stepwise site. Targeted more to advanced Cocoa programmers, Stepwise posts all kinds of informative and technical articles on Cocoa programming as well as Mac programming in general. Despite its tendency for more advanced topics, beginners can sometimes walk away with something from Stepwise. They're old-timers when it comes to Cocoa (and NEXT) programming, so if you're looking for definitive answers, Stepwise is a good place to start.

Appendix

Installing Mac OS X Developer Tools

System Requirements

To use the Mac OS X Developer Tools, you must have a corresponding version of Mac OS X installed on your Macintosh computer. Besides the 128 MB RAM minimum that Mac OS X requires, you'll also want to have at least 500 MB of free space on your hard drive. In these days of cheap hard drives, this isn't a hard requirement to meet.

Installing the Developer Tools

To install the Mac OS X Developer Tools from a CD, perform the following steps:

1. **Insert the CD.**

   Insert the Developer Tools CD into the CD or DVD drive of your Macintosh.

2. **Launch the Developer.mpkg file from the CD.**

   Double-click the Developer.mpkg file to launch the Developer Tools installer.

3. **Authenticate as a user with administrator privileges.**

   Because the Developer Tools installer places files all over your system, it needs permission to write to all those places. Only administrator accounts can perform these functions. Click the small icon with a lock on it to authenticate as an administrator.

4. **Install the Developer Tools.**

   Choose Easy Install to install all the tools that you'll need for Cocoa development.

5. **Wait until the installation is complete!**

   At the end of the installation process, the installer performs many time-consuming functions that are vital to proper installation of the Developer Tools. Be patient and wait for the installer to completely install the tools — even if the message displayed on the screen indicates that the installation should be finished already.

What to Do If You Don't Have the Developer Tools CD

If your copy of Mac OS X didn't come with a copy of the Developer Tools CD, you can still get your hands on a copy of the Developer Tools software through the Internet. Visit the Apple Developer Connection to register for a free account:

```
https://connect.apple.com
```

After you're registered as a member of the Apple Developer Connection, you can download a variety of development-related software, late-breaking documentation, and source code. Among the offerings is a full download of the Developer Tools. After you download the Developer Tools, perform the preceding steps, beginning at Step 2. The ADC also posts updates to the Developer Tools that usually correspond to a Mac OS X version update. You should download and install all recommended updates from the Apple Developer Connection to achieve the best development results.

Index

Symbols and Numerics

@ (at) sign, Cocoa string, 141, 201
\ (backslash), NSString declaration, 330
\n (newline character), 330
: (colon), Objective-C, 132
{ } (curly brackets), 38
/ (forward slash), 239
- (minus sign), method declaration, 120
%A (Weekday name), date format specifier, 187
%B (Month name), date format specifier, 187
%e (Day of the month as an integer), date format specifier, 187
%I (Hours), date format specifier, 187
%M (Minutes), date format specifier, 187
%m (Month as an integer), date format specifier, 187
%S (Seconds), date format specifier, 187
%3F, URL escape sequence, 273
%Y (Year), date format specifier, 187
+ (plus sign), method declaration, 144
? (question mark), e-mail URL, 273
; (semicolon)
  Objective-C, 132
  separating formats with, 59–60
[ ] (square brackets), 38, 132
~ (tilde), Home directory, 24
32-bit icon, 104

• A •

%A (Weekday name), date format specifier, 187
About menu, renaming, 79
accessor method, 129
action
  adding to controller class, 82
  btnAction1, 325
  btnAction2, 325
  btnAction3, 325
  calculateAnswer, 32, 36, 38, 89–90
  calculateAverage, 96
  copyTheFile, 250, 252
  createBanner, 318
  displayAString, 201
  feedAnimal, 123
  interface, connecting to, 35–36
  loadWebManually, 270
  loadWebPage, 266, 270
  moveTheFile, 252–253
  naming, 32
  openMovie, 296
  printToPDF, 262
  selectFile, 243, 248–249
  selectTheFile, 242, 251
  stopSoundFile, 287, 289
Actions tab, 32, 86
ADC. See Apple Developer Connection
Adobe Photoshop, 104
.aiff file extension, 282
AIFF file, loading into an NSMovie, 299
alloc method, 141–143
Alpha mask, 104
Animal class, 118
answerField, 52, 59
answerFormatter object, 59
AppKit. See Application Kit Framework
AppKit.h, 145
Apple Developer Connection (ADC), 346
Apple, developer Web site, 9–10
AppleScript
  btnAction1 action, 325
  btnAction2 action, 325
  btnAction2 method, 329
  btnAction3 action, 325
  btnAction3 method, 329–331
  Bundle Resources, 328
  default_voice variable, 330
  executeAndReturnError message, 326
  executeAndReturnError method, 329
  importance of, 18, 324–325
  Launch iMovie button, 324–325
  MyController class, 325
  MyController.m, 326, 331–332

AppleScript *(continued)*
  NSAppleScript, 326, 329
  NSURL, 326
  QuickTime, 325
  Record Text-to-Speech button, 324–325
  Say Hello button, 324–325
  Scripts list, 328
  speakText.applescript, 327
  speakText.scpt, 326
  speechField outlet, 325
  target_file variable, 330
AppleScript button, 77
AppleScript Studio, documentation, 64
application, building, 21–22, 66–67
application, document-based
  dataRepresentationOfType method, 311
  Document Types, Info.plist Entries, 308
  fileContents, 311
  importance of, 303
  loadDataRepresentation method, 311
  MyDocument, 304, 308
  MyDocument.h, 305, 309
  MyDocument.m, 305–306, 310
  myTextView outlet, 308
  NSTextView, 307
  OS Types box, 308
  rich text file, 308
  simple text editor, creating interface for, 307–309
  windowControllerDidLoadNib method, 311
Application Kit (AppKit) Framework
  benefits of using, 11
  color spaces, 214
  including in project, 145–146
Aqua interface, building, 17
argument, passing, 132
array
  index, 183
  inserting object into, 184–185
  loading, 177
  mutable compared to immutable, 184
  NSArray class, 182–185
arrayWithCapacity method, 184
arrayWithObjects method, 183
at (@) sign, Cocoa string, 141, 201

audio
  file formats, 282
  isPlaying method, 288
  MyAudioController class, 284
  MyAudioController.h, 287–288
  MyAudioController.m, 286–287
  NSSound class, 282
  Play Application Sound button, 284
  Play Sound File button, 284, 289
  Play System Sound button, 284
  playAppSound method, 287
  playAppSound outlet, 284
  player example, 284–289
  playSoundFile method, 287
  playSoundFile outlet, 284
  playSystemSound method, 287
  playSystemSound outlet, 284
  QuickTime, 282
  someSound.aiff, 285
  sound file types, 283
  soundNamed class method, 282
  Sounds directory, 282
  Sounds pane, 72
  stop method, 287
  Stop Sound File button, 289
  stopSoundFile action, 287, 289
  stopSoundFile method, 287–288
  system sounds, 282
  user-selected sounds, playing, 283–284
Average button, adding to interface, 94–96
AVI file, loading into an NSMovie, 299
awakeFromNib message, 128
awakeFromNib method, 128, 149–150, 179, 196–197, 338

• *B* •

%B (Month name), date format specifier, 187
backslash (\), NSString declaration, 330
banner command, 313–315
bannerField outlet, 318
base colors, mixing, 215
Basic Settings Tab
  adjusting settings, 47–48
  importance of, 45
BCC field, e-mail, 273
beginSheet, 159

benefits of programming with Cocoa, 10
bezierPath method, 229
BezierPathWithOvalInRect function, 222
BezierPathWithRect function, 221
blackColor preset color component, 214
blueColor preset color component, 214
BMP file, loading into an NSMovie, 299
bookmark, 62
Bookmarks tab
  editing bookmark, 63–64
  viewing bookmark list, 62
BOOL data type, 185
Boolean variable, 138
boot drive, 239
border, adding to window, 298
bottom-left corner, graphics, 212
breakpoint
  deleting, 61
  inserting, 56
Breakpoints tab, 62
brownColor preset color component, 214
brushed-metal look, window, 153
btnAction1 action, 325
btnAction2 action, 325
btnAction2 method, 329
btnAction3 action, 325
btnAction3 method, 329–331
Build and Debug function, keyboard
    shortcut, 66
Build and Run, 39, 53, 66, 92
Build folder, opening, 41
Build function, keyboard shortcut, 66
Build tab, 47
bundle, 111, 238
Bundle Resources, 328
button control
  AppleScript button, 77
  Average button, 94–96
  bevel button, 167
  Calculate Fare button, 135
  calculator application interface, 30
  check box, 166–167
  Cocoa Container Views button, 77
  Cocoa Data Views button, 77
  Cocoa Graphic Views button, 77
  Cocoa Menus button, 76
  Cocoa Views button, 76
  Cocoa Windows button, 77

Copy File to Desktop button, 250
Create button, 316
Custom Settings button, 47
Disconnect button, 86
dragging into application interface
    window, 28
importance of, 161–162
label, adding, 28
Launch iMovie button, 324–325
Load URL Manually button, 269
Load URL with Client button, 269
Many Windows button, 47
matrix, radio buttons, 168
Max button, Info window, 295
Move File to Desktop button, 250
Open plain text button control, 206
Open rich text button control, 206
Other Cocoa Views button, 76, 84
Play Application Sound button, 284
Play Sound File button, 284, 289
Play System Sound button, 284
popup button, 84
push button, 162–164
Record Text-to-Speech button, 324–325
round button, 165–166
Save plain text button control, 203
Save rich text button control, 203
Say Hello button, 324–325
Send Email Manually button, 276
Send Email with Client button, 276
Single Window button, 47–48
Some Windows button, 47
Stop Sound File button, 289
Task Templates button, 45

• C •

C language, 2, 250
C++ language, 250
Calculate Fare button, 135
calculateAnswer action, 32, 36, 38, 89–90
calculateAnswer function, 53, 89
calculateAnswer method, 37
calculateAverage action, 96
calculator sample application, purpose, 23
CalculatorProject.pbproj, 45, 70
calibrated color, 214–215
CC field, e-mail, 273

cells, collection of, 168
center method, 149
centerWindow, 151
CFBundleExecutable, 111–112
CFBundleIconFile entry, Info.plist, 107, 111–112
Cheeseman, Bill (*Cocoa Recipes for Mac OS X: The Vermont Recipes*), 343
class
  Animal, 118
  built-in, 117
  Controller, 82, 168
  creating, 31, 118, 133
  definition, 117
  Driver, 133, 137
  fuse box, similarity to, 30
  Fusebox, 31–33, 53
  instantiating, 32–33
  MyAudioController, 284
  MyCanvas, 218–219
  MyController, 122, 325
  MyDataController, 176–177
  MyMovieController, 295–296
  MySheetController, 157
  MyTextController, 193
  naming conventions, 143
  NSArray, 181–185
  NSCalendarDate, 185–187
  NSData, 267
  NSFileManager, 252
  NSMailDelivery, 275
  NSMovie, 289–290
  NSMovieView, 289–291
  NSNumber, 181–182
  NSObject, 31, 118, 134, 217
  NSPipe, 315
  NSSound, 282
  NSTabViewItem, 172
  NSWindow, 148, 244
  NSWorkspace, 266, 273
  numberWithBool, 185
  OpenPanel, 243–244, 251, 283
  outlets, adding to, 31–32
  printOperationWithView, 261
  SavePanel, 251
  sendEmailManually, 276
  sendEmailWithClient, 276
  sharedWorkspace, 266
  soundNamed, 282

Class Browser, 53–54, 337
class method, 144
Classes group, expanding, 52
Classes pane, 72–73
Classes tab, 31, 288
Clean function, keyboard shortcut, 66
Clipboard. *See* Pasteboard
closePath function, 230
closeSheet, 158
Cocoa Container Views button, 77
Cocoa Data Views button, 77
Cocoa Document-based Application, New Project Assistant window, 303–304
Cocoa Graphic Views button, 77
Cocoa Mailing List Archive (Web site), 342–343
Cocoa Menus button, 76
Cocoa project, development process, 11–13
Cocoa Recipes for Mac OS X: The Vermont Recipes (Bill Cheeseman), 343
Cocoa Views button, 76
Cocoa Windows button, 77
Cocoa-Data pane, Palettes window, 175
CocoaDev (Web site), 342
CocoaDev Central (Web site), 342
CocoaGraphicsView pane, 294
Cocoa.h, 146
Cocoa-Other pane, 170
code
  downloading from Web site, 257
  initializing, 338
  reuse, 129, 339
code editor, 65
colon (:), Objective-C, 132
color
  device dependent, 214–216
  device independent, 214–215
  mixing schemes, 215
  named, 214–215
  NSColor, 213
  path, filling, 222–226
  preset components, 214
  space, 215
color changes, applying to selected text, 192
ColorWell, 195
colorWithCalibratedRed method, 179
colorWithDeviceRed method, 215

command line, 238
command-line utilities *See* commands, text
commands, text
    `banner` command, 313–315
    `bannerField` outlet, 318
    Create button, 316
    `createBanner` action, 318
    `fileHandleForReading` method, 315
    hi banner output, 321
    importance of, 313
    `launch` message, 314
    `MyController`, 318
    `MyController.h`, 319
    `MyController.m`, 320
    `NSArray`, 315
    `NSButton` control, 316
    `NSFileHandle`, 315
    `NSPipe` class, 315
    `NSTask` command, 314
    `NSTextView` control, 316
    `outputField` outlet, 318
    `setArguments` method, 315
    `setLaunchPath` method, 315
    Size settings, changing, 317
    Terminal application, 314
Connections, Info window, 86
context-sensitive functions, keyboard
        shortcut, 336
Continuous mode, slider control, 171
Control-drag, 34–35
`Controller` class
    creating, 82
    entire matrix, connecting to, 168
controller, definition, 133
controls
    adding to window, 84
    bevel button, 167
    button, importance of, 161–162
    check box, 166–167
    definition, 161
    dragging into application interface
        window, 28
    dragging into window, 82
    progress bar, 174–175
    push button, 162–164
    radio, 168–170
    round button, 165–166
    slider, 170–171
    tab view, 172–173
    table, 175–180
Controls section, Info window, 28
Copy File to Desktop button, 250
`copyPath` method, 252
`copyTheFile` action, 250, 252
`count` method, 183
Create button, 316
create file, keyboard shortcut, 336
Create Files menu item, 82, 156
`createBanner` action, 318
`createDirectoryAtPath` method, 253
creating, class, 118
curly brackets ({ }), 38
Custom Class, 218
Custom Settings button, 47
`CustomView`, 218–220
`cyanColor` preset color component, 214

`darkGrayColor` preset color component,
        214
data, separating from interface, 129
data type, `NSCalendarDate` class, 185–187
data types. *See also* array
    `BOOL`, 185
    C language compared to Cocoa, 181
    `numberWithDouble` numerical type, 182
    `numberWithFloat` numerical type, 182
    `numberWithInt` numerical type, 182
    `numberWithLong` numerical type, 182
    `numberWithUnsignedShort` numerical
        type, 182
`dataRepresentationOfType` method, 311
`dataSource`, 176
`dataWithContentsOfFile` method, 208
date conversion specifier, 187
Day of the month as an integer (%e), date
        format specifier, 187
`dealloc` method, 140, 179
Debug tab, 47, 57
Debugger window
    Build Succeeded message, 40
    contents, 39
debugging
    breakpoints, inserting, 56–57
    problem detection, 55–56

default_voice variable, 330
delegate outlet, 177
delete
  bookmark, 63
  breakpoint, 61
  file, 253
  folder, 253
  text field, 84
deliverMessage method, 275
description method, 186
Description tab, PackageMaker, 109–110
descriptionWithCalendarFormat
    method, 186
Design window
  controls, laying out, 74–75
  displaying, 72
desktop, creating path to, 251
Desktop folder, 251
destination path, 251
determinate progress bar, 174–175
Developer Tools
  benefits of using, 10
  Developer.mpkg file, 345
  downloading, 9, 346
  installing, 2, 345–346
  reusable code, 11
development process, application, 11–13
device color, 214–215
device independent color, 214–215
DeviceCMYK color mixing scheme, 215
DeviceRGB color mixing scheme, 215
DeviceWhite color mixing scheme, 215
dialog window, 156–159
directory
  definition, 238
  determining whether file is, 246
disclosure triangle, 50
Disconnect button, 86
displayAString action, 201
displayNameAtPath method, 246
dissolveToPoint function, 235
distanceCheckbox, 135, 141
Document Types, Info.plist Entries, 308
documentation
  built-in Help, 64
  importance of, 336–337
  lookup, keyboard shortcut, 336
  methods, 253

document-based application
  dataRepresentationOfType method,
    311
  Document Types, Info.plist Entries, 308
  fileContents, 311
  importance of, 303
  loadDataRepresentation method, 311
  MyDocument, 304, 308
  MyDocument.h, 305, 309
  MyDocument.m, 305–306, 310
  myTextView outlet, 308
  NSTextView, 307
  OS Types box, 308
  rich text file, 308
  simple text editor, creating interface for,
    307–309
  windowControllerDidLoadNib method,
    311
doubleValue method, 182
downloading file from Web, 267–268
drag and drop feature, 337–338
drawAtPoint function, 231
drawPoint function, 231
drawRect method, 220, 225–228
drawWithPDFInsideRect, 263
Driver class, 133, 137
driver object, 141
driverDisplay, 135–136
Driver.h, 133, 137
Driver.m, 133, 137

• E •

%e (Day of the month as an integer), date
    format specifier, 187
Edit menu, 199–200
Editable attribute, 292
Editable property, Info window, 29
editing text, manually, 200–202
e-mail
  adding to MyInternetController class,
    276–278
  sending, 272–276
  server information, 275
  URL, 272–273
endSheet, 159
error
  displaying, 60
  types of, 55

escape sequence, URL, 273
executeAndReturnError message, 326
executeAndReturnError method, 329
Expert Configuration tab, 45
Expert View, 107

• F •

fareCheckbox, 136
fareDisplay, 135–136, 141
feed method, 121
feedAnimal action, 123
file
  audio, 283
  common formats, 250
  copying, 251–252
  creating interface for opening, 239–243
  deleting, 253
  determining whether it's a directory, 246
  displaying information about, 243–247
  downloading from Web, 267–268
  icon, viewing, 247–249
  manual merge, 83, 87
  moving, 252–253
  naming conventions, 143
  types, 143, 237–238
File Creation Date text field, 240
File Demo project, creating, 239
File Location text field, 239
File Modification Date text field, 240
File Name text field, 239
File Size text field, 240
fileAttributesAtPath method, 246–247
fileContents, 311
fileCreatedDisplay outlet, 242
fileDirDisplay outlet, 242
fileExistsAtPath method, 246
fileExistsDisplay outlet, 242
fileHandleForReading method, 315
fileIconDisplay outlet, 242–243
FileMerge application
  Choose both (left first) option, 100–101
  file differences, displaying, 98–99
  Fusebox.h check box, 97
  Fusebox.m check box, 97
  importance of, 83
  launching, 94
  location on hard drive, 94
fileModifiedDisplay outlet, 242

filename method, 245–246
fileNameDisplay outlet, 242, 246
filePathDisplay outlet, 242, 246
File's Owner, Instance pane, 73
Files project output, 254
Files tab, 48, 109–110
fileSizeDisplay outlet, 242
Find tab, 47
find term, keyboard shortcut, 336
First Responder, Instance pane, 73
firstName pointer, 140
firstName variable, 138
FirstResponderPerformMiniaturize, 86
Flash file, loading into an NSMovie, 299
float type, 51
floatValue method, 52, 182
folder
  copying, 251–252
  definition, 238
  deleting, 253
  determining whether file is, 246
  moving, 252–253
Font Manager object, 198
Font menu, 198–199
For Dummies Web site, 2, 45, 94, 267
format, variable, 58
forward slash (/), 239
Foundation Framework
  benefits of using, 11
  documentation, 144–146
Foundation Kit, 137
Foundation.h, 145
frame method, 149, 154
framework, benefits of using, 11
Frameworks folder, 275
function
  BezierPathWithOvalInRect, 222
  BezierPathWithRect, 221
  Build, 66
  Build and Debug, 66
  calculateAnswer, 53, 89
  Clean, 66
  closePath, 230
  dissolveToPoint, 235
  drawAtPoint, 231
  drawPoint, 231
  floatValue, 52
  moveToPoint, 229
  moving to code editor, 55

function *(continued)*
  NSButton, 121, 134, 201, 240
  NSHomeDirectory, 251
  NSNumber, 117
  NSString, 117, 141, 182–183, 205, 275
  relativeLineToPoint, 229
  set, 216
  setFloatValue, 52, 171
  setLineWidth, 226
  setShowPanels, 261
Fusebox class
  Class Browser, viewing in, 53
  creating, 31
  instantiating, 32–33
Fusebox.h
  adding mathematical functions, 88–89
  MyFirstProject code sample, 36–37
Fusebox.m
  creating, 36
  initial contents of, 37
  modifying code, 51
  MyFirstProject code sample, 38–39
  SimpleCalculator code sample, 51–52, 59,
    90–91

• G •

game programming, 343
generic class, 118
generic pointer, 126
Get Info window, Finder, 239
giveFood method, 127
GNU C, documentation, 64
GNU source-level debugger (GNB),
    documentation, 64
go method, 138
Graphic Converter, 104
graphics
  displaying, 234–235
  interface, 217–221
  NSBezierPath, 221–222
  NSColor, 213–216
  NSPoint, 212
  NSRect, 212
  NSSize, 212–213
  text, drawing, 231–233
greenColor preset color component, 214
group, 50
Groups & Files list, 52

• H •

.h file extension, 36, 119
hardware, Textured property, 153
header file. *See* interface file
Help
  documentation, 64
  keyboard shortcut, 336
  Project Builder, 65–66
hi banner output, 321
Hide NewApplication menu, 79
Hide SimpleCalculator menu, 79
hideWindow method, 148
hierarchical structure, object-oriented
    programming, 338
Home directory, 24, 251
horizontal slider control, 171
horizontal tabs, 47
Hours (%I), date format specifier, 187
Huge icon, 106
Human Interface Guidelines (Apple), 10, 17
HyperJeff Network (Web site), 344
Hypertext Markup Language (HTML) file,
    displaying in interface, 268–269

• I •

%I (Hours), date format specifier, 187
iApps, Textured property, 153
IBAction, 126
IBOutlet, 126
icns Browser, 108
.icns file extension, 103
icon file, 103
icon method, 248–249
Icon mode, Instance pane, 73
IconComposer
  components, 104
  icon file, building, 104–106
  icon template, 103
  image-editing application, 104
  Info.plist Entries list, 107
id pointer, 126
IDE (integrated development
    environment), 43
iDevGames (Web site), 343
image, displaying, 234–235
ImageRGB/Alpha (32 Bit), 104

Images pane, 72
immutable array, 184
immutable object, 231
iMovie, creating window like, 294
implementation file
  definition, 37
  merging new with existing file, 83
  modifying, 82
#import, 37, 146, 278
#include, 37, 146
indeterminate progress bar, 174–175
indeterminateProgess outlet, 174
index, zero-based, 183
IndexOfSelectItem message, 89
indexOfTabViewItem, 172
Info tab, PackageMaker, 109–110
Info window
  examples, 78
  opening, 26, 85
  purpose, 77–78
Info.plist, 107, 111
InfoPlist.strings, editing, 81
inheritance, 338
init method, 338
initFileURLWithPath method, 267
initWithContentsOfFile method, 284
initWithURL method, 290
insertObject method, 184
instance
  creating, 32–33, 118
  interface, connecting to, 34
  naming conventions, 143
  storing reference to in array, 182–183
instance method, 144
instance variable
  adding to class, 120
  definition, 117
Instances pane, 72–73
Instances tab, 33
int type, 51
integer variable, creating, 38
integrated development environment
  (IDE), 43
interface
  action, connecting to, 35–36, 87
  graphics, 217–221
  instance, connecting to, 34, 86–87
  saving, 87

separating from data, 129
testing, 79
Interface Builder
  appearance of, 17–18, 27
  Design window, 74–75
  documentation, 64
  files, copying, 69
  importance of, 13, 17, 19
  Info window, 77–78
  main windows, 71
  MainMenu.nib, 70
Interface Builder
  Menu editor window, 79–81
  nib file window, 72–74
  Palettes window, 75–77
interface file
  Fusebox.h, 37
  merging new with existing file, 83
intValue message, 38
intValue method, 182
iPhoto, Textured property, 153
Is Editable attribute, 292
isEqualToNumber method, 182
isPlaying method, 288
isVisible method, 148
iTunes, Textured property, 153

• J •

Jaguar, 22
Java, 2, 18
JPEG file
  downloading, 268
  loading into an NSMovie, 299

• K •

Key Equivalent attribute, 86
keyboard shortcuts, 335–336
keyword, locating in source code, 65

• L •

label, adding to button, 28
large text field control, calculator
  application interface, 30
Launch iMovie button, 324–325
launch message, 314

library, compared to framework, 11

`lightGrayColor` preset color component, 214

Load URL Manually button, 269

Load URL with Client button, 269

`loadDataRepresentation` method, 311

`loadResourceDataNotifyingClient` method, 268

`loadWebManually` action, 270

`loadWebPage` action, 266, 270

`longValue` method, 182

Loop mode attribute, 291

Looping Back and Forth setting, 291

lowercase letter, beginning instance name with, 143

• *M* •

%M (Minutes), date format specifier, 187

%m (Month as an integer), date format specifier, 187

.m file extension, 36, 119

Mac OS X

Developer Tools CD, 9

version 10.2, 2, 22

MacTech magazine (Web site), 341–342

MacTelligence (Web site), 342

`magentaColor` preset color component, 214

main source code file, 37

MainMenu, Instance pane, 73, 82

MainMenu.nib

Classes tab, 31, 33

opening, 25, 70, 81

saving, 36

`makeKeyAndOrderFront` method, 149

Manage Templates tab, 45

Many Windows button, 47

matrix, radio buttons, 168

Max button, Info window, 295

menu, duplicating, 82

Menu editor window

basic menu, creating, 79

purpose, 79

testing, 80–81

menu items, editing, 85

MenuWindow, 150

merging files, 83, 87. *See also* FileMerge application

message, sending to an object, 38

Message.framework file, 274

method

adding to class, 120

`alloc`, 141–143

`arrayWithCapacity`, 184

`arrayWithObjects`, 183

`awakeFromNib`, 128, 149–150, 179, 196–197, 338

`bezierPath`, 229

`btnAction2`, 329

`btnAction3`, 329–331

`calculateAnswer`, 37

`center`, 149

`colorWithCalibratedRed`, 179

`colorWithDeviceRed`, 215

`copyPath`, 252

`count`, 183

`createDirectoryAtPath`, 253

`dataRepresentationOfType`, 311

`dataWithContentsOfFile`, 208

`dealloc`, 140, 179

definition, 117

`deliverMessage`, 275

`description`, 186

`descriptionWithCalendarFormat`, 186

`displayNameAtPath`, 246

`doubleValue`, 182

`drawRect`, 220, 225–228

`executeAndReturnError`, 329

`feed`, 121

`fileAttributesAtPath`, 246–247

`fileExistsAtPath`, 246

`fileHandleForReading`, 315

`filename`, 245–246

`floatValue`, 182

`frame`, 149, 154

`giveFood`, 127

`go`, 138

`hideWindow`, 148

`icon`, 248–249

`init`, 338

`initFileURLWithPath`, 267

`initWithContentsOfFile`, 284

`initWithURL`, 290

`insertObject`, 184

intValue, 182
isEqualToNumber, 182
isPlaying, 288
isVisible, 148
loadDataRepresentation, 311
loadResourceDataNotifyingClient,
    268
longValue, 182
makeKeyAndOrderFront, 149
movePath, 252
numberOfRowsInTableView, 177, 179
numberWithBool class, 185
objectForKey, 247
objectValueForTableColumn, 177, 179
OpenPanel, 290
openURL, 266, 273
orderFront, 148
orderOut, 148, 159
playAppSound, 287
playSoundFile, 287
playSystemSound, 287
printOnePage, 258, 260–261
printOperationWithView class, 261
remainingFood, 121, 127
removeTheFileAtPath, 253
replaceCharactersInRange, 202,
    208–209
replaceObjectAtIndex, 185
resizeWithMagnification, 293, 297
resourceDataUsingCache, 267–268
RTFFromRange, 205
runModal, 205, 208, 244
runModalWithPrintInfo, 260
runOperation, 261
selectRow, 170
setAlpha, 155
setArguments, 315
setCanChooseDirectories, 244
setDoubleValue, 175
setExcludedFromWindowsMenu, 150
setFirstName, 138
setFrame, 154
setFrameOrigin, 149
setIntValue, 127, 171
setLaunchPath, 315
setSelectedRange, 202
setString, 201, 338
setStringValue, 245, 338

setTitle, 154, 208, 244
setTitleWithRepresentedFilename,
    154
sharedWorkspace class, 266
showPagePanel, 260
soundNamed class, 282
startAnimation, 174
stop, 287
stopAnimation, 175
stopSoundFile, 287–288
string, 144, 205
stringByAppendingPathComponent, 251
stringWithContentsOfFile, 208
stringWithString, 144
unsignedShort, 182
URLResourceDidFinishLoading, 268
URLs, 290
willDisplayCell, 177, 179
windowControllerDidLoadNib, 311
writeToFile, 205–206, 263, 267
writeTofilestringByExpandingTilde
    InPath, 267
zoom, 154
Microsoft Word, text formatting, 203
Minimize menu item, 85
minimize window, keyboard shortcut, 336
minus sign (-), method declaration, 120
Minutes (%M), date format specifier, 187
modal dialog, 156
modal window, 205
mode of operation, 205
model, definition, 133
Model-View-Controller (MVC), 129, 339
Month as an integer (%m), date format
    specifier, 187
Month name (%B), date format specifier,
    187
mountedVolumes array, 177, 179
.mov file extension, 299
Move File to Desktop button, 250
moveLeft, 151
movePath method, 252
moveTheFile action, 252–253
moveToPoint function, 229
movie
    border, adding to window, 298
    CocoaGraphicsView pane, 294
    Editable attribute, 292

movie *(continued)*
 initWithURL method, 290
 Is Editable attribute, 292
 Loop mode attribute, 291
 Looping Back and Forth setting, 291
 movieScreen outlet, 296
 MyMovieController class, 295–296
 MyMovieController.m, 296–297
 NSMovie class, 289–290
 NSMovieView class, 289–291
 openMovie action, 296
 OpenPanel method, 290
 player example, 294–297
 Plays Selection Only attribute, 292
 QuickTime, 289
 resizeWithMagnification method, 293, 297
 resizing window, 298
 Show Controller attribute, 291
 theWindow outlet, 296
 URLs method, 290
 window coordinate system, 298
movieScreen outlet, 296
MP3 file, loading into an NSMovie, 299
MP4 file, loading into an NSMovie, 299
MPG file, loading into an NSMovie, 299
multimedia
 audio files, opening as QuickTime movie, 298–300
 audio player example, 284–289
 movie player example, 294–298
 NSMovie class, 290
 NSMovieView class, 290–294
 NSSound class, 282
 sound files, loading, 283–284
 system sounds, 282
mutable array, 184
mutable object, 231
MVC. *See* Model-View-Controller
MyAudioController class, 284
MyAudioController.h, 287–288
MyAudioController.m, 286–287
MyCanvas subclass, 218–219
MyCanvas.h, 220
MyCanvas.m, 220
MyCanvasView outlet, 258
MyController, 318
MyController class, 122, 325
MyController.h, 125–126, 137, 319

MyController.m, 125–127, 137, 320, 326, 331–332
MyDataController class, 176–177
MyDataController.h, 177
MyDataController.m, 178–179
MyDocument, 304, 308
MyDocument.h, 305, 309
MyDocument.m, 305–306, 310
MyFileController, 241–242, 250
MyFileController.h, 251
MyFirstProject, 24, 41
MyInternetController, 269–270, 276
MyInternetController.h file, 278
MyInternetController.m file, 271, 278–280
MyMovieController class, 295–296
MyMovieController.m, 296–297
MyPrintController, 257–258
MyPrintController.h, 258–259, 262
MyPrintController.m, 259–261, 263
MySheetController class, 157
MySheetController.m, 158
MyTextController class, 193
MyTextController.h, 202, 204, 206
MyTextController.m, 202, 204, 207
myTextView outlet, 308
MyWindowController, 151
MyWindowController.m, 151–152

• *N* •

\n (newline character), 330
name parameter, 140
name, project, 24
named color, 214–215
naming conventions, Objective-C, 143
nesting methods, 133
New Project Assistant window, 303–304
New Project dialog box, 24
NeXT Interface Builder (NIB), 70
NextStep (NS), 71
.nib file extension, 70
nib file window
 Classes pane, 72–73
 displaying, 72
 Images pane, 72
 Instances pane, 72–73
 Sounds pane, 72

`nil` object, 183, 252
`NO` value, `BOOL` data type, 185
NS (NextStep), 71
`NSAppleScript`, 326, 329
`NSArray`, 315
`NSArray` class, 181–185
`NSAttributedString`, 269
`NSBezierPath`, 229
`NSButton` control, 316
`NSButton` function, 121, 134, 201, 240
NSButton Info window, 316
`NSColor`, 117, 213–216
`NSColorWell` control, 192, 196
`NSControl`, 171, 338
`NSData` class, 267
`NSDictionary`, 231–232
`NSDirectory`, 246–247
`NSFileHandle`, 315
`NSFileManager` class, 246, 252
`NSFileWrapper`, 247–248
`NSForm`, 191
`NSHomeDirectory` function, 251
`NSImage`, 234, 248
`NSImageView`, 241
`NSIndicator`, 174
`NSLog`, 186, 283
`NSMailDelivery` class, 275
`NSMakeRect`, 213
`NSMatrix`, 168–169
`NSMovie` class, 289–290
`NSMovieView` class, 289–291
`NSMutableArray`, 184
`NSMutableDictionary`, 231–232
`NSMutableDirectory`, 246–247
`NSNumber` class, 181–182
`NSNumber` function, 117
`NSNumberFormatter` object, 59
`NSObject` class, 31, 118, 134, 217
`NSOKButton`, 205, 208
`NSOpenPanel`, 208
`NSPageLayout`, printing, 255, 260
`NSPipe` class, 315
`NSPoint`, 149, 212, 234
`NSPrintInfo` object, 259
`NSPrintInfo`, printing, 256
`NSPrintOperation`, printing, 256, 261
`NSPrintPanel`, printing, 256
`NSRange` value, 205

`NSRange` variable, 202
`NSRect`, 212
`NSRect` structure, 149
`NSResponder`, 217
`NSSavePanel`, 208
`NSScaleToFit`, 248
`NSScrollView`, 176
`NSSize`, 149, 212–213
`NSSound` class, 282
`NSString` function, 117, 141, 182–183, 205, 275
`NSTableView`, 175–176
`NSTabView`, 172
`NSTabViewItem` class, 172
`NSTask` command, 314
`NSTextField`, 121, 134, 191, 239–240, 338
`NSTextView`, 192, 196–197, 208, 268–269, 316
`NSURL`, 266, 326
`NSView`, 217, 255
`NSWindow` class, 148, 244
`NSWorkspace` class, 266, 273
`NSWorkspace` object, 179
Number of Items field, 171
`numberField1`, 32
`numberField2`, 32
`numberField3`, 32
`numberOfRowsInTableView` method, 177, 179
`numberWithBool` class method, 185

 • O •

object, 115. *See also* instance
`objectForKey` method, 247
Objective-C
    C language, relationship to, 10, 19, 131–132
    compared to other programming languages, 2
    data types, 181
    framework, benefits of using, 11
    naming conventions, 143
    nesting methods, 133
    parameter, passing, 132
    Reference, 144
    return value, 133
    syntax, 132

object-oriented programming (OOP)
  benefits of using, 116
  class, 117
  importance of, 2, 10, 115
  inheritance, 338
  instance variable, 117
  method, 117
objectValueForTableColumn method, 177, 179
opacity, window, 154–155
Open dialog box, 104
open file, keyboard shortcut, 336
Open plain text button control, 206
Open rich text button control, 206
openMovie action, 296
OpenPanel class, 243–244, 251, 283
OpenPanel method, 290
OpenRichTextFile, 206
openSheet, 158
OpenTextFile, 206
openURL method, 266, 273
operationPopup control, 86, 89
Option-double-click, 65
orangeColor preset color component, 214
orderFront method, 148
orderOut method, 148, 159
origin, graphics, 212
OS Types box, 308
Other Cocoa Views button, 76, 84
Other Sources folder, 37, 52
outlet
  adding, 86, 122
  adding to controller class, 82
  bannerField, 318
  class, adding to, 31
  delegate, 177
  fileCreatedDisplay, 242
  fileDirDisplay, 242
  fileExistsDisplay, 242
  fileIconDisplay, 242–243
  fileModifiedDisplay, 242
  fileNameDisplay, 242, 246
  filePathDisplay, 242, 246
  fileSizeDisplay, 242
  indeterminateProgess, 174
  interface, connecting to, 34
  movieScreen, 296
  myTextView, 308

outputField, 318
playAppSound, 284
playSoundFile, 284
playSystemSound, 284
renaming, 32
speechField, 325
theAnimal, 124, 127
theEmailField, 276
theHTMLView, 270
theTextField, 123
theURLfield, 270
theWindow, 296
Outlet tab, 122
Outline mode, Instance pane, 73
outputField outlet, 318
oval path, 222

• P •

package, definition, 238
PackageMaker, 109–111
page orientation, selecting, 256
Page panel, 256
pageData pointer, 267, 269
Palettes window
  buttons, 76–77
  dragging controls from, 28, 82
  slider controls, 170–171
  table control, 175–180
  viewing, 75–76
Palette-Views window, 168
paper size, selecting, 256
parameter, passing, 132
Parts folder, 109
Pasteboard, 199–200
path, file
  definition, 238
  desktop, 251
path, graphics
  drawing, 226–228
  filling, 222–226
  NSBezierPath, 221
  oval, 222
  rectangular, 221
PB. *See* Project Builder
PDF file, printing to, 261–263
Photoshop Elements, 104
Photoshop format, 104

PICT file, loading into an NSMovie, 299
pinstripe background, window, 152
plain text, 203–206
Play Application Sound button, 284
Play Sound File button, 284, 289
Play System Sound button, 284
playAppSound method, 287
playAppSound outlet, 284
playback, stopping, 287
player example, 284–289
Plays Selection Only attribute, 292
playSoundFile method, 287
playSoundFile outlet, 284
playSystemSound method, 287
playSystemSound outlet, 284
plus sign (+), method declaration, 144
point, 212
pointer, 126
popup button, 84
printable area dimensions, 257
PrintInfo object, 256–257
printing
  adding print controller to project,
    257–261
  NSPageLayout, 255
  NSPrintInfo, 256
  NSPrintOperation, 256
  NSPrintPanel, 256
  NSView, 255
  Page panel, 256
  PDF file, 261–263
printOnePage method, 258, 260–261
printOperationWithView class method,
  261
printToPDF action, 262
product, 49–50
programming experience, recommended, 2
progress bar, 174–175
project
  adding more capabilities to existing,
    83–88
  duplicating, 45
Project Builder (PB)
  Basic Settings, 47–48
  bookmark, 62–64
  default set up, 45
  documentation, 64
  editing files, 51–53
  functions, 16

group, 50
Help, 65–66
importance of, 13
launching, 24
purpose, 43–44
syntax coloring, 14
Targets tab, 48–50
window examples, 14–16, 46
Project Builder Preferences window, 45
project name, 24
project window, 25
Property List Editor, 111–112
purpleColor preset color component, 214

•Q•

QTVR file, loading into an NSMovie, 299
Quartz graphic engine, 211
question mark (?), e-mail URL, 273
QuickDraw, Rect structure used in, 213
QuickTime
  AppleScript, 324
  audio files, opening as movie, 298–300
  audio player example, 284–289
  movie player example, 294–298
  multimedia files, 250
  NSMovie class, 290
  NSMovieView class, 290–294
  NSSound class, 282
  sound files, loading, 283–284
  system sounds, 282
  Textured property, 153
quit application, keyboard shortcut, 336
Quit NewApplication menu, 79
Quit SimpleCalculator menu, 79

•R•

radio control, 168–170
REALbasic, familiarity with, 2
recipient, e-mail, 275
Record Text-to-Speech button, 324–325
Rect, 212–213, 221
rectangle, 212, 221
redColor preset color component, 214
Redo menu item, enabling, 200
Reference Documentation, 144
relativeLineToPoint function, 229
remainingFood method, 121, 127

removeTheFileAtPath method, 253
renaming bookmark, 63
replaceCharactersInRange method, 202, 208–209
replaceObjectAtIndex method, 185
ResEdit, compared to Interface Builder, 25–26
Resize option, Info window, 28
resizeWithMagnification method, 293, 297
resizing window, 154, 298
Resource folder, 25
resourceDataUsingCache method, 267–268
Resources tab, PackageMaker, 109–110
return value, 133
reusable code, 11, 339
rich text file, 203–206, 308
.rtf file extension, 206
RTFFromRange method, 205
ruler, displaying, 192, 197
run application, keyboard shortcut, 336
Run tab, 47
runModal method, 205, 208, 244
runModalWithPrintInfo method, 260
runOperation method, 261
runtime error, 55

• S •

%S (Seconds), date format specifier, 187
save file, keyboard shortcut, 336
Save plain text button control, 203
Save rich text button control, 203
SavePanel class, 204–205, 251
SaveRichTextFile, 203
SaveTextFile, 203
saving text, 202–206
Say Hello button, 324–325
Scotland Software (Web site), 343
Scripts list, 328
search for term, keyboard shortcut, 336
Seconds (%S), date format specifier, 187
selectFile action, 243, 248–249
selecting text field, 84
selectRow method, 170
selectTheFile action, 242, 251

semicolon (;)
    Objective-C, 132
    separating formats with, 59–60
Send Email Manually button, 276
Send Email with Client button, 276
sendEmailManually class, 276
sendEmailWithClient class, 276
sending e-mail, 274–276
set function, 216
setAdditionMenu, 86, 90
setAlpha method, 155
setArguments method, 315
setAttributedString, 269
setCanChoosedirectories method, 244
setDivisionMenu, 86, 90
setDoubleValue method, 175
setExcludedFromWindowsMenu method, 150
setFirstName method, 138
setFloatValue function, 52, 171
setFormat message, 59
setFrame method, 154
setFrameOrigin method, 149
setImageScaling, 248
setIntValue message, 38
setIntValue method, 127, 171
setLaunchPath method, 315
setLineWidth function, 226
setMultiplicationMenu, 86, 90
setSelectedRange method, 202
setShowPanels function, 261
setString method, 201, 338
setStringValue method, 245, 338
setSubtractionMenu, 86, 90
setTheBackgroundColor, 194, 196
setTheTextColor, 194, 196
setTitle method, 154, 208, 244
setTitleWithRepresentedFilename method, 154
sharedWorkspace class method, 266
sheet, adding to project, 156–159
Show Controller attribute, 291
Show Info menu, 26, 49
showPagePanel method, 258, 260
showWindow, 151
simple text editor, creating interface for, 307–309

SimpleCalculator project
  adding more capabilities to, 84–88
  overview, 49–50
SimpleText file, 203
Single Window button, 47–48
Size settings, changing, 317
Some Windows button, 47
someSound.aiff, 285
Sosumi alert, 282
sound
  file formats, 282
  isPlaying method, 288
  MyAudioController class, 284
  MyAudioController.h, 287–288
  MyAudioController.m, 286–287
  NSSound class, 282
  Play Application Sound button, 284
  Play Sound File button, 284, 289
  Play System Sound button, 284
  playAppSound method, 287
  playAppSound outlet, 284
  player example, 284–289
  playSoundFile method, 287
  playSoundFile outlet, 284
  playSystemSound method, 287
  playSystemSound outlet, 284
  QuickTime, 282
  someSound.aiff, 285
  sound file types, 283
  soundNamed class method, 282
  Sounds directory, 282
  Sounds pane, 72
  stop method, 287
  Stop Sound File button, 289
  stopSoundFile action, 287, 289
  stopSoundFile method, 287–288
  system sounds, 282
  user-selected sounds, playing, 283–284
source code file. *See* implementation file
source path, 251
speakText.applescript, 327
speakText.scpt, 326
speechField outlet, 325
square brackets ([ ]), 38, 132
square, positioning on grid, 212
startAnimation method, 174
status 0 message, 45
Stepwise (Web site), 344
stop method, 287

Stop Sound File button, 289
stopAnimation method, 175
stop-sign-shaped path, 228–230
stopSoundFile action, 287, 289
stopSoundFile method, 287–288
string literal, assigning, 141
string method, 144, 205
stringByAppendingPathComponent
    method, 251
stringWithContentsOfFile method, 208
stringWithString method, 144
stroke commands, 230
subclass, 338
Subject field, e-mail, 273, 275
superclass, 138, 338
syntax error, 55
System Preferences, 275
system requirements, 345
system sounds, 282

● *T* ●

tab view, 172–173
table control
  connecting, 176
  MyDataController class, 177
  MyDataController.h, 177
  MyDataController.m, 178–179
  NSTableView, 175–176
  sample output, 180
target, changing name of, 49
Target Info window, 49
Target Summary settings, 49
target_file variable, 330
Targets tab, 48–49, 107
Targets window, 308
Task Templates button, 45
tasks, displaying all in one window, 47
template, filling, 106
Terminal application, 314
testing, importance of, 55
text
  displaying, 191–192
  drawing, 231–233
  Edit menu, 199–200
  Font menu, 198–199
  manual editing, 200–202
  MyTextController, 193–195
  NSColorWell, 192

text *(continued)*
  NSTextView, 192, 196–197
  Pasteboard, 199–200
  plain text format, 203–206
  rich text format, 203–206
  setTheBackgroundColor, 196
  setTheTextColor, 196
  word-processor styles, adding, 198
text commands
  banner command, 313–315
  bannerField outlet, 318
  Create button, 316
  createBanner action, 318
  fileHandleForReading method, 315
  hi banner output, 321
  importance of, 313
  launch message, 314
  MyController, 318
  MyController.h, 319
  MyController.m, 320
  NSArray, 315
  NSButton control, 316
  NSFileHandle, 315
  NSPipe class, 315
  NSTask command, 314
  NSTextView control, 316
  outputField outlet, 318
  setArguments method, 315
  setLaunchPath method, 315
  Size settings, changing, 317
  Terminal application, 314
text field control
  connecting to Fusebox instance, 34
  dragging into window, 29
  removing, 84
  types of, 29–30
text field label control, calculator
  application interface, 30
text file
  opening, 206–209
  saving, 202–206
Textured property, window, 152–153
Textured Window attribute, Info window, 294
theAnimal outlet, 124, 127
theApplySwitch, 194
theBackgroundColorWell, 194

theBaseWindow, 158
theEmailField, 276
theFileName, 284
theFileTypes, 283
theHTMLView, 270
theMenuWindow, 151
thePrintInfo, 260
theRect, 213
theSheet, 158
theShowButton, 151
theTextColorWell, 194
theTextField, 123
theTextView, 194, 206
theURLField, 266, 270
theWindow, 151, 296
32-bit icon, 104
%3F, URL escape sequence, 273
Thumbnail icon, 104–106
Thumbnail.psd, 104
Thumbnail.tiff, 104
TIFF file, loading into an NSMovie, 299
TIFF format, 104
tilde (~), Home directory, 24
title
  button, 201
  window, 26, 154
toggleTheRuler, 194–195
top-left corner, graphics, 212
transparent window, 154–155
tutorial, built-in Help
.txt file extension, 206

• U •

undo, keyboard shortcut, 336
Undo menu item, enabling, 200
uniform resource locator (URL)
  escape sequence, %3F, 273
  hard-coded, 266
  loading into Web browser, 266
Unix, Mac OS X, relationship to, 10
unsignedShort method, 182
uppercase letter, beginning class name
  with, 143
URL. *See* uniform resource locator
URL Loaded message, 266

URLResourceDidFinishLoading method, 268
URLs method, 290
URLWithString parameter, 267
user-selected sounds, playing, 283–284
/usr/bin directory, 315

• V •

Vermont Recipes (Web site), 343
Version tab, PackageMaker, 109–110
vertical slider control, 171
vertical tabs, 48
view, definition, 133
visual cues, adding to interface, 29

• W •

WAVE file, loading into an NSMovie, 299
Web browser, loading URL into, 266
Web, downloading file from, 267–268
Web sites, recommended
  Cocoa Mailing List Archive, 342–343
  CocoaDev, 342
  CocoaDev Central, 342
  cocoadevcentral.com, 342
  cocoadev.com, 342
  HyperJeff Network, 344
  iDevGames, 343
  macintelligence.com, 342
  MacTech magazine, 341–342
  MacTelligence, 342
  Scotland Software, 343
  Stepwise, 344
  Vermont Recipes, 342–343
Weekday name (%A), date format specifier, 187
what you see is what you get (WYSIWYG) editor, 13
whiteColor preset color component, 214
willDisplayCell method, 177, 179
window
  attributes, displaying, 77
  closing, 148
  count, 337
  hiding, 148

importance of, 147
keeping track of, 149–150
modal, 205
opacity, 154–155
pinstripe background, 152
positioning, 149
resizing, 154, 220
sheet, 156–159
springs, 316
Textured property, 152–153
title, 154
window contents, unalterable, 29
window coordinate system, 298
Window, Instance pane, 73–74, 84, 218
Window Title property, 26
windowControllerDidLoadNib method, 311
withAttributes, 231
word-processing styles, including in application, 198
writeToFile method, 205–206, 263, 267
writeTofile stringByExpandingTilde-InPath method, 267
WYSIWYG (what you see is what you get) editor, 13

• Y •

%Y (Year), date format specifier, 187
yellowColor preset color component, 214
YES value, BOOL data type, 185

• Z •

zero-based index, 183
zoom method, 154

FOR DUMMIES®

The easy way to get more done and have more fun

PERSONAL FINANCE & BUSINESS

0-7645-2431-3

0-7645-5331-3

0-7645-5307-0

Also available:

Accounting For Dummies
(0-7645-5314-3)

Business Plans Kit For
Dummies
(0-7645-5365-8)

Managing For Dummies
(1-5688-4858-7)

Mutual Funds For Dummies
(0-7645-5329-1)

QuickBooks All-in-One Desk
Reference For Dummies
(0-7645-1963-8)

Resumes For Dummies
(0-7645-5471-9)

Small Business Kit For
Dummies
(0-7645-5093-4)

Starting an eBay Business
For Dummies
(0-7645-1547-0)

Taxes For Dummies 2003
(0-7645-5475-1)

HOME, GARDEN, FOOD & WINE

0-7645-5295-3

0-7645-5130-2

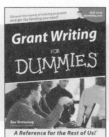

0-7645-5250-3

Also available:

Bartending For Dummies
(0-7645-5051-9)

Christmas Cooking For
Dummies
(0-7645-5407-7)

Cookies For Dummies
(0-7645-5390-9)

Diabetes Cookbook For
Dummies
(0-7645-5230-9)

Grilling For Dummies
(0-7645-5076-4)

Home Maintenance For
Dummies
(0-7645-5215-5)

Slow Cookers For Dummies
(0-7645-5240-6)

Wine For Dummies
(0-7645-5114-0)

FITNESS, SPORTS, HOBBIES & PETS

0-7645-5167-1

0-7645-5146-9

0-7645-5106-X

Also available:

Cats For Dummies
(0-7645-5275-9)

Chess For Dummies
(0-7645-5003-9)

Dog Training For Dummies
(0-7645-5286-4)

Labrador Retrievers For
Dummies
(0-7645-5281-3)

Martial Arts For Dummies
(0-7645-5358-5)

Piano For Dummies
(0-7645-5105-1)

Pilates For Dummies
(0-7645-5397-6)

Power Yoga For Dummies
(0-7645-5342-9)

Puppies For Dummies
(0-7645-5255-4)

Quilting For Dummies
(0-7645-5118-3)

Rock Guitar For Dummies
(0-7645-5356-9)

Weight Training For Dummies
(0-7645-5168-X)

Available wherever books are sold.
Go to www.dummies.com or call 1-877-762-2974 to order direct

FOR DUMMIES®

A world of resources to help you grow

TRAVEL

0-7645-5453-0

0-7645-5438-7

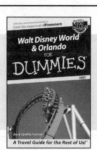

0-7645-5444-1

Also available:

America's National Parks For Dummies
(0-7645-6204-5)

Caribbean For Dummies
(0-7645-5445-X)

Cruise Vacations For Dummies 2003
(0-7645-5459-X)

Europe For Dummies
(0-7645-5456-5)

Ireland For Dummies
(0-7645-6199-5)

France For Dummies
(0-7645-6292-4)

Las Vegas For Dummies
(0-7645-5448-4)

London For Dummies
(0-7645-5416-6)

Mexico's Beach Resorts For Dummies
(0-7645-6262-2)

Paris For Dummies
(0-7645-5494-8)

RV Vacations For Dummies
(0-7645-5443-3)

EDUCATION & TEST PREPARATION

0-7645-5194-9

0-7645-5325-9

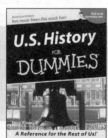

0-7645-5249-X

Also available:

The ACT For Dummies
(0-7645-5210-4)

Chemistry For Dummies
(0-7645-5430-1)

English Grammar For Dummies
(0-7645-5322-4)

French For Dummies
(0-7645-5193-0)

GMAT For Dummies
(0-7645-5251-1)

Inglés Para Dummies
(0-7645-5427-1)

Italian For Dummies
(0-7645-5196-5)

Research Papers For Dummies
(0-7645-5426-3)

SAT I For Dummies
(0-7645-5472-7)

U.S. History For Dummies
(0-7645-5249-X)

World History For Dummies
(0-7645-5242-2)

HEALTH, SELF-HELP & SPIRITUALITY

0-7645-5154-X

0-7645-5302-X

0-7645-5418-2

Also available:

The Bible For Dummies
(0-7645-5296-1)

Controlling Cholesterol For Dummies
(0-7645-5440-9)

Dating For Dummies
(0-7645-5072-1)

Dieting For Dummies
(0-7645-5126-4)

High Blood Pressure For Dummies
(0-7645-5424-7)

Judaism For Dummies
(0-7645-5299-6)

Menopause For Dummies
(0-7645-5458-1)

Nutrition For Dummies
(0-7645-5180-9)

Potty Training For Dummies
(0-7645-5417-4)

Pregnancy For Dummies
(0-7645-5074-8)

Rekindling Romance For Dummies
(0-7645-5303-8)

Religion For Dummies
(0-7645-5264-3)